ASPEN Parenteral Nutrition Handbook

THIRD EDITION

EDITORS

Phil Ayers, PharmD, BCNSP, FASHP
Elizabeth S. Bobo, CNSC, MS, RDN, LDN
Ryan T. Hurt, MD, PhD
Andrew A. Mays, PharmD, BCNSP, CNSC
Patricia H. Worthington, MSN, RN, CNSC

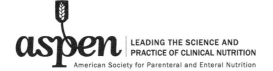

aspen | LEADING THE SCIENCE AND
PRACTICE OF CLINICAL NUTRITION
American Society for Parenteral and Enteral Nutrition

About ASPEN

The American Society for Parenteral and Enteral Nutrition (ASPEN) is a scientific society whose members are healthcare professionals—physicians, dietitians, nurses, pharmacists, other allied health professionals, and researchers—who envision an environment in which every patient receives safe, efficacious, and high-quality patient care.

ASPEN's mission is to improve patient care by advancing the science and practice of clinical nutrition and metabolism.

Print **ISBN** 978-1-889622-41-5
eBook **ISBN** 978-1-889622-42-2
PDF **ISBN** 978-1-889622-47-7

Suggested citation: Ayers P, Bobo ES, Hurt RT, Mays AA, Worthington PH, eds. *ASPEN Parenteral Nutrition Handbook, Third Edition.* Silver Spring, MD: American Society for Parenteral and Enteral Nutrition; 2020.

1 2 3 4 5 6 7 8 9 10
Printed in the United States of America.

Table of Contents

Preface

Parenteral Nutrition (PN) has been a major medical advancement over the past 50 years. The complexity of PN and the complications that can develop with its use require trained clinicians to carefully support and monitor patients receiving PN. This comprehensive handbook provides specific information on how to safely, effectively, and confidently care for patients receiving PN. In this convenient reference, the clinician will find information helpful for achieving positive patient outcomes, including step-by-step recommendations based on the most current research and a wide variety of practical tools to save time and enhance quality of care.

PN safety is a high priority for the American Society for Parenteral and Enteral Nutrition (ASPEN). Products of ASPEN committees include a PN safety summit published as a Journal of Parenteral and Enteral Nutrition supplement, PN guidelines, consensus practice recommendations, and translational tools and checklists available on the ASPEN website. The third edition of this handbook combines the best of ASPEN's evidence-based guidelines, core curriculum, nutrition support practice manual, standards, PN tutorials, and safe practices with the hands-on clinical skills necessary to deliver optimal PN therapy to patients. It has been developed primarily as a quick reference and professional resource for practitioners and trainees in dietetics, medicine, nursing, and pharmacy. Although it can function as an easy-to-access and understandable pocket guide for this very complex therapy, the handbook's best-practices format, multidisciplinary perspective, and training expertise offer something for everyone from the novice to the advanced practitioner.

This handbook provides advice on PN management and systems useful to the clinician in an easy, clear format intended to assist with answering questions related to PN therapy. With best-practice recommendations and up-to-date evidence, this handbook serves as an "Ask-the-expert" resource for clinicians responsible for PN.

Jay M. Mirtallo, MS, RPh, BCNSP, FASHP, FASPEN

We thank the many contributors who shared their knowledge, analyses of the literature, and clinical expertise in the area of PN support. It is our hope that this handbook improves the ordering, administration, and safety of PN support for patients.

Editors & Contributors

Phil Ayers, PharmD, BCNSP, FASHP
Chief, Clinical Pharmacy Services
Baptist Medical Center

Associate Clinical Professor
University of Mississippi School of Pharmacy

Jackson, MS

Elizabeth S. Bobo, CNSC, MS, RDN, LDN
Clinical Dietitian
Nemours Children's Clinic

Jacksonville, FL

Ryan T. Hurt, MD, PhD
Director, Home Parenteral and Enteral Nutrition
Department of Internal Medicine
Mayo Clinic

Associate Professor of Medicine
Mayo Clinic College of Medicine and Science

Rochester, Minnesota

Andrew A. Mays, PharmD, BCNSP, CNSC
Clinical Pharmacy Specialist – Nutrition Support
University of Mississippi Medical Center

Clinical Assistant Professor
University of Mississippi School of Pharmacy

Jackson, MS

Patricia H. Worthington, MSN, RN, CNSC
Retired
Philadelphia, PA

CHAPTER 1

Nutrition Screening, Assessment, and Plan of Care

Introduction

Nutrition screening and assessment of all patients are key components of nutrition care. Although screening and assessment have many similar concepts in regard to adult and pediatric patients, there are differences (see the section "Approach to Pediatric Malnutrition" for specifics on assessment in children). The American Society for Parenteral and Enteral Nutrition (ASPEN) defines nutrition screening as "a process to identify an individual who is malnourished or who is at risk for malnutrition to determine if a detailed nutrition assessment is indicated."[1] In the United States, The Joint Commission mandates nutrition screening within 24 hours of admission to an acute care center.[2]

Guidelines from ASPEN and the Society of Critical Care Medicine (SCCM) recommend that a determination of nutrition risk be completed on all intensive care unit (ICU) patients when there is concern about the ability to consume adequate nutrition orally.[3] Table 1-1 shows a list of validated adult nutrition screening tools and associated parameters.[4]

Table 1-1. Selected Nutrition Screening Instrument Parameters

Screening Tools	INSTRUMENT		
	Anthropometry and/ or Diet-Related	Severity of Illness	Other (Physical, Psychological Variables or Symptoms)
Modified MNA-SF (MNA-SF-BMI and MNA-SF-CC)[5-9]	Appetite, weight loss, BMI, calf circumference (if weight/height unavailable)	Acute disease in last 3 mo	Mobility, psychological stress, neuropsychological problems
SNAQ[10]	Appetite, weight loss, use of oral supplement or tube feeding		
MST[11]	Appetite, weight loss		
NRS 2002[12]	Decreased appetite, weight loss, BMI	Diagnosis (severity)	
MUST[13]	BMI, weight loss	Presence of acute disease	
MNA-SF[14-15]	Appetite, weight loss, BMI	Acute disease in last 3 mo	Mobility, psychological stress, neuropsychological problems

BMI, body mass index; CC, calf circumference; MNA-SF, Mini Nutrition Assessment Short Form; MST, Malnutrition Screening Tool; MUST, Malnutrition Universal Screening Tool; NRS, Nutritional Risk Screening 2002; SNAQ, Short Nutritional Assessment Questionnaire.

Patients identified as nutritionally at risk based on the nutrition screen should receive a nutrition assessment.[16] Criteria for the adult patient at nutrition risk include the following[17]:

- involuntary weight loss of 10% of usual body weight within 6 months or 5% within 1 month,

- involuntary loss of 10 lb within 6 months,

- body mass index (BMI) < 18.5 kg/m^2,

- increased metabolic requirements,

- altered diets or diet schedules, and

- inadequate nutrition intake, including not receiving food or nutrition products for >7 days.

Nutrition assessment has been defined by ASPEN as "a comprehensive approach to identifying the nutrition-related problems that uses a combination of the following: medical, nutrition, medication and client histories; nutrition-focused physical examination; anthropometric measurements; and biomedical data/medical diagnostic tests and procedures."[1] The goal of nutrition assessment is to document baseline nutrition parameters, determine nutrition risk factors/deficits, evaluate individual nutrition needs, and determine medical, psychosocial, and socioeconomic factors that might affect the prescription and administration of nutrition support therapy.[16]

Nutrition assessments may lead to recommendations for improving nutrition status (eg, some intervention such as change in diet), using enteral nutrition (EN) or parenteral nutrition (PN), seeking further medical assessment, or undergoing rescreening.[18-20] A nutrition assessment provides the basis for a nutrition intervention. Clinical skill, resource availability, and the care setting determine the specific methods used to perform a nutrition assessment.[21,22] In addition, reassessment and monitoring are extensions of the assessment process within overall nutrition care. As illustrated in Figure 1-1, nutrition assessment (including rescreening and reassessment) is a continuous process.[16]

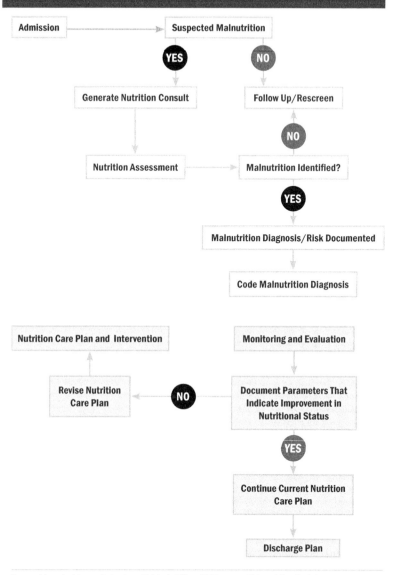

Figure 1-1. ASPEN Adult Nutrition Care Pathway (Age 18+ Years)

Admission ----→ Suspected Malnutrition

YES → Generate Nutrition Consult

NO → Follow Up/Rescreen

Generate Nutrition Consult → Nutrition Assessment ----→ Malnutrition Identified?

NO → Follow Up/Rescreen

YES → Malnutrition Diagnosis/Risk Documented

Malnutrition Diagnosis/Risk Documented → Code Malnutrition Diagnosis

Nutrition Care Plan and Intervention

Monitoring and Evaluation

Revise Nutrition Care Plan ←**NO**— Document Parameters That Indicate Improvement in Nutritional Status

Revise Nutrition Care Plan → Nutrition Care Plan and Intervention

YES → Continue Current Nutrition Care Plan

Continue Current Nutrition Care Plan → Discharge Plan

Source: Adapted with permission from Ukleja A, Gilbert K, Mogensen KM. et al. Standards for nutrition support: adult hospitalized patients. *Nutr Clin Pract.* 2018;33(6):906–920.

Table 1-2 lists nutrition assessment instruments commonly cited in the literature. The table segregates parameters used in these instruments that are primarily related to anthropometry and diet, severity of illness (disease and trauma), or other variables (including physical and psychological).[23] These instruments were generally developed to predict or assess undernutrition.

Table 1-2. Selected Nutrition Assessment Instrument Parameters

Instrument	Anthropometry and/ or Diet-Related	Severity of Illness	Other (Physical and Psychological Variables or Symptoms)
Mini Nutritional Assessment[24]	Weight data, height, mid-arm circumference, calf circumference, diet history, appetite, feeding mode	Serum albumin, prealbumin, and cholesterol levels; lymphocyte count	Self-perception of nutrition and health status
Subjective Global Assessment[25]	Weight history, diet history	Primary diagnosis, stress level	Physical symptoms (subcutaneous fat, muscle wasting, ankle edema, sacral edema, ascites), functional capacity, GI symptoms

GI, gastrointestinal.
Source: Adapted with permission from Mueller C, Compher C, Druyan ME; ASPEN Board of Directors. A.S.P.E.N. clinical guidelines—nutrition screening, assessment and intervention in adults. *JPEN J Parenter Enteral Nutr.* 2011;35(1):16–24.

In the adult population with critical illness, it is recommended that nutrition assessment include evaluation of comorbid conditions, risk for aspiration, and the functionality of the gastrointestinal (GI) tract.[3] Traditional markers of nutrition assessment, such as serum protein markers, are not reliable in this population.

Malnutrition and Inflammation

Experts define malnutrition as "an acute, subacute or chronic state of nutrition, in which a combination of varying degrees of overnutrition or undernutrition with or without inflammatory activity have led to a change in body composition and diminished function."[1,26] Parameters used to diagnose malnutrition in the screening and assessment processes reflect both nutrition intake and severity and duration of disease. These factors may lead to changes in body composition and metabolic alterations associated with poor outcome.

Inflammation and the related compensatory mechanisms associated with disease or injury may cause anorexia and alterations in body composition and stress metabolism. Metabolic alterations associated with inflammation are predominantly cytokine-mediated and persist as long as the inflammatory stimulus is present. These metabolic alterations include elevated energy expenditure, lean tissue catabolism (proteolysis), fluid shift to the extracellular compartment, acute-phase protein changes, and hyperglycemia. Decreased synthesis of negative acute-phase proteins results in reduced serum concentrations of albumin, transferrin, prealbumin, and retinol-binding protein, which are potent indicators of a poor outcome. Indeed, experts have advised against using albumin and prealbumin in isolation to assess nutrition status because they are fundamentally markers of inflammatory metabolism.[27-29] Positive acute-phase proteins such as C-reactive protein are also potent predictors of morbidity and mortality and are elevated in the presence of inflammation.[28,30] Table 1-3 outlines useful parameters for inflammation assessment.[31]

Table 1-3. Parameters Useful to Assess for Inflammation

Laboratory	Clinical
Decreased serum albumin level	Fever
Decreased serum transferrin level	Hypothermia
Decreased serum prealbumin level	Presence of infection
Elevated C-reactive protein level	Urinary tract infection
Elevated blood glucose level	Pneumonia
Decreased or increased white blood cell count	Bloodstream infection
Increased percentage of neutrophils in the cell differential	Wound or incisional infection
Decreased platelet count	Abscess
Marked negative nitrogen balance	--

Source: Reprinted with permission from Malone A, Hamilton C. The Academy of Nutrition and Dietetics/the American Society for Parenteral and Enteral Nutrition consensus malnutrition characteristics: application in practice. *Nutr Clin Pract.* 2013;28(6):639–650.

Adult Malnutrition Characteristics and Assessment

No single clinical or laboratory parameter can serve as an indicator of comprehensive nutrition status. Data must be collected from several domains. A systematic approach to assessment[32] is detailed in Table 1-4 to guide malnutrition diagnosis. The approach uses indicators of malnutrition and inflammation that include medical/surgical history and clinical diagnosis, clinical signs and physical examination, anthropometric data, laboratory results, dietary assessment, and functional outcomes. Clinically relevant micronutrient deficiencies may be detected in association with any of the malnutrition syndromes.[33]

Table 1-4. Elements of Nutrition Assessment

Assessment Elements	Results
Anthropometrics	Height, weight, BMI, weight history, skin folds.
Client history	Medical, surgical, family, and psychosocial histories.
	Review of medications and herbal supplements.
	Current clinical presentation.
Biochemical data	Caution should be used with markers that are indicative of inflammation and possible protein malnutrition (serum albumin, prealbumin).
	Interpreting laboratory values is tailored to disease.
Nutrient intake data	Data should include oral food/beverage intake, EN, parenteral infusions, and supplements.
	A modified diet history or 24-hour recall can be easily used.
	Other options include a diet record, nutrient intake analysis and food frequency questionnaire.
NFPE findings	Includes assessment of muscle and sub-cutaneous fat status; presence of edema; identification of possible micronutrient deficiencies.
Functional status	Handgrip to assess muscle strength.
	Patient-reported changes in functional status.
	Quality-of-life measures to assess functional ability.

BMI, body mass index; EN, enteral nutrition; NFPE, nutrition-focused physical examination.
Source: Adapted with permission from JeVenn AK, Galang M, Hipskin P, et al. Malnutrition screening and assessment. In: Mueller CM, ed. *ASPEN Adult Nutrition Support Core Curriculum.* 3rd ed. Silver Spring, MD: ASPEN; 2017:185–212.

Adult Malnutrition

The adult malnutrition consensus statement developed by the Academy of Nutrition and Dietetics/ASPEN Malnutrition Work Group provides a framework for diagnosing malnutrition.[30] The framework couples the etiology of a malnutrition diagnosis with specific criteria or characteristics to define malnutrition. The Academy of Nutrition and Dietetics/ASPEN Malnutrition Work Group identified 6 characteristics to assess for the presence of adult malnutrition. If a patient demonstrates ≥2 characteristics, malnutrition can be diagnosed, with its severity further defined via specific thresholds, descriptions, or both. Tables 1-5 and 1-6 outline the 6 characteristics and their respective thresholds for both severe and nonsevere (moderate) malnutrition. Gathering the respective data to determine if malnutrition is present requires a systematic approach beginning with a review of the patient's medical record and verbal discussion with the patient and/or caregiver, coupled with physical assessment. The following sections highlight each of the 6 malnutrition characteristics and offer further details specific to their use.

Table 1-5. Characteristics to Diagnose Severe Malnutrition

Characteristic	Acute Illness or In-jury	Chronic Disease	Social or Environmental Factors
Weight loss	>2%/1 wk	>5%/1 mo	>5%/1 mo
	>5%/1 mo	>7.5%/3 mo	>7.5%/3 mo
	>7.5%/3 mo	>10%/6 mo	>10%/6 mo
		>20%/1 y	>20%/1 y
Energy intake	<50% for >5 d	<75% for >1 mo	<50% for >1 mo
Body fat	Moderate depletion	Severe depletion	Severe depletion
Muscle mass	Moderate depletion	Severe depletion	Severe depletion
Fluid accumulation	Moderate to severe	Severe	Severe
Grip strength	Not recommended in ICU	Reduced for age/sex	Reduced for age/sex

Source: Reprinted with permission from White JV, Guenter P, Jensen GL, et al; Academy Malnutrition Work Group; ASPEN Malnutrition Task Force; ASPEN Board of Directors. Consensus statement: Academy of Nutrition and Dietetics and the American Society for Parenteral and Enteral Nutrition: characteristics recommended for the identification and documentation of adult malnutrition (undernutrition). *JPEN J Parenter Enteral Nutr.* 2012;36(3):275–283.

Table 1-6. Characteristics to Diagnose Nonsevere (Moderate) Malnutrition

Characteristic	Acute Illness or Injury	Chronic Disease	Social or Environmental Factors
Weight loss	1%–2%/1 wk	5%/1 mo	5%/1 mo
	5%/1 mo	7.5%/3 mo	7.5%/3 mo
	7.5%/3 mo	10%/6 mo	10%/6 mo
		20%/1 y	20%/1 y
Energy intake	<75% for >7 d	<75% for ≥1 mo	<75% for ≥3 mo
Body fat	Mild depletion	Mild depletion	Mild depletion
Muscle mass	Mild depletion	Mild depletion	Mild depletion
Fluid accumulation	Mild	Mild	Mild
Grip strength	Not applicable	Not applicable	Not applicable

Source: Reprinted with permission from White JV, Guenter P, Jensen GL, et al; Academy Malnutrition Work Group; ASPEN Malnutrition Task Force; ASPEN Board of Directors. Consensus statement: Academy of Nutrition and Dietetics and the American Society for Parenteral and Enteral Nutrition: characteristics recommended for the identification and documentation of adult malnutrition (undernutrition). *JPEN J Parenter Enteral Nutr.* 2012;36(3):275–283.

Weight Loss

Assessing weight loss in a specific patient requires knowing the patient's usual or previous body weight and his or her current weight. Admission weight is frequently obtained by the admitting clinician as either an actual or reported measurement. Caution must be exercised in evaluating admission weights in patients who have been fluid resuscitated or are demonstrating signs of dehydration. In these cases, the clinician will need to conduct further assessment to ascertain the patient's "dry" weight. When interviewing the patient and/or caregiver, the clinician must identify the patient's "usual" body weight and when that weight was measured, which may be difficult for the patient and/or caregiver to remember. Oftentimes the measurement coincides with a recent surgical procedure or prior to the patient's currently diagnosed disorder.

A clinician may be able to obtain a patient's previous weight from a recent hospitalization or from information available at the primary care physician's office. If the nutrition assessment is being conducted during the patient's hospitalization, the admission weight can be compared with the patient's current weight for evaluation.[30,34,35]

Certain factors may contribute to inaccuracies in assessing weight loss. In addition to the underlying fluid status, which can mask weight loss, other factors include the inability of the patient to recall his or her weight correctly, equipment error, and measurement/documentation error.[36]

Insufficient Energy Intake

Identifying how well a newly admitted patient has been able to consume nutrients is best achieved through questioning the patient and/or caregiver. For hospitalized patients, reviewing meal intake data, assessing "calorie counts," and/or analyzing enteral/parenteral consumption via intake and output records provides data for assessment. It should be noted that calorie counts can be problematic in providing adequate data for evaluation. For newly admitted patients who have been able to consume food orally, information should be obtained from the patient and/or caregiver on the patient's general meal intake over a specific period.[36,37] For previously or currently hospitalized patients, identifying periods of inadequate intake will assist in delineating the overall percentage of energy intake that he or she has been able to achieve.

Objective data from a medical record review and/or patient/caregiver interview can be compared with the patient's estimated energy requirements to determine the specific percentage of energy intake that the patient has achieved. This percentage indicates the severity level of inadequate intake. Energy requirements can be measured via indirect calorimetry (eg, in patients with critical illness), or they can be estimated with prediction equations such as Penn State or Mifflin St-Jeor.[38,39]

Physical Assessment Components

Completion of a nutrition-focused physical examination (NFPE) is important for determination of a patient's overall nutrition status. The techniques used to conduct an NFPE include inspection, palpation, percussion and auscultation, with inspection and palpation being the primary techniques used.[40] Aspects assessed in an NFPE include examination of muscle and fat stores, assessment of possible micronutrient deficiencies, and evaluation of fluid accumulation.[40] This examination is comprehensive and includes assessment of the skin, head, upper body, and lower body.[40,41] Fluid accumulation is assessed via examination that evaluates the presence of local and/or generalized accumulation.[30] It is important to first evaluate overall fluid status to help determine other etiologies for any fluid accumulation. Areas useful to assess include the lower and upper extremities, face and eyes, and the scrotal area as well as the abdomen for ascites. In patients with underlying disease states such as congestive heart failure or chronic kidney disease, discerning fluid accumulation due to malnutrition is difficult. The results of NFPE coupled with the patient interview can provide sufficient data for the nutrition clinician to diagnose malnutrition. Dual-energy x-ray absorptiometry may be used to further assess fat mass but is not recommended at this time as a marker of lean body mass.[42]

Hand Grip Strength

Hand grip strength has been validated as a proxy for lean body mass and was consequently chosen as an important functional parameter in assessing for malnutrition.[30,43] Assessment of grip strength is performed via a dynamometer by those experienced/trained in its use. Abnormal grip strength measurements are based on the specific dynamometer used. Diseases and/or conditions that limit a patient's ability to perform a valid hand grip strength measurement must be considered, including rheumatoid arthritis, cerebrovascular accident, neuromuscular disease, and dementia, among others. In addition, patients who are heavily sedated and/or unresponsive, such as those in the ICU, will be unable to complete hand grip measurements. Some practitioners have chosen not to use hand grip strength in assessing for malnutrition.[44] Other parameters that could be considered for functional assessment include general performance status, ability to perform activities of daily living, ability to tolerate physical therapy, and ability to wean from mechanical ventilation. Validity and usability testing of additional functional parameters will shed light on alternate parameters that may be useful in addition to grip strength.

General Considerations in Applying the Malnutrition Characteristics

In an evaluation of a patient's specific malnutrition criteria, the possible etiologies for malnutrition may not always be clear. The patient's characteristics might fit within >1 etiology; for example, malnutrition may be related to both acute illness and chronic disease. The malnutrition etiology can change as the clinical course evolves, which is why characteristics should be routinely assessed at frequent intervals. Some degree of ≥1 characteristic may be present in patients without malnutrition. Conversely, characteristics may not be present in all patients at high risk for malnutrition. These patients are likely to have been well nourished prior to admission and are considered at high risk because of the nature of their illness (eg, burns or traumatic injury). Close and frequent monitoring of these patients is essential because nutrition status may shift as clinical condition changes.[30,31,45]

Global Perspective on Malnutrition

Subsequent to the development of the Academy of Nutrition and Dietetics/ASPEN Malnutrition Work Group recommendations, the Global Leadership Initiative on Malnutrition (GLIM) developed criteria for the diagnosis of malnutrition (undernutrition).[46] The criteria are similar in some aspects to those defined by the Academy of Nutrition and Dietetics/ASPEN Malnutrition Work Group. The requirements for diagnosis include both phenotypic and etiologic criteria. Phenotypic criteria are weight loss, low BMI, and reduced muscle mass. Etiologic criteria are reduced food intake or assimilation and inflammation. To diagnose a patient with malnutrition, he or she must have at least 1 phenotypic criterion and 1 etiologic criterion. However, the severity of malnutrition is based on phenotypic criteria only. Malnutrition severity is categorized as either stage 1 (moderate) or stage 2 (severe).[46] Tables 1-7 and 1-8 provide GLIM criteria for the diagnosis of malnutrition.[47]

Table 1-7. Phenotypic and Etiologic Criteria for the Diagnosis of Malnutrition

PHENOTYPIC CRITERIA[a]			ETIOLOGIC CRITERIA[a]	
Weight Loss (%)	Low BMI (kg/m²)	Reduced Muscle Mass[b]	Reduced Food Intake or Assimilation[c,d]	Inflammation[e-g]
>5% within past 6 mo, or >10% beyond 6 mo	<20 if <70 y or <22 if >70 y **Asia:** <18.5 if <70 y or <20 if>70 y	Reduced by validated body composition measuring techniques[b]	≤50% or ER > 1 wk, or any reduction for >2 wk, or any chronic GI condition that adversely impacts food assimilation or absorption[c,d]	Acute disease/ injury[e,g] or chronic disease– related[f,g]

BMI, body mass index; ER, energy requirements; GI, gastrointestinal.

Source: Adapted with permission from Jensen G, Cederholm T, Correia MITD, et al. GLIM criteria for the diagnosis of malnutrition: a consensus report from the global clinical nutrition community. *JPEN J Parenter Enteral Nutr*. 2019;43(1):32–40.

[a]Requires at least 1 phenotypic criterion and 1 etiologic criterion for diagnosis of malnutrition.

[b]For example, fat-free mass index (kilograms per meter squared) by dual-energy absorptiometry or corresponding standards using other body composition methods such as bioelectrical impedance analysis, computed tomography, or magnetic resonance imaging. When not available or by regional preference, physical examination or standard anthropometric measures such as mid-arm muscle or calf circumferences may be used. Thresholds for reduced muscle mass need to be adapted to race (Asia). Functional assessments such as hand grip strength may be considered as a supportive measure.

[c]Consider GI symptoms as supportive indicators that can impair food intake or absorption (eg, dysphagia, nausea, vomiting, diarrhea, constipation, or abdominal pain). Use clinical judgement to discern severity based on the degree to which intake or absorption is impaired. Symptom intensity, frequency, and duration should be noted.

[d]Reduced assimilation of food/nutrients is associated with malabsorptive disorders such as short bowel syndrome and pancreatic insufficiency and after bariatric surgery. It is also associated with disorders such as esophageal strictures, gastroparesis, and intestinal pseudo-obstruction. Malabsorption is a clinical diagnosis manifest as chronic diarrhea or steatorrhea. Malabsorption in those with ostomies is evidenced by elevated volumes of output. Use clinical judgement or additional evaluation to discern severity based on frequency, duration, and quantitation of fecal fat and/or volume losses.

[e]Acute disease– or injury-related. Severe inflammation is likely to be associated with major infection, burns, trauma, or closed head injury. Other acute disease– or injury-related conditions are likely to be associated with mild to moderate inflammation.

[f]Chronic disease–related. Severe inflammation is not generally associated with chronic disease conditions. Chronic or recurrent mild to moderate inflammation is likely to be associated with malignant disease, chronic obstructive pulmonary disease, congestive heart failure, chronic renal disease, or any disease with chronic recurrent inflammation. Note that transient inflammation of a mild degree does not meet the threshold for this etiologic criterion.

[g]C-reactive protein may be used as a supportive laboratory measure.

Table 1-8. Thresholds for Severity of Grading of Malnutrition

PHENOTYPIC CRITERIA[a]

	Weight Loss	Low BMI (kg/m2)[b]	Reduced Muscle Mass[c]
Stage 1/moderate malnutrition (requires 1 phenotypic criterion that meets this grade)	5%–10% within the past 6 mo, or 10%–20% beyond 6 mo	<20 if <70 y, <22 if ≥70 y	Mild to moderate deficit (per validated assessment methods: see below)
Stage 2/severe malnutrition (requires 1 phenotypic criterion that meets this grade)	>10% within the past 6 mo, or >20% beyond 6 mo	<18.5 if <70 y, <20 if ≥70 y	Severe deficit (per validated assessment methods; see below)

BMI, body mass index.
Source: Adapted with permission from Jensen G, Cederholm T, Correia MITD, et al. GLIM criteria for the diagnosis of malnutrition: a consensus report from the global clinical nutrition community. *JPEN J Parenter Enteral Nutr.* 2019;43(1):32–40.
[a]Severity grading is based on the noted phenotypic criteria, whereas the etiologic criteria are used to provide the context to guide intervention and anticipated outcomes.
[b]Further research is needed to secure consensus reference BMI data for Asian populations in clinical settings.
[c]For example, appendicular lean mass index (kilograms per meter squared) by dual-energy absorptiometry or corresponding standards using other body composition methods such as bioelectrical impedance analysis, computed tomography, or magnetic resonance imaging. When not available or by regional preference, physical examination or standard anthropometric measures such as mid-arm muscle or calf circumferences may be used. Functional assessments such as hand grip strength may be used as a supportive measure.

Approach to Pediatric Malnutrition

Pediatric malnutrition (undernutrition) is defined by ASPEN as "an imbalance between nutrient requirement and intake, resulting in cumulative deficits of energy, protein, or micronutrients that may negatively affect growth, development, and other relevant outcomes".[48] The ages included under this definition are children ages 1 month to 18 years.[49] Based on its etiology, malnutrition is either related to illness (≥1 disease or injury that directly results in nutrient imbalance) or caused by environmental or behavioral factors associated with decreased nutrient intake, delivery, or both.[48] Environmental factors that result in malnutrition or negatively affect its remediation often involve socioeconomic conditions associated with inadequate food availability or complicating behavioral disorders such as anorexia and food aversion. Malnutrition is classified as either acute (<3 months in duration) or chronic (≥3 months in duration). Chronic malnutrition may manifest with growth deficits, especially diminished height velocity (stunting). Hospital-acquired malnutrition refers to nutrient imbalance acquired during hospitalization; it may occur with or without preexisting malnutrition (ie, malnutrition that was present prior to hospital admission).[48]

The mechanisms of nutrient imbalance in illness-related malnutrition include decreased nutrient intake, altered utilization, increased nutrient losses, or increased nutrient requirements (hypermetabolism) not matched by intake. These basic mechanisms may be interrelated, and >1 mechanism is often involved. In addition, much more remains to be learned about disease-specific disruptions of normal metabolic pathways in acute and chronic illness.

General recommendations for assessing the nutrition status of pediatric patients are presented in Table 1-9. As with adults, an NFPE should also be utilized to assess nutrition status. In fact, the NFPE is likely more crucial in the pediatric cohort secondary to the impact of malnutrition on growth and development.[50]

Table 1-9. Recommendations for Assessment of Nutritional Status of Infants and Children

Domain	Recommendations
A. Anthropometric variables: relevant variables, reference data, statistical tests to detect deviation from reference/ standard	• Record weight, height, BMI, and MUAC and consider TSF and mid-arm muscle circumference on admission and then serially using appropriate growth charts. MUAC and TSF require a trained professional to provide these measurements.
	• Head circumference must be obtained in infants <2 y of age.
	• When feasible, a single trained individual using standardized techniques and devices should perform anthropometric measurements for nutrition assessment in individual patients.
	• Measure an infant's length supine on a length board until age 2 y, after which time children should be measured upright. For children older than 2 y and unable to stand, consider utilizing an alternative measurement (eg, tibia length, knee height, arm span) for a height proxy.
	• Weigh infants and children with minimal clothing on scales accurate to at least 100 g.
	• Use existing technology (beds with accurate scales) to weigh children who are bedridden.
	• Use the 2006 WHO charts as the population standard against which individual growth and nutrition characteristics should be described for children up to 2 y of age who are measured in the supine position for length.
	• For children aged 2–20 y, use the Centers for Disease Control and Prevention 2000 charts with a standing height measurement used for plotting. Healthcare centers may utilize their electronic health records systems to develop an efficient system of documenting and plotting serial measurements against the reference or standard curves.
	• Use the z-score to express individual anthropometric variables in relation to the population reference standard.

Domain	Recommendations
A. (continued)	• When assessing nutrition status on admission or first hospital visit, anthropometric parameters should be recorded and plotted on reference or standard age-appropriate curves to obtain the z-score. • Classify severity of existing or current nutrition state based on cutoffs for individual anthropometric parameters.
B. Growth: dynamic changes	• Use dynamic changes in weight and length velocity over time as compared with a single measured parameter. • Use a decline in z-score for individual anthropometric measurement (eg, a decrease > 1), as the indication of faltering growth. This threshold must prompt investigation into the etiology of growth failure and potential interventions.
C. Chronicity of malnutrition	Use 3 mo as a cutoff to classify duration of malnutrition as acute (<3 mo) or chronic (≥3 mo).
D. Etiology of malnutrition and etiology and pathogenesis: underlying illness, mechanism of nutrient imbalance	• When malnutrition is secondary to a disease or injury, use the term *illness-related malnutrition* in the definition and include the specific disease or condition (acute or chronic) if it is directly responsible for nutrient imbalance. • Include a description of the most predominant mechanism leading to nutrient imbalance in the definition. Review and include the most common mechanisms for pediatric malnutrition: (a) decreased intake/starvation (eg, fluid-restricted cardiac failure), (b) increased requirement/hypermetabolism (eg, burn injury), (c) excessive losses (chronic diarrhea, burns, proteinuria), and (d) failure to assimilate (absorb or utilize) the delivered nutrients (eg, malabsorption states). • Include >1 mechanism if mechanisms exist simultaneously. • Recognize the role of inflammation on nutrition status. • Consider including the presence of inflammation in the definition when laboratory parameters such as C-reactive protein and cytokines are conclusive. • Hospital-acquired malnutrition in children is malnutrition that is acquired or worsens after admission to the hospital. Perform nutrition screening at admission to detect children at higher risk of nutrition deterioration during the illness course. • Awareness of nutrition deterioration during hospitalization will highlight the impact of disease on nutrition state and provide opportunities for improvement in hospital system of care. This should be documented as "worsening malnutrition" as soon as it is evident during the illness course.
E. Impact of malnutrition on functional status	• Consider developmental assessment and neurocognitive monitoring in determining the impact of chronic malnutrition in children. • Include lean body mass measurement (by body composition measurement or anthropometric techniques) with some measure of muscle strength as a meaningful and quantifiable expression of outcomes affected by malnutrition in children. • Use validated objective measures of body composition and uniform assessment techniques for muscle strength in children.

BMI, body mass index; MUAC, mid–upper arm circumference; TSF, triceps skin fold; WHO, World Health Organization.
Source: Adapted with permission from Mehta NM, Corkins MR, Lyman B, et al. Defining pediatric malnutrition: a paradigm shift toward etiology-related definitions. *JPEN J Parenter Enteral Nutr.* 2013;37(4):460–481.

The Academy of Nutrition and Dietetics and ASPEN have developed diagnostic indicators for the identification and classification of pediatric malnutrition. These indicators are intended for children 1 month to 18 years of age. They are not to be used for the neonatal population. These indicators are applicable in a variety of care settings, such as in the hospital and also in outpatient facilities.[49] See Tables 1-10 and 1-11 for diagnosing malnutrition based on a single data point or multiple data points.[49]

Table 1-10. Primary Indicators When Only a Single Data Point Is Available

Primary Indicators	Mild Malnutrition	Moderate Malnutrition	Severe Malnutrition
Weight-for-height z-score	−1 to −1.9 z-score	−2 to −2.9 z-score	≥ −3 z-score
BMI-for-age z-score	−1 to −1.9 z-score	−2 to −2.9 z-score	≥ −3 z-score
Length/height z-score	No data	No data	−3 z-score
Mid–upper arm circum-ference	≥ −1 to −1.9 z-score	≥ −2 to −2.9 z-score	≥ −3 z-score

BMI, body mass index.
Source: Adapted with permission from Becker P, Carney L, Corkins MR, et al. Consensus Statement of the Academy of Nutrition and Dietetics/American Society for Parenteral and Enteral Nutrition: indicators recommended for the identification and documentation of pediatric malnutrition (undernutrition). *Nutr Clin Pract.* 2015;30(1):147–161.

Table 1-11. Primary Indicators When ≥2 Data Points Are Available

Primary Indicators	Mild Malnutrition	Moderate Malnutrition	Severe Mal-nutrition
Weight gain velocity (<2 y of age)	<75%[a] of the norm[b] for expected weight gain	<50%[a] of the norm[b] for expected weight gain	<25%[a] of the norm[b] for expected weight gain
Weight loss (2–20 y of age)	5% usual body weight	7.5% usual body weight	10% usual body weight
Deceleration in weight for length/ height z-score	Decline of 1 z-score	Decline of 2 z-score	Decline of 3 z-score
Inadequate nutrient in-take	51%–75% estimated energy/ protein need	26%–50% estimated energy/protein need	≤25% estimated energy/protein need

Source: Adapted with permission from Becker P, Carney L, Corkins MR, et al. Consensus statement of the Academy of Nutrition and Dietetics/American Society for Parenteral and Enteral Nutrition: indicators recommended for the identification and documentation of pediatric malnutrition (undernutrition). *Nutr Clin Pract.* 2015;30(1):147–161.
[a]From Guo et al.[51]
[b]World Health Organization data for patients younger than 2 y.

Nutrition Support Care Plan

Based on data gathered from the comprehensive nutrition assessment, a nutrition diagnosis is determined, and a plan of care is established. Nutrition intervention decisions include timing, nutrient needs, route of therapy, and whether nutrition support therapy formulations are needed. See Figure 1-2 for a decision-making algorithm.[16]

Figure 1-2. Adult Route of Administration Algorithm

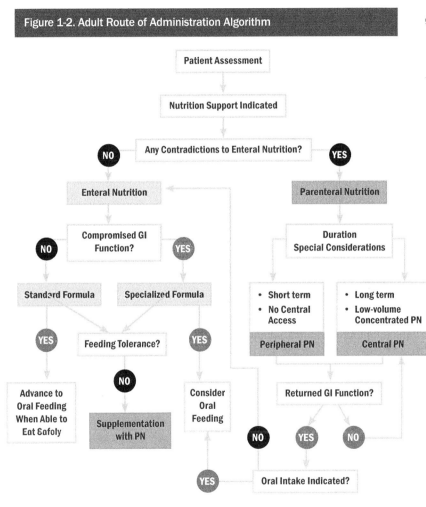

GI, gastrointestinal; PN, parenteral nutrition.

Source: Adapted with permission from Ukleja A, Gilbert K, Mogensen K, et al. Standards for Nutrition Support: Adult Hospitalized Patients. *Nutr Clin Pract.* 2018;33(6):906–920.

Timing of Nutrition Intervention

It is suggested that for well-nourished adult patients without critical illness, EN initiation may be delayed until no or inadequate oral intake reaches 7–14 days.[52] Other recommendations advise initiation of EN when there is likely to be no oral intake for >5–7 days.[53] In the adult population with critical illness, it is recommended that EN be started within 24–48 hours if oral intake is insufficient and PN is not indicated, provided that the patient is hemodynamically stable.[3]

PN should be initiated in a well-nourished, stable adult who has not been able to receive significant (≥50% of estimated requirements) oral or enteral nutrients after 7 days.[17] Adults who are nutritionally at risk and not anticipated to reach desired oral or enteral needs should have PN initiated within 3–5 days.[17] Adults with moderate or severe malnutrition in whom oral or enteral intake is not possible or sufficient should have PN initiated as soon as possible.[17] PN should not be initiated in adults with severe metabolic instability until the condition has improved.[17]

Pediatric patients have increased metabolic rate and nutrient needs for growth and lower nutrient reserves than adults. Surgery or a short-term illness can rapidly alter a child's nutrition status.[48] Guidelines for the pediatric patient with critical illness developed by SCCM and ASPEN recommend that pediatric ICU (PICU) patients receive a nutrition assessment within 48 hours of hospital admission. It is further recommended that these patients be reassessed weekly, at a minimum.[54] Early introduction of nutrition support is indicated for children at high risk of malnutrition or those who are malnourished. For those under 2 years with malnutrition prior to admission, initiation of trophic enteral feedings within 8 hours has been suggested, along with advancing to the nutrition goal within 48 hours if tolerated.[55] For older children, it is suggested that EN start within the first 18 hours and be advanced as tolerated to the goal level within 24–36 hours. If a child with critical illness has severe malnutrition or is at risk for impaired nutrition status and EN is not able to be advanced to goal, PN may be provided as adjunct therapy.[54] It is not recommended that PN be initiated within 24 hours of PICU admission.[54] PN may be started within 1–3 days for infants and within 4–5 days for older children and adolescents when it is clear that they will not be able to consume full oral nutrition or EN for an extended time.[17] Recent data suggest that withholding PN for the first week of PICU admission may improve outcomes. More randomized controlled trials in this area are needed to develop a consensus on this issue.[56]

Nutrition Support Therapy

Integral to the process of nutrition care and the administration of nutrition support therapy is the decision on route of administration. Nutrition support therapy may be needed for management of specific conditions such as renal failure, liver failure, or critical illness. Generally, EN should be given in preference to PN nutrition when nutrition requirements are not met by oral intake and there is a functional GI tract of sufficient length and condition to allow adequate nutrient absorption.[57] PN should be used when the GI tract is not functional or cannot be accessed and in patients who cannot be adequately nourished by oral diets or EN.[18] See chapter 2 for more detail on PN indications.

Nutrition Monitoring and Evaluation

Once the nutrition assessment is complete and nutrition intervention begins, monitoring is needed. Many of the assessment parameters used initially are repeated serially to assess the efficacy of therapy related to desired outcomes and for potential complications associated with the therapy. How often a patient is monitored depends on the severity of the illness, level of metabolic stress, nutrition status, and the clinical condition of the patient.[16] For example, frequent monitoring is recommended for patients who have critical illness, are at risk for refeeding syndrome, or are transitioning between nutrition support modalities. Less frequent monitoring, such as weekly, may be appropriate for patients who are clinically and metabolically stable.[16] As the patient is being monitored, the data collected should be compared with the goals established in the nutrition care plan. If the established goals are not being met, the nutrition care plan should be adjusted accordingly.[16]

References

1. ASPEN Board of Directors and Clinical Practice Committee. Definition of terms, style, and conventions used in ASPEN Board of Directors–approved documents. ASPEN website. https://www.nutritioncare.org/uploadedFiles/Documents/Guidelines_and_Clinical_Resources/ASPEN%20Definition%20of%20Terms,%20Style,%20and%20Conventions%20Used%20In%20ASPEN%20Board%20of%20Directors%E2%80%93Approved%20Documents.pdf. Published May 2018. Accessed November 14, 2019.

2. The Joint Commission. *Comprehensive Accreditation Manual for Hospitals.* Chicago, IL: The Joint Commission; 2007.

3. McClave S, Taylor B, Martindale R, et al. Guidelines for the provision and assessment of nutrition support therapy in the adult critically ill patient: Society of Critical Care Medicine (SCCM) and American Society for Parenteral and Enteral Nutrition (A.S.P.E.N.). *JPEN J Parenter Enteral Nutr.* 2016;40(2):159–211.

4. Academy of Nutrition and Dietetics. Nutrition screening adults: adult nutrition screening tool comparison. Evidence Analysis Library website. https://www.andeal.org/topic.cfm?cat=4079&highlight=Screening%20adults&home=1. Published 2018. Accessed December 30, 2019.

5. Garcia-Meseguer MJ, Serrano-Urrea R. Validation of the revised Mini Nutritional Assessment Short-Forms in nursing homes in Spain. *J Nutr Health Aging.* 2013;17(1):26–29.

6. Kaiser MJ, Bauer JM, Ramsch C et al; MNA-International Group. Validation of the Mini Nutritional Assessment short-form (MNA-SF): a practical tool for identification of nutritional status. *J Nur Health Aging.* 2009;13(9):782–788.

7. Kaiser MJ, Bauer JM, Uter W, et al. Prospective validation of the Modified Mini Nutritional Assessment Short-Forms in the community, nursing home, and rehabilitation setting. *J Am Geriatr Soc.* 2011;59(11):2124–2128.

8. Lera L, Sánchez H, Ángel B, et al. Mini Nutritional Assessment Short-Form: validation in five Latin American cities. SABE Study. *J Nutr Health Aging.* 2016;20(8):797–805.

9. Martín A, Ruiz E, Sanz A, et al. Accuracy of different Mini Nutritional Assessment reduced forms to evaluate the nutritional status of elderly hospitalized diabetic patients. *J Nutr Health Aging.* 2016;20(4): 370–375.

10. Kruizenga HM, Tulder MW, Seidell JC, Thijs A, Ader HJ, Van Bokhorst-de van der Schueren MA. Effectiveness and cost effectiveness of early screening and treatment of malnourished patients. *Am J Clin Nutr.* 2005;82(5):1082–1089.

11. Ferguson M, Capra S, Bauer J, Banks M. Development of a valid and reliable malnutrition screening tool for adult acute hospital patients. *Nutrition.* 1999;15(6):458–464.

12. Kondrup J, Rasmussen HH, Hamberg O, Stanga Z; Ad Hoc ESPEN Working Group. Nutritional risk screening (NRS 2002): a new method based on an analysis of controlled clinical trials. *Clin Nutr.* 2003;22(3):321–336.

13. Malnutrition Advisory Group, British Association for Parenteral and Enteral Nutrition. Introducing "MUST". BAPEN website. http://www.bapen.org.uk/screening-for-malnutrition/must/introducing-must. Published April 10, 2013. Accessed November 14, 2019.

14. Cohendy R, Rubenstein LZ, Eledjam JJ. The Mini Nutritional Assessment-Short Form for preoperative nutritional evaluation of elderly patients. *Aging (Milano).* 2001;13(4):293–297.

15. Rubenstein LZ, Harker JO, Salvá A. et al. Screening for undernutrition in geriatric practice: Developing the short-form mini-nutritional assessment (MNA-SF). *J Gerontol A Biol Sci Med Sci.* 2001;56(6):M366–M372.

16. Ukleja A, Gilbert K, Mogensen KM, et al. Task Force on Standards for Nutrition Support: Adult Hospitalized Patients, the American Society for Parenteral and Enteral Nutrition. Standards for nutrition support: adult hospitalized patients. *Nutr Clin Pract.* 2018;33(6):906–920.

17. Worthington P, Balint J, Bechtold M, et al. When is parenteral nutrition appropriate? *JPEN J Parenter Enteral Nutr.* 2017;41(3):324–377.

18. Ukleja A, Freeman KL, Gilbert K, et al; Task Force on Standards for Nutrition Support: Adult Hospitalized Patients, and the American Society for Parenteral and Enteral Nutrition Board of Directors. Standards for nutrition support: adult hospitalized patients. *Nutr Clin Pract.* 2010;25(4):403–414.

19. Durfee SM, Gallagher-Allred C, Pasquale JA, Stechmiller J; ASPEN Board of Directors; Task Force on Standards for Specialized Nutrition Support for Adult Residents of Long Term Care Facilities. Standards for specialized nutrition support for adult residents of long-term care facilities. *Nutr Clin Pract.* 2006;21(1):96–104.

20. Kovacevich DS, Frederick A, Kelly D, Nishikawa R, Young L; ASPEN Board of Directors; Standards for Specialized Nutrition Support Task Force. Standards for specialized nutrition support: home care patients. *Nutr Clin Pract.* 2005;20(5):579–590.

21. Pesce-Hammond K, Wessel J. Nutrition assessment and decision making. In: Merritt R, ed. *The A.S.P.E.N. Nutrition Support Practice Manual.* Silver Spring, MD: ASPEN; 2005:3–26.

22. Krystofiac Russell M, Mueller C. Nutrition screening and assessment. *The A.S.P.E.N. Nutrition Support Core Curriculum.* Silver Spring, MD: ASPEN; 2007:163–186.

23. Mueller C, Compher C, Druyan ME, ASPEN Board of Directors. ASPEN clinical guidelines: nutrition screening, assessment and intervention in adults. *JPEN J Parenter Enteral Nutr.* 2011;35(1):16–24.

24. Guigoz Y. The Mini Nutritional Assessment review of the literature-what does it tell us? *J Nutr Health Aging.* 2006;10:466-485.

25. Detsky AS, McLaughlin JR, Baker JP, et al. What is subjective global assessment of nutritional status? *JPEN J Parenter Enteral Nutr.* 1987;11:8-13

26. Soeters PB, Reijven PLM, van Bokhorst-de van der Schueren MA, et al. A rational approach to nutrition assessment. *Clin Nutr.* 2008;27(5):706–716.

27. Jensen GL. Inflammation as the key interface of the medical and nutrition universes: a provocative examination of the future of clinical nutrition and medicine. *JPEN J Parenter Enteral Nutr.* 2006;30(5):453–463.

28. Fuhrman MP, Charney P, Mueller CM. Hepatic proteins and nutrition assessment. *J Am Diet Assoc.* 2004;104(8):1258–1264.

29. Barbosa-Silva MC. Subjective and objective nutritional assessment methods: what do they really assess? *Curr Opin Nutr Metab Care.* 2008;11(3):248–254.

30. White JV, Guenter P, Jensen GL, et al.; Academy Malnutrition Work Group; ASPEN Malnutrition Task Force; ASPEN Board of Directors. Consensus statement: Academy of Nutrition and Dietetics and the American Society for Parenteral and Enteral Nutrition: characteristics recommended for the identification and documentation of adult malnutrition (undernutrition). *JPEN J Parenter Enteral Nutr.* 2012;36(3):275–283.

31. Malone A, Hamilton C. The Academy of Nutrition and Dietetics/The American Society for Parenteral and Enteral Nutrition consensus malnutrition characteristics: application in practice. *Nutr Clin Pract.* 2013;28(6):639–650.

32. JeVenn AK, Galang M, Hipskin P, et al. Malnutrition screening and assessment. In: Mueller CM, ed. *ASPEN Adult Nutrition Support Core Curriculum.* 3rd ed. Silver Spring, MD: APSEN; 2017:185–212.

33. Jensen GL, Hsiao PY, Wheeler D. Adult nutrition assessment tutorial. *JPEN J Parenter Enteral Nutr.* 2012;36(3):267–274.

34. Jensen GL, Mirtallo J, Compher C, et al. Adult starvation and disease-related malnutrition: a proposal for etiology-based diagnosis in the clinical practice setting from the International Consensus Guideline Committee. *JPEN J Parenter Enteral Nutr.* 2010;34(2):156–159.

35. Blackburn GL, Bistrian BR, Maini BS, Schlamm HT, Smith MF. Nutritional and metabolic assessment of the hospitalized patient. *JPEN J Parenter Enteral Nutr.* 1977;1(1):11–22.

36. Jensen GL, Hsaio PY, Wheeler D. Nutrition screening and assessment. In: Mueller CM, ed. *A.S.P.E.N. Adult Nutrition Support Core Curriculum.* 2nd ed. Silver Spring, MD: ASPEN; 2012:155–169.

37. Kondrup J, Johansen N, Plum LM, et al. Incidence of nutritional risk and causes of inadequate nutritional care in hospitals. *Clin Nutr.* 2002;21(6):461–468.

38. Frankenfield DC, Coleman A, Alam S, Cooney R. Analysis of estimation methods for resting metabolic rate in critically ill adults. *JPEN J Parenter Enteral Nutr.* 2009;33(1):27–36.

39. Mifflin MD, St Jeor ST, Hill LA, Scott BJ, Daugherty SA, Koh YO. A new predictive equation for resting energy expenditure in healthy individuals. *Am J Clin Nutr.* 1990;51(2):241–247.

40. Hamilton C, ed. Nutrition-Focused Physical Exam: *An Illustrated Handbook.* Silver Spring, MD: ASPEN; 2016.

41. Esper DH. Utilization of nutrition-focused physical assessment in identifying micronutrient deficiencies. *Nutr Clin Pract.* 2015;30(2):194–202.

42. Sheean P, Gonzalez MC, Prado CM, et al. American Society for Parenteral and Enteral Nutrition Clinical Guidelines: the validity of body composition assessment in clinical populations [published online June 19, 2019]. *JPEN J Parenter Enteral Nutr.* doi:10.1002/jpen.1669

43. Norman K, Stobäus N, Gonzalez MC, Schulzke JD, Pirlich M. Hand grip strength: outcome predictor and marker of nutritional status. *Clin Nutr.* 2011;30(2):135–142.

44. Nicolo M, Compher CW, Still C, Huseini M, Dayton S, Jensen GL. Feasibility of accessing data in hospitalized patients to support diagnosis of malnutrition by the Academy-A.S.P.E.N. malnutrition consensus recommended clinical characteristics. *JPEN J Parenter Enteral Nutr.* 2014;38(8)954–959.

45. Keys A, Brozek J, Henschel A, et al. *The Biology of Human Starvation*. Minneapolis, MN: University of Minnesota Press; 1950.

46. Cederholm T, Jensen GL, Correia MITD, et al. GLIM criteria for the diagnosis of malnutrition – a consensus report from the global clinical nutrition community. *J Cachexia Sarcopenia Muscle*. 2019;10(1):207–217.

47. Jensen GL, Cederholm T, Correia MITD, et al. GLIM criteria for the diagnosis of malnutrition: a consensus report from the global clinical nutrition community. *JPEN J Parenter Enteral Nutr*. 2019;43(1):32–40.

48. Mehta NM, Corkins MR, Lyman B, et al; ASPEN Board of Directors. Defining pediatric malnutrition: a paradigm shift toward etiology-related definitions. *JPEN J Parenter Enteral Nutr*. 2013;37(4):460–481.

49. Becker PJ, Carney LN, Corkins MR, et al. Consensus statement of the Academy of Nutrition and Dietetics/American Society for Parenteral and Enteral Nutrition: indicators recommended for the identification and documentation of pediatric malnutrition (undernutrition). *Nutr Clin Pract*. 2015;30(1):147–161.

50. Green Corkins K. Nutrition-focused physical examination in pediatric patients. *Nutr Clin Pract*. 2015;30(2):203–209.

51. Guo S, Roche AF, Foman SJ, et al. Reference data on gains in weight and length during the first two years of life. *Pediatrics*. 1991;119(3):355-362

52. Boullata J, Nieman Carney L, Guenter P, eds. *The ASPEN Enteral Nutrition Handbook*. Silver Spring, MD: ASPEN; 2010.

53. Stroud M, Duncan H, Nightingale J. Guidelines for enteral feeding in adult hospital patients. *Gut*. 2003;52(suppl 7):vii1–vii12.

54. Mehta NM, Skillman HE, Irving SY, et al. Guidelines for the provision and assessment of nutrition support therapy in the pediatric critically ill patient: Society of Critical Care Medicine and American Society for Parenteral and Enteral Nutrition. *JPEN J Parenter Enteral Nutr*. 2017;41(5):706–742.

55. Thureen P. Early aggressive nutrition support. *Pediatr Rev*. 1999;20(9):e45–e55.

56. Jacobs A, Verlinden I, Vanhorebeek I, Van den Berghe G. Early supplemental parenteral nutrition in critically ill children: an update. *J Clin Med*. 2019;8(6):E830. doi:10.3390/jcm8060830

57. ASPEN Board of Directors; ASPEN Clinical Guidelines Task Force. Guidelines for the use of parenteral and enteral nutrition in adult and pediatric patients, III: nutrition assessment—adults [erratum in *JPEN J Parenter Enteral Nutr*. 2002;26(2):144]. *JPEN J Parenter Enteral Nutr*. 2002;26(1 suppl):1SA–138SA.

CHAPTER 2

Overview of Parenteral Nutrition

Introduction

Parenteral nutrition (PN) is the provision of intravenous (IV) nutrients to patients whose gastrointestinal (GI) tracts are not functioning or cannot be accessed. It may also be administered to patients whose nutrition needs cannot be met with oral diets or enteral nutrition (EN). Recognized as one of the major medical advances in the past 50 years, PN has provided lifesaving therapy for patients who could not otherwise be nourished. According to US national data, patients received PN during 292,655 hospital stays in 2014.[1] Because of its complexity, PN therapy requires careful monitoring by trained clinicians to avoid serious complications. New knowledge and technological advances with PN have resulted in appropriate patient selection and therapies that have steadily improved patient safety.

PN refers to a combination of nutrients — crystalline amino acids, dextrose, fat emulsion, sterile water for injection, electrolytes, vitamins, and minerals — administered intravenously. PN was initially called IV hyperalimentation, but now the terms peripheral PN (PPN) and central PN (CPN) are preferred. There are 2 types of PN admixtures. Mixtures of dextrose, amino acids, sterile water for injection, electrolytes, vitamins, and minerals are referred to as dextrose/amino acids (2-in-1) admixtures, whereas lipid injectable emulsion (ILE) is infused separately. PN admixtures that contain ILE in the same container with dextrose, amino acids, sterile water for injection, electrolytes, vitamins, and minerals are referred to as total nutrient admixtures, or 3-in-1 or all-in-one admixtures.

Successful infusion of hypertonic parenteral nutrients by Dudrick and colleagues[2] in the late 1960s was a major advancement in providing nutrition to patients with a nonfunctioning GI tract. Although there had been interest in providing IV nutrition since the 1600s, the work of Dudrick, Vars, and Rhoads was stimulated by the observation that nutrition status played an important role in how patients fared postoperatively (wound healing, complications, morbidity, and mortality).[3]

Early problems with providing PN therapy included sources of safe IV nutrients and adequate venous access for hypertonic nutrient administration. Vascular access problems were resolved by subclavian vein catheterization, which minimized thrombotic complications associated with PPN infusions. Early PN formulations consisted of dextrose and protein hydrolysates of either casein or fibrin. Protein hydrolysates, which may contain significant preformed ammonia, were abandoned for newer formulations containing crystalline amino acids that are better used and pose less risk of hyperammonemia. Soybean-oil ILE was not available in the United States until the 1970s and then was used primarily as a source of essential fatty acids.

It was not until the 1980s that ILEs were routinely used as an energy source. This coincided with the US Food and Drug Administration (FDA) approval for ILE to be compounded in the same container as other IV nutrients. An ILE containing a mixture of soybean and olive oils was approved by the FDA in 2013 but not marketed until 2018. A 4-oil ILE containing soybean oil, medium-chain triglycerides, olive oil, and fish oil was approved for use in the United States in adults in 2016. In 2018, a fish-oil ILE received approval in the United States for PN-associated cholestasis in pediatric patients.

PN has been used in several clinical situations. Early use demonstrated a significant benefit to patients with GI fistulas who were unable to ingest nutrients by mouth.[4] Home PN has become a lifeline for patients with intestinal failure (ie, short bowel syndrome), allowing them to resume a nearly normal lifestyle. Refinement of PN will continue to make it a useful therapy for patients with complex diseases whose GI tract is nonfunctional.

PN is a complex mixture containing up to 40 different chemical (nutrient) components that may result in issues with stability and compatibility.

Serious patient harm and death have resulted from improperly compounded PN formulations. For example, 2 deaths were attributed to the infusion of calcium phosphate precipitates resulting from an improper admixture process.[5] Other complications have contributed to patient morbidity, including catheter-related infections, hepatobiliary disease, and glucose disorders.[6,7] Complications can be minimized through careful patient selection and by having experienced clinicians work as an interdisciplinary team to oversee the nutrition support program.

Nehme[8] reported that patients receiving PN who were treated by an interdisciplinary team had significantly reduced metabolic and fluid/electrolyte complications as compared with patients treated by individual clinicians. It has also been determined that interdisciplinary teams are more likely to use PN according to clinical guidelines and scientific literature.[9]

Routes of Infusion

The components of PN determine its osmolarity and infusion route. PN may be prepared for peripheral vein infusion or infusion through a central venous access device. PN admixtures are typically hypertonic to body fluids and, if administered inappropriately, may result in venous thrombosis, suppurative thrombophlebitis, and/or extravasation (leakage of IV infusions into the extravascular tissue around the site of infusion). Specifically, the osmolarity of PN is dependent primarily on the content of dextrose, amino acids, and electrolytes. Dextrose contributes approximately 5 mOsm/g, amino acids contribute approximately 10 mOsm/g, and electrolytes contribute approximately 1 mOsm/mEq per individual electrolyte additive. As outlined in Table 2-1, for example, the estimated osmolarity of a 1-L PN that provides 150 g of dextrose, 50 g of amino acids, 20 g of ILE, and 150 mEq of total electrolyte additives is 1414 mOsm/L. Central venous administration is preferred because the maximum PN osmolarity generally tolerated by a peripheral vein in adults is approximately 900 mOsm/L.[10]

PN Component	mOsm	PN Content/L[b]	mOsm/L[b]
Dextrose	5/g	150 g	750
Amino acids	10/g	50 g	500
ILE, 20%	0.71/g (product dependent)	20 g	14
Electrolytes	1/mEq	150 mEq	150
			Total = 1414

ILE, lipid injectable emulsion; PN, parenteral nutrition.
[a]Based on approximations of the osmolarity of the PN components and used as an estimate only.
[b]Based on a 1-L volume.

CPN Formulations

CPN formulations are hyperosmolar (>1000 mOsm/L) and must be delivered into a large-diameter or "central" vein such as the superior vena cava. The rate of blood flow in these large vessels rapidly dilutes the hypertonic CPN to that of body fluids, minimizing complications associated with its infusion. CPN provides nutrition in a reasonable fluid volume and may be concentrated to provide adequate energy and protein for patients requiring fluid restriction. Because central venous access can be maintained for prolonged periods (weeks to years), CPN is preferred for use in patients who will require PN support for >7–14 days.

PPN Formulations

PPN formulations have similar composition as CPN formulations, but lower concentrations of nutrient components are necessary to allow peripheral venous administration.

The use of PPN is controversial, with many advocating that the risk of complications outweighs any potential benefit, as candidates for this therapy have only minor, if any, nutrition deficits.[11] Although less concentrated than CPN admixtures, PPN admixtures are also hyperosmolar (600–900 mOsm/L), which may cause phlebitis, and require frequent peripheral IV site rotations (generally every 48–72 hours). ILE may be used to increase the energy density of PPN with less osmolarity, and this has been reported to improve peripheral vein tolerance of PPN.[12] The addition of heparin at 1–2 units per milliliter of total volume has also been shown to improve PPN tolerance in premature infants.[13] Finally, the use of midline catheters may improve the peripheral vein tolerance to PPN. These catheters are longer, and the tip is more likely to reach a larger vein, where blood flow may dilute the PPN to a more tolerable concentration. For greater detail on IV access devices, see chapter 3.

Patients considered for PPN must meet 2 criteria: (1) peripheral venous access is available and (2) the patient can tolerate increased fluid volumes (eg, up to 2–3 L/d in a 60-kg adult). The patient should require <2 weeks of PPN. Contraindications to PPN are listed in Table 2-2.

Table 2-2. Contraindications to PPN[14]

Significant malnutrition (eg, >5% weight loss in last 3 mo)

Severe metabolic stress (eg, hypercatabolic, hypermetabolic)

Large nutrient or electrolyte needs (potassium is a strong vascular irritant)

Fluid restriction

Need for prolonged PN (>2 wk)

Renal or hepatic compromise

PN, parenteral nutrition; PPN, peripheral PN.

Indications for PN

General Guidelines

Malnutrition is associated with increased patient complications and mortality.[15] Although PN has been shown to improve several markers of nutrition status, prospective randomized trials have rarely shown PN to improve patient outcomes.[16,17] However, many of these trials have been criticized for inadequate study designs, including inconsistent control for nutrition status and extent or type of underlying disease as well as a lack of consistency in nutrient type and dose.[17,18] PN has been shown to be of benefit in the following circumstances: perioperative support of patients with moderate to severe malnutrition, GI fistulas, or short bowel syndrome; patients with critical illness who will have nothing by mouth for prolonged periods (eg, >5–7 days); and patients with severe acute necrotizing pancreatitis.[16,17,19,20]

PN is costly and may result in serious complications if used inappropriately.[21] The costs of PN include not only the admixture but also the placement and maintenance of a vascular access device, laboratory monitoring, and treatment for complications.[21] As such, the use of PN is scrutinized[16] and should only be used in patients who will demonstrate benefit.[22] Identifying these patients is not always an easy task because nutrition care may be confounded by the underlying disease process and its treatment. Fortunately, specific guidelines for implementation of PN have been developed by the American Society for Parenteral and Enteral Nutrition (ASPEN).[23] Criteria that may be used in determining the appropriate application of PN are outlined in Table 2-3. ASPEN published a consensus recommendation in 2017 to provide additional guidance regarding appropriate use of PN.[20] Considerations for PN use include the patient's nutrition status, GI function, and extent and severity of the underlying disease process.

GI function. Symptoms including nausea, vomiting, diarrhea, and abdominal distention or cramps may preclude the use of the GI tract for prolonged periods. The duration of inadequate oral nutrition and partial or complete starvation that impacts a patient's outcome is highly variable. Generally, treatment toxicities in patients with cancer that preclude adequate oral intake for >1 week are an indication for PN.[20] In patients with critical illness, PN is indicated if EN is not possible and hypermetabolism is expected to last >5 days.[16] For the patient with severe malnutrition, PN is indicated when an impairment of the GI tract occurs. PN is indicated in other conditions precluding the use of the GI tract for >7–10 days in adults, >5–7 days in pediatric patients, and >1–2 days in high-risk or premature neonates.[20,23-25] PN is often used when EN is unsuccessful or inadequate as evidenced by high gastric residual volumes or pulmonary aspiration. In some cases, enteral access is contraindicated or attempts at achieving enteral access may have failed. Finally, there may be certain conditions in which the GI tract should not be used until the underlying problem is treated (Table 2-3).

Table 2-3. Indications for PN

Guidelines	Considerations for PN Use
ASPEN guidelines[8,23]	1. Patients who are unable to meet nutrition requirement with EN. These patients already have, or have the potential of developing malnutrition. 2. PPN may be used in selected patients to provide partial or total nutrition support for up to 2 wk in patients who cannot ingest or absorb oral or enteral tube-delivered nutrients or if CPN is not feasible. 3. CPN support is necessary when parenteral feeding is indicated for >2 wk, peripheral venous access is limited, nutrient needs are large, or fluid restriction is required and the benefits of PN support outweigh the risks.

General guidelines	Use CPN when
	
	1. Patient has failed EN trial with appropriate tube placement (postpyloric).
	
	2. EN is contraindicated or the intestinal tract has severely diminished function because of underlying disease or treatment. Specific applicable conditions are as follows:
	
	  • Paralytic ileus
	
	  • Mesenteric ischemia
	
	  • Small bowel obstruction
	
	  • GI fistula, except when enteral access may be placed posterior to the fistula, or the volume of output (<200 mL/d) supports a trial of EN.
	
	3. A prolonged period without enteral feeding is anticipated (eg, postoperatively). As the exact duration of starvation that can be tolerated without increased morbidity is unknown, expert opinion suggests that wound healing would be impaired if PN is not started within 5-10 days after operation for patients unable to eat or tolerate enteral feeding.[2]
	
	CPN is withheld or withdrawn during clinical conditions in which the patient has a compromised ability to metabolize the infusion of energy substrate and nutrients and/or to process metabolic byproducts. Conditions in which nutrition support should be withheld until better tolerated are severe hyperglycemia, azotemia, encephalopathy and hyperosmolality, and severe fluid and electrolyte disturbances.

ASPEN, American Society for Parenteral and Enteral Nutrition; CPN, central PN; EN, enteral nutrition; GI, gastrointestinal; PN, parenteral nutrition; PPN, peripheral PN.

Clinical status. PN should only be initiated in patients who are hemodynamically stable and able to tolerate the fluid volume and protein, carbohydrate, and ILE doses necessary to provide adequate nutrient substrate. Table 2-4 shows examples of situations in which PN warrants caution.

Table 2-4. Clinical Conditions Warranting Cautious Use of PN[20]

Condition	Suggested Criteria[a]
Hyperglycemia	Glucose > 300 mg/dL
Azotemia	BUN > 100 mg/dL
Hyperosmolality	Serum osmolality > 350 mOsm/kg
Hypernatremia	Na > 150 mEq/L
Hypokalemia	K < 3 mEq/L
Hyperchloremic metabolic acidosis	Cl > 115 mEq/L
Hypophosphatemia	Phosphorus < 2 mg/dL
Hypochloremic metabolic alkalosis	Cl < 85 mEq/L

[a]There is no evidence in the literature of the specific criteria noted in this column. These values are suggestions by the authors and should be modified based on the specific patient in question or environment in which PN is being administered, such as intensive care, a general medical ward, a long-term care facility, or at home. These recommendations are not a substitute for the exercise of such judgment by the health professional but rather are a tool to be used by the health professional in the exercise of such judgment. These recommendations are voluntary and should not be deemed inclusive of all proper methods of care or exclusive of methods of care reasonably directed toward obtaining the same result.

The use of a nutrition consult form can be an educational tool for clinicians requesting PN for a specific patient to address the variables that may identify the potential PN candidate (Figure 2-1).

Figure 2-1. Nutrition Assessment and Recommendation Form

DATE	TIME	CONSULTING SERVICE	

IBW (KG)	ACTUAL WEIGHT (KG)	DOSING WEIGHT (KG)	RECENT WEIGHT LOSS (KG)

INDICATION

○ Acute pancreatitis   ○ SBO   ○ Ileus   ○ Fistula   ○ Short bowel syndrome
○ Intractable vomiting/diarrhea   ○ Other: _____

PHM

○ DM1   ○ DM2   ○ CHF   ○ CRI   ○ ESRD-HD   ○ Liver disease
○ Other: _____

CURRENT MEDICAL PROBLEMS

○ Hyperglycemia   ○ Sepsis   ○ Pregnancy   ○ Hyper TG   ○ ARF
○ Other: _____

CURRENT MEDICATIONS

Glucose Control

○ Insulin drip: _____
○ ICU–sliding scale (insulin) every: _____
○ Sliding scale (insulin) ( ) every: _____
○ Oral Hypoglycemics: _____
○ Octreotide: _____
○ Steroids: _____

Sedation

○ Propofol drip: _____

GI Meds

○ PPI (IV, by mouth, tube)

○ H2 blocker: _____

NUTRITION ACCESS

○ PICC   ○ Central line   ○ NG/OG-tube

ESTIMATED DAILY NEEDS

Energy: _____ kcal/d   Protein: _____ g/d

BASELINE NUTRITION STATUS

○ Acute malnutrition (acute injury/illness)   ○ Chronic disease-related malnutrition
○ Chronic malnutrition (starvation)   ○ Well-nourished at baseline
○ Nothing by mouth for 24–72 h   ○ Nothing by mouth for >72 h
○ Currently receiving EN meeting ____% of goals

REFEEDING RISK

○ Low   ○ Moderate   ○ High

BASELINE LABS

Na	K+	Cl	Bicarb	BUN	CR	Gluc	Ca	Alb
Mg	Phos	Chol	Trig	WBC	PLT	Hgb	HCT	PAB

CRCL: _____ mL/min   CBGs: _____

IMPRESSION

Recommendation/Formula: ○ Modified/special diet   ○ Enteral/tube feeding   ○ PN

Goals of Therapy: _____
_____
_____

Consult Completed by: _____

Sample/simulated form that may facilitate nutrition assessment including key components required to diagnose malnutrition, determine the indications for EN or PN, and establish a nutrition care plan that is documented for the patient. Alb, albumin; ARF, acute renal failure; Bicarb, bicarbonate; BUN, blood urea nitrogen; Ca, calcium; CBGs, complete blood gases; CHF, congestive heart failure; Chol, cholesterol; Cl, chloride; Corr Ca, corrected Ca; CR, creatinine; CRCL, CR clearance; CRI, chronic renal insufficiency; DM1, type 1 diabetes; DM2, type 2 diabetes; EN, enteral nutrition; ESRD-HD, end-stage renal disease on hemodialysis; GI, gastrointestinal; Gluc, glucose; H2 blocker, H-2 receptor antagonist; HCT, hematocrit; Hyper TG, hypertriglyceridemia; IBW, ideal body weight; ICa, ionized Ca; ICU, intensive care unit; IV, intravenous; K+, potassium; Labs, laboratory values; Meds, medications; Mg, magnesium; Na, sodium; NG/OG, nasogastric/orogastric; PAB, prealbumin; Phos, phosphorus; PICC, peripherally inserted central catheter; PLT, platelets; PMH, previous medical history; PN, parenteral nutrition; PPI, proton-pump inhibitor; SBO, small bowel obstruction; Trig, triglycerides; WBC, white blood cell count.

Specific Guidelines

GI disorders. PN has not been shown to improve patient outcomes as the primary management of acute exacerbations of Crohn's disease or ulcerative colitis.[16,17] Retrospective analysis of PN use in patients with small bowel fistulas suggests an improvement in mortality rates and spontaneous and surgical closures except when the fistula arises from a bowel affected by active Crohn's disease.[16] Data suggest that bowel rest is not necessary to achieve remission in Crohn's disease.[17]

PN is unlikely to benefit patients with mild, acute, or chronic relapsing pancreatitis when the condition lasts for <1 week.[16,20,23,25-28] A recent systematic review found that PN was not beneficial and was associated with net harm in patients with mild pancreatitis.[16] Other reviews discuss the favorable response observed with EN in severe acute pancreatitis.[29-31] Patients who have a protracted course of pancreatitis or those with severe disease or complications often may require PN; however, there is a paucity of clinical trials determining the optimal route, dose, or nutrient mix.[23,31-33]

Perioperative malnutrition. Malnutrition is associated with an increase in operative complications during the perioperative period. During this time, disturbances of the GI tract often occur in surgical patients, triggering consideration of PN support. Outcomes from PN are influenced by the patient's duration of inadequate intake and his or her nutrition status and comorbidities.[19] A beneficial effect of PN has been difficult to demonstrate in surgical patients who are well-nourished or have mild malnutrition. In fact, PN has been associated with net harm in these patients.[16] However, in patients with moderate malnutrition undergoing surgery for upper GI cancer, patient outcomes were improved with PN support.[16] In addition, patients with severe malnutrition benefited from perioperative PN in the Veterans Affairs cooperative study.[34] The potential benefits compared with risks should be considered when deciding to use PN in the perioperative period. In general, routine use of PN during the perioperative period should be avoided[19]; however, patients with moderate to severe malnutrition who are expected to have a prolonged period of GI dysfunction may benefit from PN.

Critical illness. The rate of malnutrition is accelerated in patients with critical illness; therefore, nutrition is an important component of critical care. Gut failure, most often due to mesenteric ischemia, in patients with critical illness is common. The presence of critical illness also impedes the effectiveness of PN. Hemodynamic stability is generally required to improve the risk-to-benefit ratio of PN. Although it is accepted that early EN is better than PN, the benefit may not be achieved if EN is delayed.[32,35] In general, patients with critical illness requiring PN are those who are hemodynamically stable and have a paralytic ileus, acute GI bleed, or bowel obstruction.

Cancer. Routine PN use in patients receiving chemotherapy or radiation is associated with increased infectious complications and no improvement in clinical response, survival, or toxicity to chemotherapy.[16] ASPEN guidelines for providing nutrition support in adult patients receiving anticancer therapy recommend a thorough assessment of a patient's nutrition status and the use of PN only in those who have malnutrition and are anticipated to be unable to ingest and absorb adequate nutrients for a period of 7–14 days.[36] EN is preferred in patients with cancer who have functional GI tracts. EN is also preferred in patients undergoing a hematopoietic cell transplant.[36,37] Until more specific data are available, indications for these patients are similar to those for other conditions.

Home PN. In general, indications for home PN are the same as for hospitalized patients, but with careful consideration of the capabilities of the patient and family members, as well as the safety of the home environment for PN. (For greater detail on home PN support, please see chapter 10.)

ASPEN developed clinical guidelines for various disease and clinical states. These publications can be accessed via the society at http://www.nutritioncare.org/Clinical_Practice_Library/.

Specific Indications for PN in Pediatric Patients

High-Risk and Premature Infants

High-risk and preterm infants are at nutrition risk due to reduced nutrient stores, increased energy requirements for metabolism and growth, immature intestinal motility, and an uncoordinated and/or undeveloped suck/swallow reflex. Because the suck/swallow reflex develops late in gestation (around 35 weeks), most premature infants are unable to successfully take oral feedings postdelivery. To prevent catabolism, premature infants of <32 weeks' gestation are given PN support initially, which is gradually weaned as EN is initiated and advanced. Because the maturation of intestinal motility and development of the suck/swallow reflex are directly related to postconceptional age, infants born at <30 weeks' gestation may not reach full EN goals for a week or longer. In addition, concerns about necrotizing enterocolitis developing can further delay advancement of EN in premature infants. In preterm infants, initiating PN support early (within 24 hours of delivery), and providing protein in particular, has been shown to improve nitrogen balance, energy intake, and glucose tolerance without adverse metabolic effects.[38]

Pediatric Patients

PN should be used when the GI tract is not functional or cannot be accessed or when the patient's nutrient needs are greater than those that can be met through the GI tract.[39]

PN support is indicated in infants with congenital or acquired bowel anomalies (eg, intestinal atresia, intestinal stricture, gastroschisis, omphalocele, tracheoesophageal fistula, Hirschsprung's disease) until the anomaly can be surgically corrected. PN is also indicated for the medical management of necrotizing enterocolitis and following small bowel resection for intestinal anomalies resulting in intestinal failure. In addition, PN support is used in infants with failure to thrive and in any pediatric patient with protracted vomiting and/or diarrhea.[40,41]

Appropriate Use of PN

ASPEN guidelines and consensus recommendations provide practical advice for appropriate PN use as well as safe practices.[20,23] Pace and colleagues[42] were concerned with the overuse of PN, underuse of EN, and the need to update hospital policies and procedures to reflect recent advances and changes in nutrition support practice. A performance model was used to revise policies and procedures and educate staff.[42] This process resulted in a 52% decrease in PN use over a 4-year period, an increase in appropriate PN use from 74% to 95%, and elimination of PPN use.

In a tertiary care teaching hospital, PN use was evaluated in 209 patients treated by either individual medical or surgical services or a metabolic support service.[9] Indications for PN were derived from ASPEN guidelines.[23] PN therapy was considered to be preventable if there was a functional small bowel but no suitable enteral access. Therapy was considered to be contraindicated if the patients were classified as well-nourished and had inadequate EN for <7 days, had a "do not resuscitate" status, and were deemed to warrant comfort measures only or were terminally ill, or were receiving adequate EN. Of the PN regimens initiated, 62% were indicated, 23% were preventable, and 15% were not indicated. Compliance with established guidelines was improved when patients were treated by the metabolic support service.[9]

Summary

ASPEN guidelines are useful in identifying patients likely to benefit from PN. PPN may be useful for limited periods of time in maintaining nutrition status until the GI tract is functional. CPN provides adequate nutrients to maintain and make replete the patient's nutrition stores. Favorable physiologic effects have been observed, and patient outcomes such as comparable outcomes with EN[43] and improvements in body composition[44] and performance[45] have been recently reported. Therefore, PN should be used to prevent or improve malnutrition in patients in whom the enteral route is contraindicated or in whom a trial of enteral feeding has failed.

References

1. Agency for Healthcare Research and Quality (AHRQ). National (Nationwide) Inpatient Sample (NIS) of the Healthcare Cost and Utilization Project (HCUP). Available at: https://www.hcup-us.ahrq.gov/nisoverview.jsp. Accessed October 29, 2019.

2. Dudrick SJ, Wilmore DW, Vars HM, Rhoads JE. Long-term total parenteral nutrition with growth, development, and positive nitrogen balance. *Surgery*. 1968;64(6):134–142.

3. Dudrick SJ. Early developments and clinical applications of total parenteral nutrition. *JPEN J Parenter Enteral Nutr*. 2003;27(4):291–299.

4. Rhoads JE, Dudrick SJ. History of intravenous nutrition. In: Rombeau JL, Caldwell MD, eds. *Clinical Nutrition. Parenteral Nutrition*. 2nd ed. Philadelphia, PA: WB Saunders; 1993:1–10.

5. Lumpkin MM. Safety alert: hazards of precipitation associated with parenteral nutrition. *Am J Hosp Pharm*. 1994;51(11):1427–1428.

6. Btaiche IF, Khalidi N. Metabolic complications of parenteral nutrition in adults, part 2. *Am J Heath Syst Pharm*. 2004;61(19):2050–2057; quiz 2058–2059.

7. McCowen KC, Bistrian BR. Hyperglycemia and nutrition support: theory and practice. *Nutr Clin Pract*. 2004;19(3):235–244

8. Nehme AE. Nutritional support of the hospitalized patient. *JAMA*. 1980;243(19):1906–1908.

9. Trujillo EB, Young LS, Chertow GM, et al. Metabolic and monetary costs of avoidable parenteral nutrition use. *JPEN J Parenter Enteral Nutr*. 1999;23(2):109–113.

10. Mirtallo J, Canada T, Johnson D, et al.; Task Force for the Revision of Safe Practices for Parenteral Nutrition. Safe practices for parenteral nutrition [erratum in *JPEN J Parenter Enteral Nutr*. 2006;30(2):177]. *JPEN J Parenter Enteral Nutr*. 2004;28(6):S39–SS70.

11. Doglietto GB, Gallitelli L, Pacelli F, et al.; Protein-Sparing Therapy Study Group. Protein-sparing therapy after major abdominal surgery: lack of clinical effects. *Ann Surg*. 1996;223(4):357–362.

12. Anderson ADG, Palmer D, MacFie J. Peripheral parenteral nutrition. *Br J Surg.* 2003;90(9):1048–1054.

13. Alpan G, Eyal F, Springer C, Glick B, Goder K, Armon J. Heparinization of alimentation solutions administered through peripheral veins in premature infants: a randomized, controlled study. *Pediatrics.* 1984;74(3):375–378.

14. Pittruti M, Hililton H, Biffi R, MacFie J, Pertkiewicz M; ESPEN. ESPEN guidelines on parenteral nutrition: central venous catheters (access, care, diagnosis and care of complications). *Clin Nutr.* 2009;28(4):365–377.

15. Dempsey DT, Mullen JL, Buzby GP. The link between nutritional status and clinical outcome. Can nutritional intervention modify it? *Am J Clin Nutr.* 1988;47(2 suppl):352–356.

16. Klein S, Kinney J, Jeejeebhoy K, et al. Nutrition support in clinical practice: review of published data and recommendations for future research directions. Summary of a conference sponsored by the National Institutes of Health, American Society for Parenteral and Enteral Nutrition, and American Society for Clinical Nutrition. *JPEN J Parenter Enteral Nutr.* 1997;66(3):683–706.

17. Koretz RL, Lipman TO, Klein S; American Gastroenterological Association. AGA technical review on parenteral nutrition. *Gastroenterology.* 2001;121(4):970–1001.

18. Detsky AS, Baker JP, O'Rourke K, Goel V. Perioperative parenteral nutrition: a meta-analysis. *Ann Intern Med.* 1987;107(2):195–203.

19. Compher CW, Spencer C, Kinosian B. Perioperative parenteral nutrition: impact on morbidity and mortality in surgical patients. *Nutr Clin Pract.* 2005;20(4):460–467.

20. Worthington P, Balint J, Bechtold M, et.al. When is parenteral nutrition appropriate? *JPEN J Parenter Enteral Nutr.* 2017;41(3):324–377.

21. Twomey PL, Patching SC. Cost effectiveness of nutritional support. *JPEN J Parenter Enteral Nutr.* 1985;9(1):3–10.

22. Mullen JL, Buzby GP, Matthews DC, Smale BF, Rosato EF. Reduction of operative morbidity and mortality by combined preoperative and postoperative nutrition support. *Ann Surg.* 1980;192(4):604–613.

23. ASPEN Board of Directors and the Clinical Guidelines Task Force. Guidelines for the use of parenteral and enteral nutrition in adult and pediatric patients [erratum in *JPEN J Parenter Enteral Nutr.* 2002;26(2):144]. *JPEN J Parenter Enteral Nutr.* 2002;26(1 suppl):1SA–138SA.

24. Valentine CJ, Puthoff TD. Enhancing parenteral nutrition therapy for the neonate. *Nutr Clin Pract.* 2007;22(2):183–193.

25. Herrmann KR, Herrmann KR. Early parenteral nutrition and successful postnatal growth of premature infants. *Nutr Clin Pract.* 2010;25(1):69–75.

26. Kalfarentzos F, Kehagias J, Mead N, Kokkinis K, Gogos CA. Enteral nutrition is superior to parenteral nutrition in severe acute pancreatitis: results of a randomized prospective trial. *Br J Surg.* 1997;84(12):1665–1669.

27. McClave SA, Greene LM, Snider HL, et al. Comparison of the safety of early enteral vs parenteral nutrition in mild acute pancreatitis. *JPEN J Parenter Enteral Nutr.* 1997;21(1):14–20.

28. Windsor AC, Kanwar S, Li AG, et al. Compared with parenteral nutrition, enteral feeding attenuates the acute phase response and improves disease severity in acute pancreatitis. *Gut.* 1998;42(3):431–435.

29. Avgerinos C, Delis S, Rizos S, Dervenis C. Nutritional support in acute pancreatitis. *Dig Dis.* 2003;21(3):214–219.

30. Alsolaiman MM, Green JA, Barkin JS. Should enteral feeding be the standard of care for acute pancreatitis? *Am J Gastroenterol.* 2003;98(11):2565–2567.

31. Al-Omran M, Groof A, Wilke D. Enteral versus parenteral nutrition for acute pancreatitis. *Cochrane Database Syst Rev.* 2003;(1):CD002837. doi:10.1002/14651858. CD002837

32. McClave SA, Martindale RG, Vanek VW, et al.; A.S.P.E.N. Board of Directors; American College of Critical Care Medicine; Society of Critical Care Medicine. Guidelines for the

provision and assessment of nutrition support therapy in the adult critically ill patient: Society of Critical Care Medicine (SCCM) and American Society for Parenteral and Enteral Nutrition (A.S.P.E.N.). *JPEN J Parenter Enteral Nutr.* 2009;33(3):277-316.

33. Tenner S, Baillie J, DeWitt J, Vege SS; American College of Gastroenterology. American College of Gastroenterology guideline: management of acute pancreatitis. *Am J Gastroenterol.* 2013;108(9):1400-1415, 1416.

34. Veterans Affairs Total Parenteral Nutrition Cooperative Study Group. Perioperative total parenteral nutrition in surgical patients. *N Engl J Med.* 1991;325(8):525-532.

35. Simpson F, Doig GS. Parenteral vs. enteral nutrition in critically ill patient: a meta-analysis of trials using the intention to treat principle. *Intensive Care Med.* 2005;31(1):12-23.

36. August DA, Huhmann MB; American Society for Parenteral and Enteral Nutrition (A.S.P.E.N.) Board of Directors. A.S.P.E.N. clinical guidelines: nutrition support therapy during adult anticancer treatment and in hematopoietic cell transplantation. *JPEN J Parenter Enteral Nutr.* 2009;33(5):472-500.

37. Arfons LM, Lazarus HM. Total parenteral nutrition and hematopoietic stem cell transplantation: an expensive placebo? *Bone Marrow Transplant.* 2005;36(4):281-288.

38. Denne SC, Poindexter BB. Evidence supporting early nutritional support with parenteral amino acid infusion. *Semin Perinatol.* 2007;31(2):56-60.

39. Corkins MR, Griggs KC, Groh-Wargo S, et al.; Task Force on Standards for Nutrition Support: Pediatric Hospitalized Patients; American Society for Parenteral and Enteral Nutrition Board of Directors; American Society for Parenteral and Enteral Nutrition. Standards for nutrition support: pediatric hospitalized patients. *Nutr Clin Pract.* 2013;28(2):263-276.

40. Koletzko B, Goulet O, Hunt J, Krohn K, Shamir R; Parenteral Nutrition Guidelines Working Group; European Society for Clinical Nutrition and Metabolism; European Society of Paediatric Gastroenterology, Hepatology and Nutrition (ESPGHAN); European Society of Paediatric Research (ESPR). Guidelines on paediatric parenteral nutrition of the European Society of the European Society of Paediatric Gastroenterology, Hepatology and Nutrition (ESPGHAN) and the European Society for Clinical Nutrition and Metabolism (ESPEN), supported by the Society of Paediatric Research. *J Ped Gastroenterol Nutr.* 2005;41(suppl 2):S1-S87.

41. Mehta NM, Compher C; A.S.P.E.N. Board of Directors. A.S.P.E.N. Clinical Guidelines: nutrition support of the critically ill child. *JPEN J Parenter Enteral Nutr.* 2009;33(3):260-276.

42. Pace NM, Long JB, Elerding S, et al. Performance model anchors successful nutrition support protocol. *Nutr Clin Pract.* 1997;12(6):274-279.

43. Klek S, Sierzega M, Szykinski P, et al. Perioperative nutrition in malnourished surgical cancer patients – a prospective, randomized, controlled clinical trial. *Clin Nutr* 2011;30(6):708-713.

44. Pelzer U, Arnold D, Govercin M, et al. Parenteral nutrition support for patients with pancreatic cancer. Results of a phase II study. *BMC Cancer.* 2010;10:86. doi:10.1186/1471-2407-10-86

45. Chermish I, Mashiach T, Annil A, et al. Home parenteral nutrition (HTPN) for incurable patients with cancer with gastrointestinal obstruction. Do the benefits outweigh the risks? *Med Oncol.* 2011;28(1):83-88.

Parenteral Nutrition Access Devices

Introduction

Despite their essential role in parenteral nutrition (PN) administration, vascular access devices (VADs) are a leading cause of serious adverse events related to PN therapy. A variety of peripheral and central VADs are available, some better suited to PN delivery than others.[1-5] When choosing a VAD for PN administration, an individualized approach that incorporates pertinent clinical information with an appraisal of the risk/benefit profile of the device promotes optimal outcomes. Healthcare organizations must implement PN protocols that address VAD insertion and maintenance, including measures aimed at reducing contamination that happens during manipulation of the catheter hub. In many ways, maintaining trouble-free vascular access is as challenging as providing the primary therapy. The greatest benefit of successful vascular access is its translation to fewer complications and improved quality of life for many patients. Table 3-1 provides an overview of VADs that highlights specific considerations for PN administration.

Table 3-1. Selection of Vascular Access Devices for PN

Type	Insertion	Dwell Time	Therapeutic Applications	PN Considerations
PVCs	Bedside insertion; <3 in long, usually inserted in veins of forearm or hand.	72–96 h. Site rotation based on clinical indication is not recommended.	Use is limited by osmolarity restrictions. Not suitable for home care because of high failure rates. Not suited for home PN.	May be used for peripheral PN for short-term therapy. Requires careful assessment of venous integrity. Peripheral PN may increase the incidence of phlebitis, particularly in pediatric patients.
Peripheral midline catheters	Requires ultrasound guided placement; 3–8 in long; inserted via the antecubital fossa into proximal basilic or cephalic veins—does not reach the central veins.	For therapies lasting >6 d; can remain in place up to 29 d.	Same restrictions for osmolarity as those for other PVCs. Not suited for home PN.	As above, associated with lower rates of phlebitis than short peripheral devices, but safety with peripheral PN is unknown.
Percutaneous nontunneled central catheters	Bedside insertion; subclavian, internal jugular sites; femoral approach is possible but suboptimal for PN because of high infection risk.	5 d to a few wk.	Appropriate for acute care settings; not suited for home care.	Not designed for self-care by patient, easily dislodged, especially in children. Preferred over PICC for access up to 14 d.
PICCs	Bedside insertion into basilic, cephalic, or brachial veins; tip rests in superior vena cava; easily removed at bedside. In difficult cases, may require fluoroscopic placement by interventional radiologist.	Maximum dwell time is unknown	Suitable for acute care, and short-term and medium-term PN for both adults and pediatric patients.	CLABSI rates are similar to percutaneous nontunneled devices. Associated with an increased risk for DVT, limiting use for indefinite PN therapy and situations in which vessel preservation is a priority. Antecubital location of exit site hinders self-care and activity. Clothing may not always cover insertion site, potentially having a negative impact on body image. May be easily removed when infected or when PN is no longer needed.
Tunneled catheters (Hickman or Broviac type)	Surgical or fluoroscopic insertion; bedside or outpatient removal.	3 mo to years.	Suitable for long-term PN; the presence of a cuff within the tunnel inhibits microbial migration and decreases risk of dislodgement.	No restrictions on upper extremity activity. Position on chest facilitates self-care; catheter can be easily hidden under clothing.

Type	Insertion	Dwell Time	Therapeutic Applications	PN Considerations
Implanted ports	Surgical or fluoroscopic insertion via subclavian, internal jugular, or peripheral veins; a port (single or double) is implanted in a subcutaneous pocket; requires surgical removal.	6 mo to years.	Primarily intended for low-frequency, intermittent access. Associated with lowest risk for CLABSI because of reduced manipulation. The presence of an indwelling needle for continuous or frequent access offsets the reduced infection benefit.	Suitable for PN in selected circumstances; motivated patients can learn access procedures; body image remains intact; requires no local site care when device is not accessed. PN may increase risk for CLABSI and occlusion in children with cancer.
Special purpose catheters (sheath introducers; pulmonary artery catheters, apheresis catheters)	Bedside or fluoroscopic insertion techniques.	Dwell time varies with the device and indication for use.	Generally, large-bore devices; subject to manipulation when hemodynamic monitoring is performed; associated high levels of microbial contamination.	Pose increased risks of CLABSI and thrombosis. Use of these devices for PN should be decided on a case-by-case basis, weighing the potential for complications against the risk of placing an additional line. PN should never be administered through a pressure-monitoring circuit.
Percutaneous femoral central venous catheters	Similar to upper extremity catheters, but relatively simple bedside insertion.	Not appropriate for long-term use. Should be removed as soon as feasible.	Tip position should rest in the inferior vena cava.	PN administration is discouraged because of high rate of complications associated with femoral vein insertion site. No data specific to osmolarity limits or PN administration are available.
Umbilical catheters	Surgical bedside insertion in neonates with critical illness.	Arterial catheters: 5 d; venous catheters: 14 d.	Provides reliable, short-term venous access in acute care.	PN has been identified as a risk factor for infection with umbilical vein catheters. Catheters should be removed and not replaced is signs of infection or thrombosis develop

CLABSI, central line–associated bloodstream infection; DVT, deep vein thrombosis; PICC, peripherally inserted central catheter; PN, parenteral nutrition; PVC, peripheral venous catheter. Adapted with permission from Worthington P, Balint J, Bechtold M, et al. When is parenteral nutrition appropriate? *JPEN J Parenter Enteral Nutr.* 2017 Mar;41(3):324–377.

Physiologic Principles and Vascular Anatomy

Venous blood flow is influenced by several physiologic principles promoting the return of blood to the heart and lungs.[6,7] Negative thoracic pressure occurs during inspiration, and muscle contractions and valves within peripheral veins assist in blood return. In the upper and lower extremities, the system of paired valves prevents retrograde blood flow against gravity. In the large central veins, such as the inferior vena cava (IVC) and superior vena cava (SVC), blood flow is not dependent on valves but relies on negative intrathoracic pressure and abdominal and diaphragmatic muscle movement. Veins, as opposed to arteries, are able to compensate for occlusions through collateral circulation.

The superficial veins of the upper extremity are visible and palpable within the superficial fascia. As shown in Figure 3-1, these vessels include the basilic, cephalic, and median cubital veins. The SVC is the main vessel for venous return from the upper trunk emptying into the right atrium.[6,7] The subclavian vessels receive the external jugular veins and join with the internal jugular vein to form the brachiocephalic vein. The SVC is formed by the joining of the right and left brachiocephalic veins. The SVC is approximately 7 cm long and 20–30 mm in diameter. The estimated blood flow is 2000 mL/min, making it the preferred site for the infusion of vesicant (potentially irritating) and hyperosmolar fluids.[6,7] Figure 3-1 also shows the location of the SVC, as well as the internal jugular and subclavian veins, which may serve as the insertion site for accessing the SVC.

Figure 3-1. Selected Vascular Anatomy

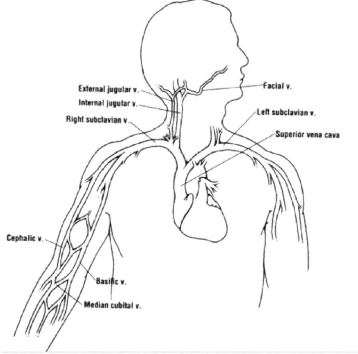

Rt., right; SVC, superior vena cava; v., vein. Reprinted from Neal AM, Drogan K. Parenteral access devices. In: Mueller CM, ed. *The ASPEN Adult Nutrition Support Core Curriculum.* 3rd ed. Silver Spring, MD: ASPEN; 2017. **Original Source**: Bennett JD, Papadouris D, Rankin RN, et al. Percutaneous inferior vena caval approach for long-term central venous access. *J Vasc Interv Radiol.* 1997;8(5):851–855.

Nomenclature: Peripheral vs Central Access

The distinction between peripheral and central venous access is based not on the initial point of entry into the vascular system but rather on the position of the distal catheter tip.[8] A peripheral venous catheter (PVC) enters and terminates in a peripheral vein in the hand; arm; or, in infants, the scalp or foot.[2,9] Examples of peripheral catheters include short peripheral intravenous cannulas and midline catheters.

The term central VAD applies to a variety of devices in which the catheter tip reaches the central circulation. Insertion sites for central VAD include peripheral veins; the subclavian, internal jugular, or femoral veins; or the vessels of the umbilical cord.[9] Regardless of insertion site, the tip of the central VAD must terminate in the lower one-third of the SVC or cavoatrial junction or, for lines placed via the femoral vein, within the IVC above the level of the diaphragm.[2] Clinicians commonly refer to central VADs by the insertion site of the device, for example, "subclavian line," "internal jugular line," or "femoral line."[8] Each of these sites is associated with a varying degree of risk for infectious, thrombotic, and mechanical complications, with the subclavian site preferred for reducing central line–associated bloodstream infection (CLABSI) risk.[10] Femoral lines allow rapid cannulation in emergency situations, but overall, femoral catheters should be avoided because of the risk of infection.[11]

Examples of central VADs are primarily central venous access devices (CVADs), such as percutaneous nontunneled catheters, peripherally inserted central catheters (PICCs), implanted ports, tunneled catheters, dialysis catheters, and umbilical catheters[9,12] However, there are instances in which an artery is used for an umbilical catheter. Figure 3-2 shows examples of central VADs that are appropriate for long-term PN administration.

Figure 3-2. Long-Term Vascular Access for Parenteral Nutrition

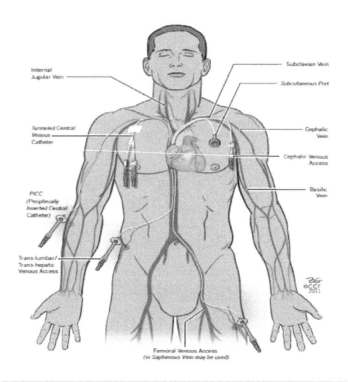

Source: Reprinted with permission, Cleveland Clinic Center for Medical Art & Photography ©2011–2017.

Peripheral Venous Catheters

One of the simplest ways to access the vascular system is to place a cannula into a peripheral vessel. Although PVCs can be used to administer dilute (<900 mOsm/L) nutrient admixtures, a high rate of technical failure stands out as the chief disadvantage of these devices.[9,13] A large database search of complications associated with PVCs over a 9-year period identified infiltration as the leading complication of peripheral access, followed by phlebitis.[9] The hallmark symptoms of infusion phlebitis include pain, erythema, tenderness, or a palpable cord.[2] This phenomenon has been related to a number of risk factors including catheter material, size, operator skill, type of infusate, and duration of cannulation.

PVCs are intended for short-term use, and the need for frequent reinsertion is an important limitation of these devices. Policies governing dwell time for PVCs vary. Guidelines issued by the US Centers for Disease Control suggest rotating insertion sites every 72–96 hours, whereas the Infusion Therapy Standards of Practice recommend replacing PVCs only when clinically indicated based on regular inspection of the site for evidence of phlebitis or extravasation (leakage into the extravascular tissue around the site of infusion).[1,2]

Recently, a large multicenter prospective study found an increase in phlebitis in PVCs after 96 hours in situ, supporting recommendations for scheduled site rotation.[14] Other research that examined data related to primary bloodstream infection (BSI) in adult hospitalized patients suggested a link between BSI and PVCs left in place >72 hours.[15] These findings call into question the safety of allowing PVCs to remain in place until warning signs of malfunction appear. Until further research delineates the optimal dwell time for PVCs, scheduled rotation of PVC sites for peripheral PN may be the most prudent policy, given the elevated risk for infectious and thrombotic complications associated with PN. Regardless of the policy for rotating the site of the peripheral intravenous catheters, the device should be removed promptly when evidence of phlebitis develops.[2] Focused surveillance for complications related to PVCs is needed to guide organizational policies and procedures related to PVC care.[9]

The dubious reliability of PVCs is frequently cited as a reason for avoiding peripheral PN.[13] Yet strategies for reducing CLABSI uniformly recommend limiting the use of central VADs in acute care settings, thus increasing pressure to rely on PVCs whenever possible.[1,2,9,16,17] In this setting, peripheral midline catheters, which can remain in place for 29 days, have emerged as an alternative to conventional PVCs.[18,19] A recent multicenter study of midline catheters found a relatively low rate of complications associated with midline devices, despite wide variation in care practices.[20]

As with all PVCs, midline catheters are prone to causing phlebitis, and no researchers, to our knowledge, have studied the use of these devices for peripheral PN.[8,21] Moreover, the location of these devices in a deeper vein may mask signs and symptoms of phlebitis such as redness or pain.

Central Venous Access Devices

Conceptually, CVADs, a type of central VAD, fall into 3 broad categories: nontunneled catheters, tunneled catheters, and implanted ports.[2,12,21,22] This general classification guides catheter selection according to factors such as the type and duration of therapy and the location of the healthcare setting in which care takes place.

Percutaneous Nontunneled Catheters

Nontunneled CVADs are most commonly used in the acute care setting for therapies of short duration.[1,2,17,22] Traditionally, these devices are inserted percutaneously into large veins (eg, subclavian, internal jugular, or femoral) and then threaded into the vena cava.[1,17] (Figure 3-3). The percutaneous approach for insertion of these CVADs carries an increased risk for pneumothorax and arterial puncture compared with other insertion methods used for central venous access.[1]

Figure 3-3. Percutaneous Nontunneled Catheter

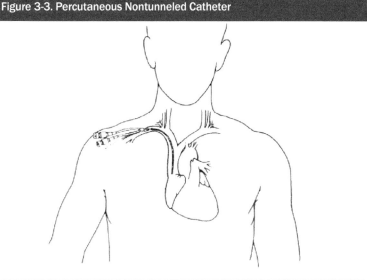

Reprinted from Krzywda EA, Adris DA, Edmiston CE, Wallace JR. Parenteral Access Devices. In: Gottschlich M, ed. *The A.S.P.E.N. Nutrition Support Core Curriculum: A Case-Based Approach—The Adult Patient.* Silver Spring, MD: ASPEN; 2007:300–322.

Peripherally Inserted Central Catheters

PICCs represent another type of nontunneled CVAD. Compared with other types of CVAD, insertion procedures for PICCs are more convenient and safer. These advantages have led to substantial increases in the use of PICCs in both acute care and home settings.[23] Although PICCs have a lower incidence of infectious complications than nontunneled CVADs, they appear to carry a higher risk for infection as compared with tunneled catheters in patients who receive home PN.[24] PICCs pose an increased risk for deep vein thrombosis (DVT) compared with other types of CVAD, a complication with important ramifications for long-term PN recipients.[25-27]

PICC placement is accomplished using the antecubital vessels of the arm, (ie, the basilic, cephalic, and brachial veins). This approach decreases the risks of a thoracic approach to catheter placement. Nurses and physicians with specialized training may place these catheters. The setting for PICC placement varies and can occur in the patient's home, at the bedside, or in a surgical or interventional radiology suite. (Figure 3-4).

Figure 3-4. Peripherally Inserted Central Venous Catheter

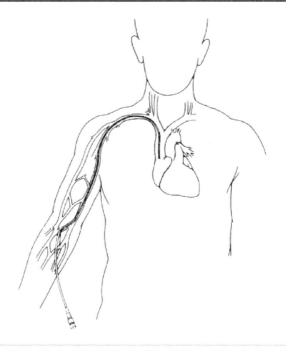

Reprinted from Krzywda EA, Adris DA, Edmiston CE, Wallace JR. Parenteral Access Devices. In: *The A.S.P.E.N. Nutrition Support Core Curriculum: A Case-Based Approach: The Adult Patient.* Gottschlich M, ed. Silver Spring, MD: A.S.P.E.N.; 2007; 300-322.

Tunneled Catheters

Tunneled CVADs, such as Broviac and Hickman catheters, were first developed for administration of long-term PN but are now also used for long-term administration of parenteral antibiotics and chemotherapies[21] (Figure 3-5). These devices lower the risk of infection by means of a subcutaneous tunnel that separates the exit site from the venipuncture location. A Dacron cuff attached to the extravascular segment of the catheter acts as a mechanical barrier that inhibits migration of microbes along the external tract of the device.[1,17] The procedure for placing and removing tunneled catheters is more invasive than that for nontunneled devices.

Figure 3-5. Tunneled Central Venous Catheter

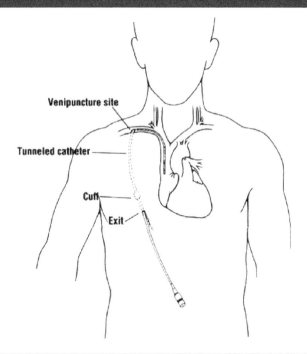

Reprinted from Krzywda EA, Adris DA, Edmiston CE, Wallace JR. Parenteral Access Devices. In: *The A.S.P.E.N. Nutrition Support Core Curriculum: A Case-Based Approach: The Adult Patient.* Gottschlich M, ed. Silver Spring, MD: A.S.P.E.N.; 2007; 300-322.

Implanted Catheters

Implanted catheters, often called ports, overcome many of the problems inherent in external lumen catheters. Implanted ports consist of a silicone elastomer catheter attached to a chamber or port that is placed in the subcutaneous tissue during a procedure performed by a surgeon or interventional radiologist (Figure 3-6). The anterior chest is the most common location for implanted ports, but peripherally inserted ports, for which the chamber rests under the skin of the arm, are also available. Access to the port is achieved by palpating the port and inserting a noncoring needle into a silicone septum located on the port. Advances in port design include models with a larger septum, double-lumen ports, and side-entry ports.

Implanted ports offer a number of advantages over external catheters. Implanted ports that are not accessed require little routine care (eg, no dressing changes and flushing with heparin only once a month to maintain patency). In addition, the totally implanted nature of the device has little impact on body image or participation in activities, such as swimming or other sports. In general, implanted devices are ideal for low-frequency, intermittent access. When continuous or frequent access is required, the presence of the needle may offset the advantage of the device by creating a portal for contamination.[22,28]

In general, studies report lower rates of infection for implanted ports than for devices with an external segment. A systematic review of >200 studies found that compared with other types of CVAD, implanted ports posed the lowest risk of infection.[29] But not all studies support this finding, particularly with respect to PN recipients.[22,30-32] Questions about the safety of PN administration through implanted ports requires further study.

Figure 3-6. Implanted Port for Central Venous Access

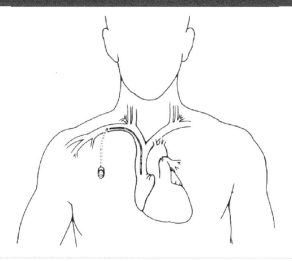

Reprinted from Krzywda EA, Adris DA, Edmiston CE, Wallace JR. Parenteral Access Devices. In: *The A.S.P.E.N. Nutrition Support Core Curriculum: A Case-Based Approach: The Adult Patient.* Gottschlich M, ed. Silver Spring, MD: A.S.P.E.N.; 2007; 300-322.

Umbilical Catheters

Primarily a site of central access in newborns, an umbilical catheter is an intravenous line placed through the umbilical vein in the umbilical stump. It may be threaded through the ductus venous and liver into the IVC. These are used for PN, exchange transfusions, monitoring of central venous pressure, and emergency access. Generally, umbilical catheters are used <7–14 days. If PN is required for >7 days, a longer-lasting central VAD should be placed. Risks include vascular embolization, thrombosis, spasm of the vessel, perforation, ischemia, hemorrhage, infection, or portal hypertension later in life from portal vein thrombosis.[2,33]

Assessment for Central Vascular Access

Evaluating Risk vs Benefit

Central venous PN administration circumvents many of the technical problems inherent to peripheral PN. However, for both adult and pediatric patients, CLABSI and DVT rank among the most common complications associated with the use of CVADs.[23,29,34] CLABSI and DVT may cause acute harm from sepsis or pulmonary embolism, respectively. But the cumulative impact of CVAD complications also jeopardizes long-term outcomes of PN therapy. Recurrent episodes of sepsis increase the risk for PN-associated liver disease, a potentially devastating complication of long-term PN, especially among infants.[35-39] Eventually, infectious and thrombotic events related to the CVAD can deplete central venous access sites. For long-term PN recipients, complications of CVADs interrupt life-preserving therapies, cause frequent hospitalizations, and add billions of dollars to healthcare costs annually.[4] Recurrent episodes of CLABSI and/or loss of central venous access may ultimately lead to referral for small intestine transplantation.[39-41] Risk factors for CLABSI and DVT appear in Table 3-2. Note that PN administration independently raises the risk for both infectious and thrombotic complications, underscoring the importance of careful CVAD selection when initiating PN.[42-44]

Table 3-2. Factors Associated with Complications of Central VADs

Central Line–Associated Bloodstream Infection	Deep Vein Thrombosis
Parenteral nutrition	Parenteral nutrition
Prolonged catheter dwell time	Prolonged catheter dwell time
Multilumen devices	Multilumen devices
Femoral insertion site in adults with obesity	Femoral insertion site
Lengthy hospitalization before central VAD insertion	Multiple insertion attempts
Heavy microbial colonization at insertion site (favors upper extremity sites over neck or groin)	Left sided insertion
Microbial colonization at the catheter hub	Catheter tip proximal to the cavoatrial junction
Multiple concurrent central VADs	Prior catheterization at same puncture site
Excessive manipulation of the catheter	Peripherally inserted central catheters
Prematurity (early gestational age)	Central line–associated bloodstream infection
Transfusion of blood products in children	

VAD, vascular access device. Adapted with permission from Worthington P, Balint J, Bechtold M, et al. When is parenteral nutrition Appropriate? *JPEN J Parenter Enteral Nutr.* 2017 Mar;41(3):324–377.

Individualizing CVAD Selection

A thorough evaluation of candidates for vascular access serves as the foundation of safe, cost-effective care. This process aligns patient characteristics and the intended therapy with the appropriate catheter.[3,4,23,34] Other factors that influence the selection of a VAD for PN include the patient's medical condition, developmental stage, and need for concurrent intravenous therapies; the anticipated duration of PN therapy; the setting in which PN is administered; and the impact on body image and the complexity of post-insertion care.[1-5] In all care settings, the patient's lifestyle and views concerning vascular access also play a role in the decision-making process for VAD selection. The patient assessment must also take into consideration the patient's cognitive ability, educational needs, and willingness to perform post-insertion care.[2,3] The need for an additional caregiver to assist with maintenance tasks impacts cost as well as the need for long-term nursing assistance.

A vascular access history and focused physical examination are also components of the selection/preoperative assessment process[3,4,6-7] A comprehensive preoperative assessment may decrease the rate of insertion-related complications. The vascular access history identifies previous devices, documenting the type of device, location, and length of time it was in place. Prior device-associated complications, such as thrombosis, infection, withdrawal occlusion, or difficult placements, should be noted. Previous clavicular fracture, chest, neck, or breast surgical procedures should be identified because anatomic landmarks used during insertion may be altered.

A physical examination should focus on identifying any lesions, tumors, previous surgical procedures, venous abnormalities, or breaks in skin integrity near the intended placement site. A complete blood and platelet count is the only laboratory work-up necessary. Coagulation parameters may be indicated if the patient is receiving therapeutic anticoagulation or has a history of liver disease. When any concern exists regarding venous patency, venous duplex ultrasonography should be performed.

Contraindications to elective placement of a long-term CVAD include sudden clinical deterioration with a change in the treatment plan, a new unexplained fever, or neutropenia (absolute neutrophil count < 1000/mm3) or the presence of blood cultures with positive results. When platelet counts are <50,000 per microliter, the efficacy of platelet administration within 2 hours of catheter insertion should be considered to prevent bleeding after the procedure.

Enhancing the Safety of CVAD Insertion and Maintenance

Pathogenesis of CLABSI

The presence of a CVAD is the most frequently reported cause of nosocomial BSIs, with an attributed mortality of 12%–25%.[11] Most instances of CLABSI originate from 1 of 2 pathways: an extraluminal route stemming from skin flora at the entrance site of the catheter or an intraluminal route arising from the hub of the device.[1,11,16,17] Both pathways play a role in the pathogenesis of CLABSI. In the days following insertion, the extraluminal route of infection is most common, whereas the intraluminal pathway is predominant with longer dwell time.[45]

Calculating CLABSI Rates

Historically, CLABSI rates have been reported as the number of infections per 1000 device days.[1] More recently, the US Centers for Disease Control and Prevention (CDC) and the National Healthcare Safety Network began reporting CLABSI data as standardized infection ratios (SIRs). The SIR compares the number of observed CLABSIs with the number of predicted infections based on a national baseline. When the SIR is <1, fewer infections were observed than predicted, indicating progress in the prevention of healthcare-associated infection.[46] In addition to these calculations, an analysis of CLABSI data submitted to the Pennsylvania Patient Safety Authority revealed that the 71.7% of CLABSIs occurred 5 days or more after device insertion.[47,48]

This led the authors to divide CLABSIs into 2 categories based on time to infection: (1) early onset or insertion-related CLABSIs, which occur ≤5 days after insertion and (2) late-onset or maintenance-related CLABSIs, which occur after the fifth day. Early infections are thought to occur through contamination that takes place during line insertion, whereas late-onset infections originate through contamination of the catheter hub. Classifying CLABSIs as either insertion-related or maintenance-related can help organizations to prioritize efforts to reduce CLABSI rates.[48]

CVAD Insertion Bundles

Over the past 2 decades, a focus on patient safety has brought the problem of CLABSI under intensive scrutiny by quality improvement organizations, regulatory agencies, and consumer groups. The Institute for Healthcare Improvement initiated these efforts by endorsing of a set of evidence-based guidelines for CVAD insertion, known as a bundle.[49] The US Centers for Medicare and Medicaid Services now mandate public disclosure of hospital-acquired infections, including central line infection rates, and no longer reimburse hospitals for CLABSIs that occur during an inpatient stay.

Patterned after CDC guidelines, the CVAD insertion bundle has 5 components: hand hygiene, maximal barrier precautions, chlorhexidine (CHG) skin antisepsis, optimal catheter site selection, and daily review of line necessity, with prompt removal of unnecessary VADs.[49] According to the bundle concept, these measures are considered a single intervention rather than a set of individual processes. Failure to complete 1 element of the bundle amounts to noncompliance with the entire protocol. A landmark study using this approach reported a 66% sustained reduction in CLABSI rates, spurring widespread implementation of the insertion bundle.[50] Additional measures have been suggested as new or stronger evidence has emerged. Examples of enhancements to the original insertion bundle include all-inclusive catheter insertion carts, sutureless catheter stabilization devices, antimicrobial catheters, and CHG bathing for patients who have critical illness or are undergoing hemodialysis.[16,49,51] In a further effort to reduce insertion-related complications, recommendations for CVAD insertion now expand the use of ultrasound guidance for the placement of CVADs inserted at the bedside.[11]

CVAD Maintenance Bundles

The elements of the original central line bundle aimed to reduce contamination of the extraluminal catheter pathway. The success of this approach led many organizations to adopt additional interventions geared toward protecting against intraluminal contamination that results from manipulation of the catheter hub. Evidence suggests that this route of contamination accounts for PN in the majority of CLABSI events.[30,48]

Known as CVAD maintenance bundles, these protocols typically emphasize appropriate hand hygiene, aseptic management of the catheter hub ("scrub the hub"), cap and tubing changes at scheduled intervals, and limiting the degree of manipulation of the device.[17,49] Table 3-3 provides a summary of measures typically included in CVAD maintenance bundles.

Table 3-3. CVAD Maintenance Bundle[1,3,11,16,49,90]

Component	Recommendations
Review of line necessity	• Daily review of ongoing need for central venous access (acute care). • Prompt transition to oral or enteral intake to limit PN therapy days.
Management of infusion system	• Consistent adherence to hand hygiene practices. • Avoid manipulation of disconnection of line for routine care. • Change PN administration tubing every 24 h. • Consider prohibition of blood drawing from CVAD for PN recipients.
Insertion site care	• Skin antisepsis with CHG. • Sterile dressing—transparent: change every 7 d; gauze: change every 2 d or if compromised or moist. • Consider using a securement device rather than sutures. • For patients ≥18 y of age, use a CHG-impregnated dressing with an FDA-cleared label that specifies a clinical indication for reducing CLABSI for short-term nontunneled catheter unless the facility is demonstrating success with baseline prevention practices.
Injection ports; catheter hub	• Scrub the needle-less adaptor or hub immediately before use with an appropriate antiseptic, such as 70% alcohol or CHG. • Consider using alcohol port caps for passive disinfection if infection rates are elevated.
Flushing and locking	• Follow flushing procedures with saline or heparinized saline per organizational policy. • Flush before and after administration of PN or other medication. • Consider using an ethanol lock for selected PN recipients with high risk for CLABSI.

CHG, chlorhexidine; CLABSI, central line–associated bloodstream infection; CVAD, central venous access device; FDA, US Food and Drug Administration; PN, parenteral nutrition.

PN CLABSI Risk in the Era of Bundles

Efforts to the prevent CLABSI have produced impressive reductions in CLABSI in the past decade.[52-54] But despite the steep downward trend in CLABSI rates, PN remains an independent risk factor for this complication.[1,17,55-57] Most importantly, exposure to PN also increases the risk for fungemia, which carries a mortality rate exceeding 30%.[1,58-61]

The factors underlying this increased risk of complications are not clear, but an interplay among patient-related issues, characteristic of the CVAD, and properties of the PN formulation itself likely play a role. Patients who require PN often have underlying medical/surgical conditions, such as intestinal failure or cancer, which leave them vulnerable to infections.[62-64] Factors related to the CVAD itself appear to play a role. PN recipients often require long-term vascular access, and the type of device, including the size and number of lumens, also influences infection risk.[31,32,65-69] Another concern is that the intravenous lipid emulsion (ILE) component of the PN formulation could promote CLABSI by serving as media for microbial growth or by altering immune function.[70-72]

In the past, hyperglycemia was widely accepted as the source of the problem, but later studies have refuted this hypothesis[73,74] More recent research points to a link between overfeeding and the risk for CLABSI, independent of blood glucose levels.[75] Questions concerning the CLABSI risk associated with PN administration require further research to delineate mechanisms and develop strategies for prevention.

Elements of CVAD Care

Vascular Access Considerations for PN Administration

Single-lumen vs multilumen devices. As noted earlier, the optimal choice of CVAD for PN administration is the smallest device with the fewest lumens necessary for the patient's needs. Although multilumen CVADs have facilitated complex intravenous therapy, additional lumens add to the risk of CLABSI and DVT.[16,17,69] Multilumen devices receive more frequent manipulation than single-lumen catheters, which most likely accounts for the increased rates of CLABSI reported with multilumen CVADs.[1,16,17,65]

Studies of adult and pediatric home PN patients have identified multilumen catheters as a risk for CLABSI, leading several researchers to recommend using single-lumen catheters for home PN when feasible.[68,76-79] One meta-analysis determined that for every 20 single-lumen catheters placed in lieu of multilumen versions, 1 CLABSI would be avoided, a difference that the authors deemed to be clinically relevant.[80] Similarly, a recent simulation study of PICCs concluded that hospitals could improve outcomes and decrease costs by instituting policies that stipulate single-lumen PICCs as the default option.[81] This information takes on greater significance when considering the elevated risk for CVAD complications that accompanies PN administration and intestinal failure.[36,37,82]

Larger-caliber CVADs are also more likely than smaller-caliber devices to create conditions that lead to thrombus formation, such as endothelial trauma, inflammation, stasis, and turbulent blood flow.[43] The risk for DVT is especially pronounced with PICCs as compared with other types of CVADs, particularly for patients who are critically ill, who are pregnant, or who have cancer.[25,26] One analysis of 2014 PICCs revealed that triple-lumen devices carried a 20-fold increase in risk for DVT when compared with single-lumen PICCs.[27]

A long-recognized link exists between thrombosis and CLABSI.[83,84] Microbial colonization occurs readily in the presence of a thrombus, setting the stage for subsequent CLABSI. In deciding to insert a multilumen central VAD for PN administration, the risk for CLABSI and DVT must be weighed against the benefits provided by the device.

Dedicated lumen. When multilumen central VADs must be used for PN, 1 lumen of the device should be dedicated exclusively for the PN administration[2,17,85,86] This recommendation stems from a single study that showed a strong association between violations of a CVAD used to administer PN and infectious complications.[87] Although the strength of the evidence supporting this recommendation is modest, the dedicated lumen policy remains a reasonable precaution. By limiting the frequency of manipulation, the dedicated lumen reduces the potential for microbial contamination. In addition, policies that restrict the use of the PN lumen offer the added benefit of avoiding co-infusion of potentially incompatible medications with the complex PN admixture.

Insertion of new central VAD for PN. The question of whether it is acceptable to administer PN through a lumen that has been used for other infusions remains unanswered; no researchers, to our knowledge, have examined this issue. A decision to insert a new central VAD for PN administration must take into consideration the risks and costs associated with the procedure. The presence of multiple simultaneous CVADs also exerts a strong influence over CLABSI rates, which may offset any potential advantage of inserting a "clean" line in cases in which existing CVADs must remain in place.[88,89]

Catheter Dressing

Appropriate care of the catheter site and hub plays a pivotal role in decreasing the risk for CLABSI. General site care principles apply regardless of the type of catheter. Guidelines support using either sterile gauze or a transparent dressing to cover the catheter exit site.[1,16] The catheter site should be monitored visually when changing the dressing or by palpation through an intact dressing on a regular basis. If tenderness develops at the insertion site, fever develops without obvious source, or other manifestations suggesting local infection or BSI develop, the dressing should be removed to allow thorough examination of the site.[1] Schedules for dressing change appear in Table 3-4. A damp, loose, or soiled dressing requires prompt replacement.

CHG-impregnated Dressings

In a 2017 revision of guidelines for prevention of CLABSI, the CDC strengthened guidelines in favor of using CHG-impregnated dressings.[90] For patients ≥18 years of age, current guidelines recommend using a CHG-impregnated patch or dressing with an FDA-cleared label that specifies a clinical indication for reducing CLABSI.[90] (CHG-impregnated dressings are not recommended to protect the site of short-term, nontunneled CVADs for premature neonates because of the risk of serious adverse skin reactions.) The CDC makes no recommendation about the use of CHG-impregnated dressings to protect the site of short-term, nontunneled central venous catheters for pediatric patients <18 years of age and nonpremature neonates because of the lack of sufficient evidence from published, high-quality studies about efficacy and safety in this age group.[90]

Hub Care

Aseptic management of the catheter hub is as critical to preventing CLABSI as emphasizing care of the site.[11,17,47] In most cases, the catheter hub is covered with a connector that allows direct access to the port without using needles (needle-less connector). Current CDC guidelines conclude that split septum needle-less connectors may be preferred over some mechanical valves because of infection risk.[1] Regardless of the type of adaptor used, accessing these devices for infusion of fluids or medication presents an opportunity to introduce microbes to the system.[11]

CVAD maintenance bundles uniformly include provisions to scrub the hub of the device before accessing the system.[11,17,48,49] Studies have demonstrated that decontaminating the needle-less connector with 70% alcohol for 5–15 seconds is an effective step in preventing bacteria from being introduced into the fluid path when accessing the system.[11] Although the degree of disinfection varies with the duration of the cleansing, the optimal scrub time is not known.[11,91]

Novel hub protectors containing 70% alcohol are available to cover the needle-less adaptor. Data pertaining to these hub protectors, which provide continuous passive disinfection, have shown a reduction in line contamination and CLABSIs with their use.[92-95] Continuous disinfecting caps avoid problems related to inconsistent or ineffective adherence to scrub-the-hub protocols, making them an attractive addition to catheter maintenance strategies.[11]

Tubing and Cap Changes

Guidelines for the frequency of tubing changes for PN admixtures often make a distinction between admixtures that contain ILE (every 24 hours) and those that contain only dextrose and amino acids (no more frequently than 96 hours).[1,2] However, these recommendations overlook the potential for contamination that could occur by changing the PN container and filter every 24 hours but leaving the administration tubing in place for 96 hours. Therefore, administration sets and filters should be changed with each new PN container.[85] For continuous infusions, this interval will typically be every 24 hours; cycled PN will require tubing and filter changes based on the hours of the infusion. Administration sets used for ILE infused separately should also be changed with each new infusion (hang time of 12 hours). In cases in which a prolonged ILE infusion is desirable to promote tolerance, the daily fat emulsion dose should be divided into 2 parts, with a new container and tubing used every 12 hours. The needleless components of the system should be changed at least as frequently as the administration set.[1]

Use of CVADs for Obtaining Blood Samples

One frequent reason for manipulating CVADs is to obtain blood samples for laboratory tests in both patients who are critically ill and patients undergoing home PN.[77,96] A number of reports have linked the use of CVADs for collecting blood samples to the risk for CLABSI.[77,96-101] The heightened risk for CLABSI led some organizations to establish a policy of not using VADs to obtain blood samples unless no peripheral access is available.[77,97] Recognizing the potential benefits of limiting manipulation of CVADs, The Joint Commission has highlighted the use of VADs for blood sampling as a "practice to avoid."[17]

The use of CVADs for blood withdrawal not only increases the risk for microbial contamination of the line and hub, but samples drawn incorrectly from a CVAD during PN infusion can also lead to spurious laboratory values. Binkley et al first drew attention to the danger of this phenomenon in a report of a 10-month quality assurance study.[102] Further evidence was collected during a year-long prospective cohort study in an academic medical center, in which 63 incidents of spurious blood work were reported in 34 PN recipients.[103] In both studies, investigators recounted incidents of patient harm—typically hypoglycemia or hypokalemia—that resulted from unnecessary medical intervention for falsely elevated laboratory values. Another study reported a decline in the number of contaminated blood cultures after decreasing the proportion of blood samples obtained for culture from CVADs by 10.9%. This result let to substantial cost savings and may have reduced the number of reportable CLABSIs.[104] Organizational protocols that discourage the use of CVADs for obtaining blood samples for PN recipients may be warranted, particularly in cases in which CLABSI rates remain elevated despite adherence to basic prevention measures.[5]

Routine Flushing

CVADs require regular flushing with saline or heparinized saline to maintain patency.[2] Catheter patency describes both the ability to infuse without resistance and the ability to aspirate blood without resistance (also referred to as withdrawal occlusion). If either of these conditions exist, the catheter is occluded. Current guidelines recommend using saline to clear the line between medications and to use saline or heparinized saline as a lock when the CVAD is idle.[2] Specific flushing procedures vary with the type of CVAD, the needle-less connector used, and the patient population. A systematic review involving adult patients found that CVADs that are intermittently locked with heparin develop fewer occlusions than catheters locked with normal saline; however, the quality of the evidence for this effect was low.[105] Although concerns about heparin induced thrombocytopenia raise questions about the safety of using heparin as a routine flushing agent, the existing trials lack the power to detect such adverse events.

Occlusions may arise from mechanical problems such as an overlooked clamp or a kink in the tubing. Precipitates or the build-up of ILE residue over time can also block catheters. If a thrombus or fibrin deposit causes the occlusion, instillation of a thrombolytic agent may restore patency.[2]

Antimicrobial Catheter Flush and Catheter Lock Prophylaxis

The use of prophylactic antimicrobial locking solutions is recommended in patients with long-term (tunneled) CVADs who have a history of multiple episodes of CLABSI despite adherence to aseptic technique.[1,4] A wide variety of antibiotic and antiseptic solutions have been used to flush or lock CVADs. However, because of concerns about the rise of antibiotic-resistant microbial strains, ethanol flushes are more widely used in both pediatric and adult home PN populations.[106-112] However, a recent prospective double-blind randomized controlled study on the routine prophylactic use of ethanol locks in patients newly started on home PN failed to show an improvement with ethanol lock therapy, leading the researchers to conclude that this therapy may be most beneficial to high-risk patients.[113]

Currently, ethanol use is limited to silicone catheters, and some reports suggest a link between ethanol locks and thrombosis.[39,114-116] A number of unresolved questions surround the use of ethanol locks. Data are needed standardize ethanol lock procedures: the optimal concentration of ethanol, frequency of use, the appropriate dwell time of the flush, and whether the best practice is flushing the ethanol through the catheter or withdrawing it after the instillation time.[39,116]

CVAD Removal

CVADs should be removed promptly when PN therapy ends.[1,4,17] Although the risk of catheter colonization and CLABSI increase with time, scheduled exchange of CVADs does not reduce CLABSI rates.[1,11] Guidelines recommend against using guidewires to replace CVADs.[1,11] Clinical judgment should guide decisions about removing the catheter in patients with fever alone.[4] When a CVAD-related infection that cannot be successfully treated with the catheter in situ occurs, including *Staphylococcus aureus*, Gram-negative *Enterococcus*, and catheter-associated fungemia, the catheter should be removed.[1,4] In patients with symptoms of sepsis, including cardiovascular instability, organ failure, and blood cultures with positive results, the catheter should be removed unless another source of infection is identified.[1,4]

Procedures for CVAD removal vary with the type of device and organizational policies regarding the healthcare providers permitted to remove CVADs. Removal of many percutaneous devices takes place at the bedside, whereas implanted and tunneled devices require a procedure by a surgeon or interventional radiologist. Complications of CVAD removal include bleeding and catheter fracture, but air embolism is the most serious and potentially fatal complication linked to CVAD termination.[117] Table 3-5 shows steps recommended for safe removal of CVADs.

Table 3-4. Steps to Prevent Air Embolism When Removing CVADs[117]

- Place the patient in a supine position with the head down or Trendelenburg position.

- Instruct patients to perform the Valsalva maneuver during catheter removal, if possible.

- If this is not possible, remove the catheter during exhalation.

- Cover the site with an impermeable dressing and maintain pressure on the site for 5–10 min to promote hemostasis and prevent air from entering the catheter tract.

- Instruct the patient to maintain supine position for 30 min after central VAD removal.

VAD, vascular access device.

Education and Engagement

Positive clinical CVAD outcomes can be achieved through robust catheter care protocols, supported by a multidisciplinary team of physicians, nurses, pharmacists, radiologists, psychologists, and surgeons.[4,118] Ongoing education and competency assessment for both clinicians and patients forms the cornerstone of safe CVAD management.[1-3,17,48,49]

A wealth of tools for effective CVAD education are available online.[119-121] At a minimum, education and competency validation should occur in the following circumstances: as part of orientation for newly hired employees or, for patients, at initiation of intravenous therapy; when a change in protocol or procedure takes place, with the introduction of new equipment or technology; and when quality improvement monitoring or other data sources reveal a gap in skills or knowledge related to CVAD care.[2,85]

Quality Improvement

Strategies to reduce complications related to the VAD hold a central place in programs to improve PN safety. Multifaceted interdisciplinary approaches must foster a culture of safety, clarify problem areas, involve key stakeholders, test change strategies, remove barriers, and maintain channels of communication.[122] Pertinent quality indicators include not simply CLABSI rates but also other factors that could shed light on factors contributing to infection: appropriateness of the device for PN therapy, adherence to insertion and maintenance bundles, dwell time of the catheter, and days to blood culture with positive results. Proactive and reactive methodologies, failure mode effects analysis, root cause analysis, and the Plan-Do-Study-Act model should all serve as the framework for identifying and closing practice gaps and engendering continuous process improvement.

Summary

Expertise in managing VADs represents a critical component of PN therapy. This process begins with selection of a device that is appropriate for the patient's clinical condition, the expected duration of therapy, and the healthcare setting. Strict adherence to evidence-based guidelines for VAD insertion and maintenance promotes positive outcomes and limits complications associated with nutrition therapy. Education for clinicians and patients alike forms the foundation for safe and effective care, whereas quality improvement detects gaps in performance and identifies corrective interventions.

References

1. O'Grady NP, Alexander M, Burns LA, et al. Guidelines for the prevention of intravascular catheter-related infections. *Clin Infect Dis.* 2011;52(9):e162–e193.

2. Infusion Nurses Society. Infusion therapy standards of practice. *J Infus Nurs.* 2016;39(1 suppl):S11–S159.

3. Moureau NL, Carr PJ. Vessel health and preservation: a model and clinical pathway for using vascular access devices. *Br J Nurs.* 2018;27(8):S28–S35.

4. Baskin K, Mermel LA, Saad TF, et al. Evidence based strategies and recommendations for preservation of central venous access in children. *JPEN J Parenter Enteral Nutr.* 2019;43(5):591–614.

5. Worthington P, Balint J, Bechtold M, et al. When is parenteral nutrition appropriate? *JPEN J Parenter Enteral Nutr.* 2017 Mar;41(3):324–377.

6. Sansivero GE. Venous anatomy and physiology: considerations for vascular access device placement and function. *J Intravenous Nurs.* 1998;21(5 suppl):S107–S114.

7. Sansivero GE. Features and selection of vascular access devices. *Semin Oncol Nurs.* 2010;26(2):88–101.

8. Simonov M, Pittiruti M, Rickard CM, Chopra V. Navigating venous access: a guide for hospitalists. *J Hosp Med.* 2015;10(7):471–478.

9. Hadaway L, Magee MC. Risky business: peripheral and central venous catheters both pose risks. *Patient Safety.* 2019;1(1):12. doi:10.33940/vascular/2019.9.4

10. Parienti JJ, Mongardon N, Megarbane B, et al. Intravascular complications of central venous catheterization by insertion site. *N Engl J Med.* 2015;373(13):1220–1229.

11. Bell T, O'Grady NP. Prevention of central line-associated bloodstream infections. *Infect Dis Clin North Am.* 2017;31(3):551–559. doi:10.1016/j.idc.2017.05.007

12. Patel AR, Patel AR, Singh S, Singh S, Khawaja I. Central line catheters and associated complications: a review. *Cureus.* 2019;11(5):e4717. doi:10.7759/cureus.4717

13. Gura KM. Is there still a role for peripheral parenteral nutrition? *Nutr Clin Pract.* 2009;24(6):709–717.

14. Cicolini G, Manzoli L, Simonetti V, et al. Phlebitis risk varies by peripheral venous catheter and increases after 96 hours: a large multi-centre prospective study. *J Adv Nurs.* 2014;70(11):2539–2549.

15. Davis J. Peripheral vascular catheter–related infection: dwelling on dwell time. *Pa Patient Saf Advis.* 2014;11(1):30–35.

16. Marschall J, Mermel LA, Fakih M, et al. Strategies to prevent central line-associated bloodstream infections in acute care hospitals: 2014 update. *Infect Control Hosp Epidemiol.* 2014;35(7):753–771.

17. The Joint Commission. Central line-associated bloodstream infections toolkit and monograph. The Joint Commission website. https://www.jointcommission.org/topics/clabsi_toolkit.aspx. Published 2012. Accessed November 1, 2019.

18. Anderson NR. Midline catheters: the middle ground of intravenous therapy administration. *J Infus Nurs.* 2004;27(5):313–321.

19. Dawson RL. Midline catheters: an essential tool in CLABSI reduction. *Infection Control Today.* March 15, 2013. https://www.infectioncontroltoday.com/clabsi/midline-catheters-essential-tool-clabsi-reduction. Accessed June 24, 2018.

20. Chopra V, Kaatz S, Swaminathan L, et al. Variation in use and outcomes related to midline catheters: results from a multicentre pilot study. *BMJ Qual Saf.* 2019;28(9):714–72.

21. Micic D, Semrad C, Chopra, V. Choosing the right central venous catheter for parenteral nutrition. *Am J Gastroenterol.* 2019;114(1):4–6.

22. Pittiruti M, Hamilton H, Biffi R, MacFie J, Pertkiewicz M. ESPEN guidelines on parenteral nutrition: central venous catheters (access, care, diagnosis and therapy of complications). *Clin Nutr.* 2009;28(4):365–377.

23. Chopra V, Flanders SA, Saint S, et al; Michigan Appropriateness Guide for Intravenous Catheters (MAGIC) Panel. The Michigan Appropriateness Guide for Intravenous Catheters (MAGIC): results from a multispecialty panel using the RAND/UCLA appropriateness method. *Ann Intern Med.* 2015.15;163(6 suppl):S1–S40.

24. Christensen LD, Holst M, Bech LF, et al. Comparison of complications associated with peripherally inserted central catheters and Hickman™ catheters in patients with intestinal failure receiving home parenteral nutrition. Six-year follow up study. *Clin Nutr.* 2016;35(4):912–917.

25. Chopra V, Anand S, Hickner A, et al. Risk of venous thromboembolism associated with peripherally inserted central catheters: a systematic review and meta-analysis. *Lancet.* 2013;382(9889):311–325.

26. Cape AV, Mogensen KM, Robinson MK, et al. Peripherally inserted central catheter complications during pregnancy. *JPEN J Parenter Enteral Nutr.* 2014;38(5):595–601.

27. Evans RS, Sharp JH, Linford LH, et al. Risk of symptomatic DVT associated with peripherally inserted central catheters. *Chest.* 2010;138(4): 803–810.

28. Kovacevich DS, Corrigan M, Ross V, McKeever L, Hall AM, Braunschweig C. American Society for Parenteral and Enteral Nutrition guidelines for the selection and care of central venous access devices for adult home parenteral nutrition administration. *JPEN J Parenter Enteral Nutr.* 2019;43(1):15–31.

29. Maki DG, Kluger DM, Crnich CJ. The risk of bloodstream infection in adults with different intravascular devices: a systematic review of 200 published prospective studies. *Mayo Clin Proc.* 2006;81(9):1159–1171.

30. Elfassy S, Kassam, Z, Amin F, Khan KJ, Haider S, Armstrong D. Epidemiology and risk factors for bloodstream infections in a home parenteral nutrition program. *JPEN J Parenter Enteral Nutr.* 2015;39(2):147–153.

31. Shenep MA, Tanner MR, Sun Y, et al. Catheter-related complications in children with cancer receiving parenteral nutrition: change in risk is moderated by catheter type. *JPEN J Parenter Enteral Nutr.* 2017;41(6):1063–1071.

32. Ross VM, Guenter P, Corrigan ML, et al. Central venous catheter infections in home parenteral nutrition: outcomes from Sustain: American Society for Parenteral and Enteral Nutrition's national patient registry for nutrition care. *Am J Infect Control.* 2016;44(12):1462–1468.

33. Baillie CT. Neonatal vascular access. In: Losty PD, Flake AW, Rintala RJ, Houston JM, Iwai N, eds. *Rickman's Neonatal Surgery.* London, England: Springer; 2018:213–226.

34. Cotogni P, Pittiruti M. Focus on peripherally inserted central catheters in critically ill patients. *World J Crit Care Med.* 2014;3(4):80–94.

35. Male C, Chait P, Andrew M, Hanna K, Julian J, Mitchell L; PARKAA Investigators. Central venous line-related thrombosis in children: association with central venous line location and insertion technique. *Blood.* 2003;101(11):4273–4278.

36. Tillman EM. Review and clinical update on parenteral nutrition-associated liver disease. *Nutr Clin Pract.* 2013;28(1):30–39.

37. Squires RH, Duggan T, Teitelbaum DH, et al. Natural history of pediatric intestinal failure: initial report from the Pediatric Intestinal Failure Consortium. *J Pediatr.* 2012;161(4):723–728.e2.

38. Pironi L, Arends J, Bozzetti F, et al. ESPEN guidelines on chronic intestinal failure in adults [erratum in *Clin Nutr.* 2017;36(2):619]. *Clin Nutr.* 2016;35(2):247–307.

39. Wales PW, Allen N, Worthington P, et al. A.S.P.E.N. clinical guidelines: support of pediatric patients with intestinal failure at risk of parenteral nutrition-associated liver disease. *JPEN J Parenter Enteral Nutr.* 2014;38(5):538–557.

40. Mercer DF, Iverson AK, Culwell KA. Nutrition and small bowel transplantation. *Nutr Clin Pract.* 2014;29(5):615–620.

41. Fishbein TM. Intestinal transplantation. *N Engl J Med.* 2009;361(10):998–1008.

42. Kucher N. Deep venous thrombosis of the upper extremities. *N Engl J Med.* 2011;364(9):861–869.

43. Grant JD, Stevens SM, Woller SC, et al. Diagnosis and management of upper extremity deep-vein thrombosis in adults. *Thromb Haemost.* 2012;108(6):1097–1108.

44. Marnejon T, Angelo D, Abu Abdou A, Gemmel D. Risk factors for upper extremity venous thrombosis associated with peripherally inserted central venous catheters. *J Vasc Access.* 2012;3(2):231–238.

45. Mermel LA. What Is the predominant source of intravascular catheter infections? *Clin Infect Dis.* 2011;52(2):211–212.

46. Centers for Disease Control and Prevention. The NHSN standardized infection ratio (SIR). https://www.cdc.gov/nhsn/pdfs/ps-analysis-resources/nhsn-sir-guide.pdf. Updated March 2019. Accessed November 10, 2019.

47. Davis J. Central-line-associated bloodstream infection: comprehensive, data-driven prevention. *Pa Patient Saf Advis.* 2011;89(3):100–105.

48. Davis J, Finley E. Calculation of outcome rates that diagnose bedside performance: central-line-associated bloodstream infection. *Pa Patient Saf Advis.* 2013;10(3):107–109.

49. Goss L (Ed). *APIC Implementation Guide: Guide to Preventing Central Line-Associated Bloodstream Infections.* Washington, DC: Association for Professionals in Infection Control and Epidemiology; 2015. https://apic.org/Resource_/TinyMceFileManager/2015/APIC_CLABSI_WEB.pdf. Accessed November 1, 2019.

50. Pronovost P, Needham D, Berenholtz S, et al. An intervention to decrease catheter-related bloodstream infections in the ICU [erratum in *N Engl J Med.* 2007;356(25):2660]. *N Engl J Med.* 2006;355(26):2725–2732.

51. Chopra V, Krein SL, Olmsted RL, Safdar N, Saint S. Prevention of central line-associated bloodstream infections: brief update review. In: Shekelle PG, Wachter RM, Pronovost PJ, et al. *Making Health Care Safer II: An Updated Critical Analysis of the Evidence for Patient Safety Practices. Comparative Effectiveness Review No. 211.* (Prepared by the Southern California-RAND Evidence-based Practice Center under Contract No. 290-2007-10062-I.) Rockville, MD: Agency for Healthcare Research and Quality; 2013. AHRQ Publication No. 13-E001-EF. www.ahrq.gov/research/findings/evidence-based-reports/ptsafetyuptp.html.

52. Centers for Disease Control and Prevention. Vital signs: central line-associated blood stream infections—United States, 2001, 2008, and 2009. *Morb Mortal Wkly Rep.* 2011;60(8):243–248.

53. Centers for Disease Control and Prevention. Healthcare-associated infections (HAIs). *Winnable Battles.* https://www.cdc.gov/winnablebattles/report/HAIs.html. Published 2016. Accessed November 4, 2019.

54. Centers for Disease Control and Prevention. 2018 national and state healthcare-associated infections progress report. https://www.cdc.gov/hai/pdfs/progress-report/2018-Progress-Report-Executive-Summary-H.pdf. Updated November 1, 2019. Accessed November 4, 2019.

55. Beghetto MG, Victorino J, Teixeira L, de Azevedo MJ. Parenteral nutrition as a risk factor for central venous catheter-related infection. *JPEN J Parenter Enteral Nutr.* 2005;29(5):367–373.

56. Ippolito P, Larson E L, Furuya EY, Liu J, Seres DS. Utility of electronic medical records to assess the relationship between parenteral nutrition and central line–associated bloodstream infections in adult hospitalized patients. *JPEN J Parenter Enteral Nutr.* 2015;39(8):929–934.

57. Fonseca G, Burgermaster M, Larson, E, Seres, DS. The relationship between parenteral nutrition and central line–associated bloodstream infections: 2009–2014. *JPEN J Parenter Enteral Nutr.* 2018;42(1):171–175.

58. Reitzel RA, Rosenblatt J, Chaftari AM, Raad II. Epidemiology of infectious and noninfectious catheter complications in patients receiving home parenteral nutrition: a systematic review and meta-analysis. *JPEN J Parenter Enteral Nutr.* 2019;43(7):832–851.

59. Stratman RC, Martin CA, Rapp RP, Berger R, Magnuson B. Candidemia in recipients of parenteral nutrition. *Nutr Clin Pract.* 2010;25(3):282–289.

60. Zilberberg MD, Shorr AF. *Fungal infections in the ICU.* Infect Dis Clin North Am. 2009;23(3):625–642.

61. Phua AI, Hon KY, Holt A, O'Callaghan M, Bihari S. Candida catheter-related bloodstream infection in patients on home parenteral nutrition - rates, risk factors, outcomes, and management. *Clin Nutr ESPEN.* 2019;31:1–9.

62. Wylie MC, Graham DA, Potter-Bynoe G, et al. Risk factors for central line–associated bloodstream infection in pediatric intensive care units. *Infect Control Hosp Epidemiol.* 2010;31(10):1049–1056.

63. Seddik TB, Tian L. Nespor C, Kerner J, Maldonado Y, Gans H. Risk factors of ambulatory central line–associated bloodstream infection in pediatric short bowel syndrome [published online June 9. 2019]. *JPEN J Parenter Enteral Nutr.* doi:10.1002/jpen.1667

64. Brandt CF, Tribler S, Hvistendahl M, et al. Home parenteral nutrition in adult patients with chronic intestinal failure: catheter-related complications over 4 decades at the main Danish tertiary referral center. *JPEN J Parenter Enteral Nutr.* 2018;42(1):95–103.

65. Dimick JB, Swoboda S, Talamini MA, Pelz RK, Hendrix CW, Lipsett PA. Risk of colonization of central venous catheters: catheters for total parenteral nutrition vs other catheters. *Am J Crit Care.* 2003;12(4):328–335.

66. Gapany C, Tercier S, Diezi M, Clement C, Lemay K, Joseph JM. Frequent accesses to totally implanted vascular ports in pediatric oncology patients are associated with higher infection rates. *J Vasc Access.* 2011;12(3):207–210.

67. LaRusso K, Schaack G, Fung T, et al. Should you pick the PICC? Prolonged use of peripherally inserted central venous catheters in children with intestinal failure *J Pediatr Surg.* 2019;54(5):999–1004.

68. Gillanders L, Angstmann K, Ball P, et al. A prospective study of catheter-related complications in HPN patients. *Clin Nutr.* 2012;31(1):30–34.

69. Chopra V, Ratz D, Kuhn L, Lopus T, Chenoweth C, Krein S. PICC-associated bloodstream infections: prevalence, patterns, and predictors. *Am J Med.* 2014;127(4):319–328.

70. Wanten GJ, Calder PC. Immune modulation by parenteral lipid emulsions. *Am J Clin Nutr.* 2007;85(5):1171–1184.

71. Kuwahara T, Shimono K, Kaneda S, Tamura T, Ichihara M, Nakashima Y. Growth of microorganisms in total parenteral nutrition solutions containing lipid. *Int J Med Sci.* 2010;7(3):101–109.

72. Mitsuboshi S, Yamada H, Nagai K. Lipid emulsion increases the risk of central line infection in Japanese adult inpatients: a retrospective study. *Can J Infect Control.* 2017; 32(2):115–118.

73. Beghetto MG, Victorino J, Teixeira L, de Azevedo MJ. Parenteral nutrition as a risk factor for enteral venous catheter-related infection. *J Parenter Enteral Nutr.* 2005;29(5):367–373.

74. Matsushima K, Cook A, Tyner T, et al. Parenteral nutrition: a clear and present danger unabated by tight glucose control. *Am J Surg.* 2010;200(3):386–390.

75. Dissanaike S, Shelton M, Warner K, O'Keefe GE. The risk for bloodstream infections is associated with increased parenteral caloric intake in patients receiving parenteral nutrition. *Crit Care.*2007;11(5):R114. doi:10.1186/cc6167

76. Chopra V, Ratz D, Kuhn L, Lopus T, Lee A, Krein S. Peripherally inserted central catheter-related deep vein thrombosis: contemporary patterns and predictors. *J Thromb Haemost.* 2014;12(6):847–854.

77. Buchman AL, Opilla M, Kwasny M, Diamantidis TG, Okamoto R. Risk factors for the development of catheter-related bloodstream infection in patients receiving home parenteral nutrition. *JPEN J Parenter Enteral Nutr.* 2014;38(6):744–749.

78. Moreau N, Chopra V. Indications for peripheral, midline and central catheters: summary of the MAGIC recommendations. *Br J Nurs.* 2016;25(8):S15–S24.

79. Larsen-Narth C, Goday PS. No light at the end of the tunneled central line. *JPEN J Parenter Enteral Nutr.* 2014;38(5):534–537.

80. Zürcher M, Tramèr MR, Walder B. Colonization and blood-stream infection with single- versus multi-lumen central venous catheters: a quantitative systematic review. *Anesth Analg.* 2004;99(1):177–182.

81. Ratz D, Hofer T, Flanders SA, Saint S, Chopra V. Limiting the number of lumens in peripherally inserted central catheters to improve outcomes and reduce cost: a simulation study. *Infect Control Hosp Epidemiol.* 2016;37(7):811–817.

82. Rodrigues AF, van Mourik IDM, Sharuf K, et al. Management of end-stage central venous access in children referred for possible small bowel transplantation. *J Pediatr Gastroenterol Nutr.* 2006;42(4):427–433.

83. Raad II, Luna M, Khalil SM, Costerton JW, Lam C, Bodey GP. The relationship between the thrombotic and infectious complications of central venous catheters. *JAMA.* 1994;271(13):1014–1016.

84. Timsit JF, Farkas JC, Boyer JM, et al. Central vein catheter-related thrombosis in intensive care patients: incidence, risks factors, and relationship with catheter-related sepsis. *Chest.* 1998;114(1):207–213.

85. Ayers P, Adams S, Boullata J, et al. A.S.P.E.N. parenteral nutrition safety consensus recommendations. *JPEN J Parenter Enteral Nutr.* 2014;38(3):296–333.

86. Rupp SM, Apfelbaum JL, Blitt C, et al.; American Society of Anesthesiologists Task Force on Central Venous Access. Practice guidelines for central venous access: a report by the American Society of Anesthesiologists Task Force on Central Venous Access. *Anesthesiology.* 2012;116(3):539–573.

87. Snydman DR, Murray SA, Kornfeld SJ, Majka JA, Ellis CA. Total parenteral nutrition-related infections. Prospective epidemiologic study using semiquantitative methods. *Am J Med.* 1982;73(5):695–699.

88. Scheithauer S, Häfner H, Schröder J, et al. Simultaneous placement of multiple central lines increases central-line associated bloodstream infection rates. Am J Infect Control. 2013;41(2):113–117.

89. Concannon C, Wijngaarden E, Stevens V, Dumyati G. The effect of multiple central venous catheters on central line-associated bloodstream infections. *Infect Control Hosp Epidemiol.* 2014;35(9):1140–1146.

90. Centers for Disease Control and Prevention. Updated recommendations on the use of chlorhexidine-impregnated dressings for prevention of intravascular catheter-related infections (2017). https://www.cdc.gov/infectioncontrol/guidelines/bsi/c-i-dressings/index.html. Accessed November 4, 2019.

91. Moureau NL, Flynn J. Disinfection of needleless connector hubs: clinical evidence systematic review. *Nurs Res Pract.* 2015:796762. doi:10.1155/2015/796762

92. Sweet MA, Cumpston A, Briggs F, Craig M, Hamadani M. Impact of alcohol-impregnated port protectors and needleless neutral pressure connectors on central line-associated bloodstream infections and contamination of blood cultures in an inpatient oncology unit. *Am J Infect Control.* 2012;40(10):931–934.

93. Wright MO, Tropp J, Schora DM, et al. Continuous passive disinfection of catheter hubs prevents contamination and bloodstream infection. *Am J Infect Control.* 2013;41(1):33–38.

94. Merrill KC, Summer S, Linford L, Taylor C, Macintosh C. Impact of universal disinfectant cap implementation on central line-associated bloodstream infections. *Am J Infect Control.* 2014;42(12):1274–1277.

95. Voor In 't Holt AF, Helder OK, Vos MC, et al. Antiseptic barrier cap effective in reducing central line-associated bloodstream infections: a systemic review and meta-analysis. *Int J Nurs Stud.* 2017;69:34–40.

96. O'Malley CH. The frequency and reasons for central line accesses in critical care units. *Can J Infect Control.* 2018;33(3):165–167.

97. Hughes AA, Vannello C, Bingeman C, Gilbert M. Reducing CLABSI by prohibiting routine blood draws through central lines [abstract]. *Am J Infect Control.* 2011;39(5):E50–E51.

98. Freeman J, Goldmann DA, Smith NE, Sidebottom DG, Epstein MF, Platt R. Association of intravenous lipid emulsion and coagulase-negative staphylococcal bacteremia in neonatal intensive care units. *N Engl J Med.* 1990;323(5):301–308.

99. Mahieu LM, De Dooy JJ, Lenaerts AE, Ieven MM, De Muynck AO. Catheter manipulations and the risk of catheter-associated bloodstream infection in neonatal intensive care unit patients. *J Hosp Infect.* 2001;48(1):20–26.

100. Callister D, Limchaiyawat P, Eells SJ, Miller LG. Risk factors for central line–associated bloodstream infections in the era of prevention bundles. *Infect Control Hosp Epidemiol.* 2015;36(2):214–216.

101. Williamson K, Gonzalez L, Neusbaum A, Messing J. Reducing the risk of central line–associated bloodstream infections. *Am Nurse Today.* 2017;2(5):42, 44, 46.

102. Binkley JE, Mills B, Roy MA, Diaz JJ, Jensen GL. Spurious laboratory values from improper sampling of blood containing parenteral nutrition. *Nutr Clin Pract.* 2004;19(5):540–541.

103. Fairholm L, Saqui O, Baun M, Yeung M, Fernandes G, Allard JP. Monitoring parenteral nutrition in hospitalized patients: issues related to spurious bloodwork. *Nutr Clin Pract.* 2011;26(6):700–707.

104. Boyce JM, Nadeau J, Dumigan D, Miller D, Dubowsky C, Reilly L, Hannon CV. Obtaining blood cultures by venipuncture versus from central lines: impact on blood culture contamination rates and potential effect on central line–associated bloodstream infection reporting. *Infect Control Hosp Epidemiol.* 2013;34(10):1042–1047.

105. López-Briz E, Ruiz Garcia V, Cabello JB, Bort-Martí S, Carbonell Sanchis R, Burls A. Heparin versus 0.9% sodium chloride locking for prevention of occlusion in central venous catheters in adults. *Cochrane Database Syst Rev.* 2018;7:CD008462. doi:10.1002/14651858

106. Opilla MT, Kirby DF, Edmond MB. Use of ethanol lock therapy to reduce the incidence of catheter-related bloodstream infections in home parenteral nutrition patients. *JPEN J Parenter Enteral Nutr.* 2007;31(4):302–305.

107. Cober MP, Kovacevich DS, Teitelbaum DH. Ethanol-lock therapy for the prevention of central venous access device infections in pediatric patients with intestinal failure. *JPEN J Parenter Enteral Nutr.* 2011;35(1):67–73.

108. Gundogan K, Dave NJ, Griffith DP, et al. Ethanol lock therapy markedly reduces catheter-related blood stream infections in adults requiring home parenteral nutrition: a retrospective study from a tertiary medical center [published online August 27, 2019]. *JPEN J Parenter Enteral Nutr.* doi:10.1002/jpen.1698

109. Wolf J, Shenep JL, Clifford V, Curtis N, Flynn PM. Ethanol lock therapy in pediatric hematology and oncology. *Pediatr Blood Cancer.* 2013;60(1):18–25.

110. Rahhal R, Abu-El-Haija MA, Fei L, et al. Systematic review and meta-analysis of the utilization of ethanol locks in pediatric patients with intestinal failure. *JPEN J Parenter Enter Nutr.* 2018;42(4):690–701.

111. Tan M, Lau J, Guglielmo BJ. Ethanol locks in the prevention and treatment of catheter-related bloodstream infections. *Ann Pharmacother.* 2014;48(5):607–615.

112. John BK, Khan MA, Speerhas R, et al. Ethanol lock therapy in reducing catheter-related bloodstream infections in adult home parenteral nutrition patients: results of a retrospective study. *JPEN J Parenter Enteral Nutr.* 2012;36(5):603–610.

113. Salonen BR, Bonnes SL, Vallumsetia N, Varayil JE, Mundi MS, Hurt RT. A prospective double blind randomized controlled study on the use of ethanol locks in HPN patients. *Clin Nutr.* 2018;37(4):1181–1185.

114. Crnich C, Halfmann JA, Crone WC, Maki DG. The effects of prolonged ethanol exposure on the mechanical properties of polyurethane and silicone catheters used for intravascular access. *Infect Control Hosp Epidemiol.* 2005;26(8):708–714.

115. Lopes BC, Borges PSGN, Gallindo RM, Tenório TBS, Machado LB, de Orange FA. Lock therapy for the prevention of nontunneled catheter-related bloodstream infection in pediatric patients. *JPEN J Parenter Enteral Nutr.* 2019;43(8):1044–1052.

116. Zhang J, Wang B, Wang J, Yang Q. Ethanol locks for the prevention of catheter-related infection in patients with central venous catheter: a systematic review and meta-analysis of randomized controlled trials. *PLoS One.* 2019;14(9):e0222408. doi:10.1371/journal.pone.0222408

117. McCarthy CJ, Behravesh S, Naidu SG, Oklu R. Air embolism: practical tips for prevention and treatment. *J Clin Med.* 2016;5(11):E93. doi:10.3390/jcm5110093

118. Dibb M, Lal S. Home parenteral nutrition: vascular access and related complications. *Nutr Clin Pract.* 2017;32(6):769–776.

119. Centers for Disease Control and Prevention. Central line associated bloodstream infection (CLABSI). https://www.cdc.gov/hai/bsi/bsi.html. Accessed November 2019.

120. Agency for Healthcare Research and Quality. Toolkit for reducing central line associated bloodstream infections. https://www.ahrq.gov/hai/clabsi-tools/index.html. Reviewed March 2018. Accessed November 5, 2019.

121. The Joint Commission. Preventing Central line–associated bloodstream infections: useful tools, an international perspective. https://www.jointcommission.org/assets/1/6/CLABSI_Toolkit_Tools_Directory_linked.pdf. Published November 20, 2013. Accessed November 5, 2019.

122. McAlearney AS. *Final Report. High-Performance Work Practices in CLABSI Prevention Interventions: Executive Summary.* (Prepared under Contract No. #HHSA2902010000221, Task Order No. 5.). Rockville, MD: Agency for Healthcare Research and Quality; 2015. AHRQ Publication No. 15-0044-EF.

Parenteral Nutrition Access Devices

Parenteral Nutrition Formulations and Managing Component Shortages

Introduction

This chapter on parenteral nutrition (PN) formulations provides information on the components and preparation of a PN admixture. It also presents strategies for managing shortages of PN components.

Formulation Components

Components used in formulating PN typically include macronutrients such as protein, carbohydrates, and fat. The PN formulation also includes electrolytes, vitamins, minerals, and trace elements. Sterile water for injection is added to provide necessary volume to the PN admixture. Various combinations of these components are incorporated into the regimen for intravenous (IV) administration based on the patient's individual requirements.

Energy Substrates

Carbohydrates. The most commonly used carbohydrate energy substrate is dextrose, which provides 3.4 kcal/g in its hydrated form. Dextrose is commercially available in concentrations ranging from 2.5% to 70%, in partially filled containers, as well as in combinations with other components of the PN admixture. According to the United States Pharmacopeia (USP), dextrose solutions are acidic, with a pH ranging from 3.5 to 6.5, and vary in osmolarity depending on their concentration. Higher dextrose concentrations (>10%) are generally reserved for central vein administration because of the propensity to cause thrombophlebitis in peripheral veins.[1]

Another carbohydrate energy substrate used less frequently is glycerol, a sugar alcohol that provides 4.3 kcal/g. Glycerol, or glycerin, is contained in certain commercially available PN products marketed for peripheral vein administration. These products have been shown to be protein-sparing and have been reported to induce less insulin response than dextrose-based regimens, although another study found the opposite to be true.[2-4]

Lipids. Lipid injectable emulsions (ILEs) provide energy as well as essential fatty acids for PN admixtures. ILEs approved for use in the United States are long-chain fatty acid emulsions of soybean oil 100%, a 2-oil mixture of olive oil (80%) and soybean oil (20%),[5,6] or a 4-oil mixture of soybean oil (30%), medium-chain triglycerides (30%), olive oil (25%), and fish oil (15%).[7] There is a fish oil 100% ILE for use in pediatric patients.[8]

Soybean oil–based ILEs are commercially available in 10% (1.1 kcal/mL), 20% (2 kcal/mL), and 30% (3 kcal/mL) concentrations. The 30% ILE formulation is approved for compounding of PN admixtures and not for direct IV administration. The olive oil and soybean oil–based ILE is available as a 20% concentration and is indicated for adults requiring PN. This product is not indicated for neonatal and pediatric patients because of the reports of deaths in preterm infants and the uncertainty of whether the product provides sufficient amounts of essential fatty acids for these patient populations.[9] The 4-oil ILE is available as a 20% concentration and should be dosed in adults at 1–2 g/kg/d with a maximum dose of 2.5 g/kg/d.[7] The fish oil 100% ILE is approved as a source of energy and fatty acids in pediatric patients with PN-associated cholestasis and is available as a 10% concentration.[8]

Other components in these ILEs are egg yolk phospholipid to act as an emulsifier, glycerin (glycerol) to render the formulation isotonic, and sodium hydroxide to adjust the final pH (range: 6–9).[10] Soybean oil–based ILEs also contain a small amount of vitamin K. Each gram of fat provides 9 kcal, and glycerol can also be metabolized for energy. This is why the nutrient density of each gram of fat in 10% ILE is equivalent to 11 kcal, whereas each gram of fat in 20% and 30% ILE is equivalent to 10 kcal.

The US Centers for Disease Control and Prevention recommend a 12-hour hang time for ILEs because of enhanced microbial growth potential with dextrose/amino acid (2-in-1) PN admixtures.[11] The USP also endorsed using ILE products within 12 hours of opening the original manufacturer's container if ILEs are infused as separate preparations from dextrose and amino acids.[12] A PN mixture containing ILE, dextrose, and amino acids in the same container (ie, a total nutrient admixture [TNA]) may be administered over 24 hours. The hang time and infusion of this admixture is extended because bacterial growth is inhibited as a result of reduced pH (approximately 5.6–6) and because of the increased total osmolarity of the TNA compared with infusing ILE separately. Whether infused separately or as a TNA admixture, the ILE infusion rate should not exceed 0.11 g/kg/h.[13] Faster infusion rates are associated with an increased risk of adverse effects, such as hypertriglyceridemia and infectious complications.

In neonates and infants, using a separate infusion of ILE is recommended (ie, a dextrose/amino acid [2-in-1] PN solution with ILE infused separately). This is because of the increased risk of calcium phosphate precipitation in neonate and infant PN admixtures.[14,15] Furthermore, the American Academy of Pediatrics (AAP) recommended that ILE be infused over 24 hours in infants and children to promote lipid tolerance.[15] It is also recommended that the ILE infusion rate not exceed 0.15 g/kg/h in neonates. Soybean oil–based ILE may be safely used in neonates with hyperbilirubinemia (ie, physiologic jaundice). The AAP recommends that ILE use be limited to meeting essential fatty acid needs (0.5–1 g/kg/d) in neonates with serum total bilirubin concentrations >8–10 mg/dL.[15]

Mixed-oil ILEs and 100% fish oil–based ILE may be useful in patients with critical illness or metabolic stress, sepsis, atopic dermatitis, or severe ulcerative colitis and in those undergoing elective surgery[16-19] Other advantages over soy oil–based ILEs are decreased peroxidation and lack of in vitro inhibition of lymphocyte function.[20,21] Data with fish oil–based ILEs have demonstrated reversal of intestinal failure–associated liver disease.[22] See Table 4-1 for a comparison of ILEs.

Table 4-1. Lipid Injectable Emulsions

Brand Name	Fat Composition	Concentration of Emulsion (%)
Intralipid[5]	Soybean oil 100%	20 or 30
Nutralipid	Soybean oil 100%	20
Clinolipid[6]	Olive oil 80%; soybean oil 20%	20
SMOFlipid[7]	Soybean 30%; medium-chain triglycerides 30%; olive oil 25%; fish oil 15%	20
Omegaven[8]	Fish oil 100%	10

Protein

Standard amino acid products. Crystalline amino acids provide protein and energy (4 kcal/g) when oxidized for energy. Nitrogen content varies depending on the concentration of the amino acid product and mixture of individual amino acids. For nitrogen-balance calculations, amino acid products are generally assumed to be 16% nitrogen (6.25 g of protein = 1 g of nitrogen). Standard or balanced amino acid products are mixtures of essential and nonessential amino acids. They are available from different manufacturers in stock solutions with concentrations ranging from 3% to 20%, although 8.5%, 10%, and 15% are most frequently used for PN compounding. The concentrated 15% and 20% products may be used when fluid restriction is necessary. Modified or specialty amino acid products are formulated for certain diseases or clinical conditions.[1] See Table 4-2 for a list of commercially available amino acid solutions. Commercially available amino acid products may also contain various concentrations and combinations of electrolytes and/or buffers, in addition to the inherent or endogenous electrolyte content of the individual amino acids.

Pediatric amino acid products. Compared with standard amino acid products, the pediatric amino acid products contain greater amounts of branched-chain amino acids (BCAAs) and decreased amounts of methionine and phenylalanine.[23] The pediatric formulations were developed to produce plasma amino acid concentrations similar to those of term-breastfed infants.[23] They have a lower pH, which enhances calcium and phosphate solubility, thereby allowing for greater administration of these minerals. Cysteine is important in the synthesis of taurine and may be considered a conditionally essential amino acid in neonates. Because it is unstable in solution over prolonged periods, cysteine must be added to PN admixtures at the time of compounding. The pediatric amino acid solutions are intended to be supplemented with cysteine hydrochloride, which further decreases solution pH and enhances calcium phosphate solubility.

Modified amino acid products. Specialty amino acid products were developed for use in certain disease states or clinical conditions. The American Society for Parenteral and Enteral Nutrition (ASPEN) published guidelines for use of these products in clinical practice.[24]

Modified amino acid products designed for use in hepatic encephalopathy contain increased amounts of BCAA and decreased amounts of aromatic amino acid (AAA) compared with standard amino acid solutions.[25] Altered metabolism in patients with hepatic failure can result in a high serum ratio of AAA to BCAA. This imbalance is thought to cause increased transport of AAAs into the brain, where they serve as precursors to neurotransmitters that may be responsible for an altered mental status. As shown in Table 4-2, 1 product is available, and its indication is limited to hepatic encephalopathy.

Although use has declined, glutamine is an amino acid known to be conditionally essential during periods of metabolic stress. Crystalline amino acids do not contain glutamine. As such, there has been considerable interest in adding glutamine to PN admixtures either as a separate entity or as part of the amino acid stock formulations. However, because of stability and compatibility limitations, no IV form of glutamine is currently commercially available for adding to PN admixtures. Studies of glutamine-supplemented PN have used extemporaneous preparations of powdered L-glutamine sterilized by filtration.[26,27] Benefits vs risk and cost-effectiveness must be carefully evaluated, given this situation.

Table 4-2. Commercially Available Crystalline Amino Acid Solutions

Brand Name	Type/Indication	Stock Concentrations (%)
Aminosyn II	Standard	8.5, 10, 15
Clinisol	Standard/fluid restriction	15
FreAmine III	Standard	10
Prosol	Standard/fluid restriction	20
Travasol	Standard	10
HepatAmine	Hepatic failure	8
Aminosyn-PF	Neonates	7, 10
PremaSol	Neonates	10
TrophAmine	Neonates	10

aContains essential amino acids + arginine.
bContains essential amino acids only.

Volume

The total volume of a PN admixture is typically estimated based on weight for adults, with the goal to maintain a urine output of 0.5–2 mL/kg/h. The volume is adjusted with sterile water for injection added to bring the PN admixture to a final volume. Intake and output for each patient can dictate the need for additional fluids. Some typical fluid losses are gastric losses through a nasogastric tube, ostomies, enterocutaneous fistulas, and chyle leaks. In pediatric patients, the volume of the PN admixture can often be used to meet maintenance fluid requirements. (See chapter 5 for daily fluid requirements for pediatric patients.)

Electrolytes

Electrolytes are available commercially as individual salts. They are also added by the manufacturer in specified amounts to certain crystalline amino acid solutions or multichamber-bag PN (MCB-PN) products. Maintenance or therapeutic amounts of various electrolytes are added to PN admixtures depending on a patient's requirements. A common question in prescribing PN is whether the sodium and potassium should be prescribed as the acetate or chloride salt. Acetate and chloride do not have specific ranges for intake, but they are adjusted as needed to maintain acid-base balance. Calcium gluconate and magnesium sulfate are the preferred salts for use in PN admixtures because they are less likely to produce physiochemical incompatibilities as compared with calcium chloride and magnesium chloride. See Table 4-3 for commercially available parenteral electrolyte salts.

Table 4-3. Commercially Available Parenteral Electrolyte Salts

Electrolyte	Salt Form
Sodium	Chloride, acetate, phosphate
Potassium	Chloride, acetate, phosphate
Chloride	Sodium, potassium
Acetate	Sodium, potassium
Calcium	Gluconate,[a] gluceptate, chloride
Magnesium	Sulfate,[a] chloride

Source: Adapted with permission from Patel R. Parenteral nutrition formulations. In: Mueller CM, et al, eds. *The ASPEN Adult Nutrition Support Core Curriculum.* 3rd ed. Silver Spring, MD: American Society for Parenteral and Enteral Nutrition; 2017:297–320.
[a]Preferred salt form for use in PN admixtures.

Vitamins

Commercially available vitamin products for PN supplementation include single-vitamin entities and multivitamin products that include both fat-soluble and water-soluble vitamins. Parenteral products for single vitamins are not commercially available for biotin, pantothenic acid, riboflavin, vitamin A, and vitamin E. Available parenteral multivitamin products for adults contain 13 vitamins. Table 4-4 lists the composition of adult parenteral multivitamin products available in the United States.

Table 4-4. Composition of Adult IV Multivitamin Products in the United States

Vitamin	Dose
C (ascorbic acid)	200 mg
A (retinol)	1 mg (3300 USP units)
D (cholecalciferol)	0.005 mg (200 USP units)
B$_1$ (thiamin)	6 mg
B$_2$ (riboflavin)	3.6 mg
B$_6$ (pyridoxine)	6 mg
B$_3$ (niacinamide)	40 mg
B$_5$ (dexpanthenol)	15 mg
E (dl-α-tocopheryl acetate)	10 mg (10 USP units)
B$_7$ (Biotin)	0.06 mg
B$_9$ (Folic acid)	0.6 mg
B$_{12}$ (Cyanocobalamin)	0.005 mg
K (Phylloquinone)	0.15 mg

IV, intravenous; USP, United States Pharmacopeia.

Parenteral multivitamin products are available for pediatric patients who are up to 11 years of age or weigh up to 40 kg. The products are formulated to comply with the guidelines outlined by the Subcommittee on Pediatric Parenteral Nutrient Requirements of the Committee on Clinical Practice Issues of the American Society for Clinical Nutrition.[28] Table 4-5 lists the composition of pediatric parenteral multivitamin products available in the United States.

Table 4-5. Composition of Pediatric IV Multivitamin Products in the United States

Vitamin	Multi-Vitamin Infusion Pediatric (Pfizer) (5 mL)	Infuvite Pediatric (Baxter) (5 mL)
A (retinol)	0.7 mg[a]	2300 IU (0.7 mg)
D (ergocalciferol)	0.01 mg[b]	400 IU (cholecalciferol)
E (dl-α-tocopheryl acetate)	7 mg[c]	7 IU (7 mg)
K (phytonadione)	0.2 mg	0.2 mg
C (ascorbic acid)	80 mg	80 mg
B_1 (thiamin)	1.2 mg	1.2 mg
B_2 (riboflavin)	1.4 mg	1.4 mg
Niacinamide	17 mg	17 mg
Dexpanthenol	5 mg	5 mg
B_6 (pyridoxine)	1 mg	1 mg
B_{12} (cyanocobalamin)	0.001 mg	0.001 mg
Biotin	0.02 mg	0.02 mg
Folic acid	0.14 mg	0.14 mg
Other		
Aluminum	0.042 mg/L	0.03 mg/L
Polysorbate 80	50 mg	50 mg
Polysorbate 20	0.8 mg	None

[a]0.7 mg vitamin A = 2300 USP units.
[b]0.01 mg ergocalciferol = 400 USP units.
[c]7 mg vitamin E = 7 USP units.

Trace Elements

Commonly used trace elements in PN formulations include zinc, copper, chromium, manganese, and selenium. These are commercially available as single-entity products and in various multiple trace element combinations and concentrations for adult, pediatric, and neonatal patients. It should be noted that the commercially available multiple trace element combinations in the United States contain 3–5 times the recommended dosages for manganese and may contribute to complications in long-term patients. See Table 4-6 for trace element supplementation for PN.[29-31] Other trace elements that may be supplemented in PN include molybdenum, iodine, and iron.[29] Three injectable iron products are available, all as single-entity products. Only iron dextran is approved for addition to PN admixtures, but this should only be considered for dextrose/amino acid (2-in-1) formulations because ILEs are disrupted by iron.[30]

Table 4-6. Daily Trace Element Supplementation in PN Formulations[a]

Trace Element	Preterm Neonates < 3 kg (mcg/kg/d)	Term Neonates 3–10 kg (mcg/kg/d)	Children 10–40 kg (mcg/kg/d)	Adolescents > 40 kg (mcg)	Adults (mcg)
Chromium	0.05–0.2	0.2	0.14–0.2	5–15	10–15
Copper	20	20	5–20	200–500	300–500
Iron	Not routinely added	Not routinely added	Not routinely added	Not routinely added	Not routinely added
Manganese	1	1	1	40–100[b]	60–100[b]
Selenium	1.5–2	2	1–2	40–60	20–60
Zinc	400	50–250	50–125	2000–5000	2500–5000

PN, parenteral nutrition.

Source: Adapted with permission from Mirtallo J, Canada T, Johnson D, et al. Safe practices for parenteral nutrition [erratum in *JPEN J Parenter Enteral Nutr.* 2006;30:177]. *JPEN J Parenter Enteral Nutr.* 2004;28(suppl 2):S39 S70.

[a]Standard intake ranges based on generally healthy individuals with normal losses.
[b]The aluminum contamination level in various components of the PN admixture can significantly contribute to total intake. Serum concentrations should be monitored with long-term use.

Other Additives

Carnitine. Carnitine is necessary for proper transport and metabolism of long-chain fatty acids. Carnitine is not present in any component of PN admixtures. An IV form of L-carnitine is commercially available for treatment of carnitine deficiency and is sometimes added to PN admixtures for selected patients who have a documented deficiency or are susceptible to a deficiency.[32]

Medication additives to PN. On occasion, some medications may need to be infused concurrently or added directly to the PN admixture. Common medication additives to PN admixtures include H2-receptor antagonists, regular insulin, or unfractionated heparin. For further information on medications, please refer to chapter 10.

PN Preparation

Admixtures: Dextrose/Amino Acids (2-in-1) vs Dextrose/Amino Acids/ILE (3-in-1, TNA)

PN admixtures may be prepared for administration in 1 of 2 types. The dextrose/amino acid, or 2-in-1, admixture incorporates dextrose and amino acid base solutions along with the prescribed electrolytes, minerals, vitamins, and trace elements in 1 or multiple containers each day. ILE is administered separately as a piggyback infusion. In contrast, the TNA incorporates dextrose, amino acids, and ILE along with the other prescribed micronutrients in the same container for final administration. Specific advantages and disadvantages are associated with the use of each PN admixture system and are discussed in chapter 6.[33-37]

Central venous access is the preferred route for PN administration. If the PN admixture is to be administered via a peripheral vein (as opposed to via a peripherally inserted central catheter), certain criteria are important for decreasing the risk of thrombophlebitis and damage to peripheral veins. Osmolarity should generally be below 900 mOsm/L. Calcium and potassium concentrations should be kept low (for some institutions, this may translate to calcium not to exceed 5 mEq/L and potassium not to exceed 40 mEq/L), and ILE is generally given daily to provide adequate energy.[27,29]

In addition, it has been speculated that using daily ILE along with the dextrose/amino acid admixtures may confer a modest protective effect on venous tolerance by diluting the dextrose/amino acid admixture and/or by some buffering action in the vein.[34] There has also been some success in reducing or preventing thrombophlebitis through the addition of small amounts of hydrocortisone sodium succinate to the PN admixture, although this practice is variable.[33] Another technique to minimize thrombophlebitis includes the use of a low-dose nitroglycerin patch at the venous insertion site. See Table 4-7 for estimating the osmolarity of PN admixtures.

Table 4-7. Estimating Osmolarity of PN Admixtures[a]

PN Component	Osmolarity (mOsm/g)	Example, 1-L Volume	
		PN Content	mOsm
Dextrose	5 mOsm/g	170 g	850
Amino acids	10 mOsm/g	60 g	600
Fat emulsion, 20%	1.3–1.5 mOsm/g[b]	20 g	26–30
Electrolytes	1 mOsm/mEq	243 mEq	243
Total			1719–1723

PN, parenteral nutrition.
Source: Adapted with permission from Mirtallo JM, Canada TW, Johnson D, et al. Safe practices for parenteral nutrition [erratum in *JPEN J Parenter Enteral Nutr.* 2006;30:177]. *JPEN J Parenter Enteral Nutr.* 2004;28:S39–S70.
[a]Based on approximations of the osmolarity of the PN components and used as an estimate only.
[b]Product-dependent.

PN Admixture Compounding

PN admixtures may be compounded manually or using automated compounding devices (ACDs). With manual compounding, the base admixture (ie, dextrose, amino acids, and sterile water for injection) may be mixed by hand or, more typically, by using a gravimetric compounder. After the base solution has been made, all other additives are drawn up in individual syringes prior to being added to the PN admixture. ACDs were originally developed to assist with streamlining the manufacturing sequence for PN admixtures. The main advantage of ACDs is enhanced accuracy of the dosage form, thereby enabling clinicians to provide more precise and safer PN admixtures to patients. (See chapter 6 for additional information on compounding.)

Multichamber-Bag PN

(See chapter 12 on MCB-PN for more detailed information.)

Several MCB-PN products are available for both central and peripheral vein administration. The products for central venous infusion generally contain final dextrose concentrations of 15%–25% and final amino acid concentrations of 3.5%, 4.25%, or 5% with or without a standard package of electrolytes. The products for peripheral vein infusion include those with final dextrose concentrations of 5%–10% and final amino acid concentrations of 2.75%, 3.5%, or 4.25% with or without electrolytes. MCB-PN products require manipulation of the container to break the seal between the chambers and mix the components prior to use. Activation of these PN products is critical to administering all PN components. All commercially available MCB-PN products require addition of IV multivitamins shortly before administration because vitamins are essential components of PN that are not stable when added >24 hours prior to use.

PN Product Shortages

PN product shortages have occurred in the United States because of a variety of factors, including manufacturing or quality issues, raw material acquisition issues, discontinuations, natural disasters, and consolidation of the market. Sources for information about PN component shortages include the US Food and Drug Administration (FDA) Drug Shortage Program Web page, the American Society for Health-System Pharmacists Drug Shortage Web page, and the ASPEN Nutrition Product Shortage Web page. Shortages of PN components affect the entire PN process and have been associated with patient harm and suboptimal patient outcomes.[38]

Strategies for managing shortages of PN components include developing the following: policies and procedures for communicating shortages and outages to prescribers, written protocols for PN component substitution and/or conservation strategies, a process to communicate PN component substitution and/or conservation strategies to prescribers, a process to implement PN component substitution and/or conservation strategies, a process to evaluate alternative PN components procured from sterile compounding facilities or imported from outside the United States, a process to modify the PN order to reflect component outages and/or conservation strategies, a process to modify the PN label to reflect changes in the PN order because of outages and/or conservation strategies, a process to modify PN compounding including ACDs to reflect change in components due to outages and/or conservation strategies, and a process to track and analyze errors associated with PN component outages and/or conservation strategies.[39]

General guidelines for managing PN component shortages and outages are listed in Table 4-8.

Table 4-8. General Strategies for PN Component Shortages

- Implement conservation strategies early.
- Assess the indication for PN.
- Switch to oral or enteral nutrients (excluding malabsorption syndromes).
- Reserve IV products for those receiving PN or those with a therapeutic medical need for IV nutrients.
- Reserve supply for those vulnerable populations (neonates, pediatric patients, or patients with malabsorption syndromes).
- Reserve age-specific products for designed patient populations.
- Observe for deficiencies with ongoing shortages.
- Purchase only as much as needed—no hoarding or stockpiling.
- Compound PN in a single, central location (either in a centralized pharmacy or as outsourced preparation) to decrease waste.
- Consider supply outreach to other facilities.
- Observe and be compliant with product labeling, USP <797>, and federal and state Boards of Pharmacy rules and regulations.
- During prolonged shortages, the FDA may approve the temporary importation of alternative products, which may have different profiles, ratios (does), packaging, and labeling than US products—carefully evaluate these products.
- Assess your PN patient population to determine whether MCB-PN products[40] may be appropriate for a portion of your patient population.
- Be cognizant of the safety concerns during shortages, and develop and implement policies and procedures to avoid areas.
- Report patient problems related to shortages to ISMP Medication Errors Reporting Program (http://www.ismp.org/merp).

FDA, US Food and Drug Administration; ISMP, Institute for Safe Medication Practices; IV, intravenous; MCB-PN, multichamber-bag PN; PN, parenteral nutrition; USP, United States Pharmacopeia.
Source: Adapted with permission from ASPEN Clinical Practice Committee Nutrition Product Shortage Subcommittee. Parenteral nutrition electrolyte and mineral product shortage considerations. ASPEN website. http://www.nutritioncare.org/News/General_News/Parenteral_Nutrition_Electrolyte_and_Mineral_Product_Shortage_Considerations/. Published 2015. Accessed November 10, 2019.

ASPEN's Clinical Practice Committee's Nutrition Product Shortage Subcommittee[41-46] developed recommendations to help clinicians manage PN therapy during shortages of amino acids, ILE, multivitamins, trace elements, electrolytes/minerals and cysteine (see Tables 4-9 to 4-18). These recommendations should only be used in the event of a shortage of these PN components and should not be employed during routine (nonshortage) clinical practice. Furthermore, when adequate supplies of a PN component become readily available and the shortage resolves, dosing of the PN component should return to regimens used prior to the shortage.

Table 4-9. Shortage Considerations for IV Amino Acid Products

- ONLY use neonatal/pediatric-specific amino acids or disease-specific amino acids for the indicated patient populations.

- Reserve high-concentration amino acids products (eg, >10%) for fluid-restricted patients requiring PN.

- Consider reviewing the entire portfolio of amino acid products available nationally. There may be a shortage in 1 concentration but availability in another.

- Different brands of amino acid products are not always directly substitutable, especially for TNA (3-in-1) vs dextrose/amino acid (2-in-1) PN formulations. They may have different pH values, different calcium-phosphorus solubility, and different amounts of phosphorus, as well as other characteristics that should be considered.

- Assess your PN patient population to determine if MCB-PN products may be appropriate for a portion of your patient population.

IV, intravenous; MCB-PN, multichamber-bag PN; PN, parenteral nutrition; TNA, total nutrient admixture.
Source: Adapted with permission from ASPEN Clinical Practice Committee Nutrition Product Shortage Subcommittee. Parenteral nutrition amino acids product shortage considerations. ASPEN website. http://www.nutritioncare.org/News/General_News/Parenteral_Nutrition_Amino_Acids_Product_Shortage_Considerations. Published 2016. Accessed November 10, 2019.

Table 4-10. Shortage Considerations for Parenteral Electrolyte/Mineral Products

- Consider switching to oral or enterally administered electrolyte or mineral supplement products when oral/enteral intake is initiated (excluding patients with malabsorption syndromes or a nonfunctioning gastrointestinal tract). Consult a pharmacist for product information.

- Eliminate the use of parenteral electrolyte/mineral injections as a supplemental additive in enteral nutrition products.

- Limit the use of electrolyte/mineral additives in IV fluids to patients with disease states and clinical conditions for which they are appropriate.

- Reconsider the use of serum electrolyte algorithms/protocols as "automatic" IV electrolyte-replacement therapies in otherwise asymptomatic patients.

- Use commercially available IV multielectrolyte/multimineral products as much as possible for replacement therapy.

- Review the entire portfolio of PN electrolyte and mineral products available nationally. There may be a shortage in one concentration or salt form but availability in another form. See Table 4-9 for alternative electrolyte and mineral salts.

- Consider decreasing or eliminating the daily amount of electrolyte added to the PN.

- Monitor serum electrolyte concentrations closely.

- Observe for an increase in deficiencies with the ongoing shortages. Increase your awareness and assessment for signs and symptoms of electrolyte and mineral deficiencies.

IV, intravenous.
Source: Adapted with permission from ASPEN Clinical Practice Committee Nutrition Product Shortage Subcommittee. Parenteral nutrition electrolyte and mineral product shortage considerations. ASPEN website. http://www.nutritioncare.org/News/General_News/Parenteral_Nutrition_Electrolyte_and_Mineral_Product_Shortage_Considerations/. Published 2015. Accessed November 10, 2019.

Table 4-11. Electrolytes and Minerals Available/Alternative Salts

Electrolyte/Mineral	Available/Alternative Salts
Calcium	Gluconate,[a] chloride
Magnesium	Sulfate,[a] chloride
Phosphate	Potassium, sodium
Potassium	Acetate, chloride, phosphate
Sodium	Acetate, chloride, phosphate, bicarbonate,[b] lactate[b]

Source: Adapted with permission from ASPEN Clinical Practice Committee Nutrition Product Shortage Subcommittee. Parenteral nutrition electrolyte and mineral product shortage considerations. http://www.nutritioncare.org/News/General_News/Parenteral_Nutrition_Electrolyte_and_Mineral_Product_Shortage_Considerations/. Published 2015. Accessed November 10, 2019.
[a]Preferred salt for parenteral nutrition admixtures.
[b]Avoid adding parenteral nutrition admixtures.

Table 4-12. Shortage Considerations for Parenteral Trace Element Products

- Consider switching to oral or enterally administered multivitamin/multimineral/multi-trace element supplement products when oral/enteral intake is initiated (excluding patients with malabsorption syndromes). Supplements may not have a full spectrum of trace elements nor contain a daily enteral maintenance dose.

- If IV multi-trace element products are no longer available, administer individual parenteral trace element entities. Dosing guidelines for individual trace elements can be found in the 2012 ASPEN position paper "Recommendations for Changes in Commercially Available Parenteral Multivitamin and Multi-Trace Element Products."[47]

- Observe for deficiencies when your institution is experiencing ongoing shortages. Increase your awareness and assessment for signs and symptoms of trace element deficiencies. Monitor serum trace element concentrations or other appropriate serum biochemical markers to evaluate trace element status.

ASPEN, American Society for Parenteral and Enteral Nutrition; IV, intravenous.
Source: Adapted with permission from ASPEN Clinical Practice Committee Nutrition Product Shortage Subcommittee. Parenteral nutrition trace element product shortage considerations. ASPEN website. http://www.nutritioncare.org/News/General_News/Parenteral_Nutrition_Trace_Element_Product_Shortage_Considerations/. Published 2016. Accessed November 10, 2019.

Table 4-13. Shortage Considerations for ILEs

Prioritize supply of soybean oil–based ILE as follows:

- Neonatal and pediatric hospitalized patients should continue the same ILE therapy as before the shortage to minimize risk of adverse effects associated EFAD in this high-risk patient population.

- Adult, hospitalized patients who are mildly to moderately malnourished receiving PN for <2 wk may have ILE withheld during a shortage unless it is considered essential in the judgment of the healthcare professional.

- Adult, hospitalized patients receiving PN for >2 wk should receive a total of 100 g of a soybean oil–based ILE weekly for EFAD prevention.

- Adult, hospitalized, patients with critical illness who are receiving propofol should not require additional ILE for EFAD prevention because the soybean oil in the medication will supply needed essential fatty acids.

- Home or long-term care patients receiving PN should continue to receive the same ILE therapy as before the shortage. However, ILE should be minimized when clinically feasible. At a minimum, patients should receive a total of 100 g of a soybean oil–based ILE weekly for EFAD prevention, which should be provided by the safest and most efficient method that minimizes waste.

- Increase awareness and assessment for signs and symptoms of EFAD. Signs and symptoms of EFAD include, but are not limited to, diffuse, dry, scaly rash; alopecia; thrombocytopenia; anemia; and impaired wound healing. Biochemical evidence of ω-6 EFAD is confirmed by a triene-to-tetraene ratio > 0.2. Using topical oils for prevention and treatment of EFAD has produced mixed results. Safflower and sunflower seed oils had beneficial results, whereas vegetable oil (corn oil) did not.

- Consider using an alternative ILE product such as a 4-oil ILE (soybean oil, medium-chain triglycerides, olive oil, and fish oil) during a soybean oil–based ILE shortage. This product is only approved for use in adults in the United States. The doses and frequency of administration to meet essential fatty acid needs for adults may be different from those for soybean oil–based ILE.

EFAD, essential fatty acid deficiency; ILE, lipid injectable emulsion; PN, parenteral nutrition.
Source: Adapted with permission from ASPEN Clinical Practice Committee Nutrition Product Shortage Subcommittee. Parenteral nutrition lipid injectable emulsion product shortage considerations. ASPEN website. http://www.nutritioncare.org/News/General_News/2017_Parenteral_Nutrition_Lipid_Injectable_Emulsion_Product_Shortage_Considerations/. Published 2017. Accessed November 10, 2019.

Table 4-14. Shortage Considerations for IV Adult Multivitamins

- The use of pediatric IV multivitamins for adults is not recommended.

- Consider switching to oral or enterally administered multivitamins when oral/enteral intake is initiated (excluding patients with malabsorption syndromes). The vitamin profile should be reviewed, and missing components should be supplemented, if available. Consult a pharmacist for assistance with selecting an appropriate oral multivitamin product.

- When supplies are limited, ration IV multivitamins in PN, such as by reducing the daily dose by 50% or giving 1 multivitamin infusion dose 3 times a wk.

- If IV multivitamins are no longer available, administer individual parenteral vitamin entities.

IV, intravenous.
Source: Adapted with permission from ASPEN Clinical Practice Committee Nutrition Product Shortage Subcommittee. Parenteral nutrition multivitamin product shortage considerations. ASPEN website. http://www.nutritioncare.org/News/Product_Shortages/Parenteral_Nutrition_Multivitamin_Product_Shortage_Considerations/. Published 2016. Accessed November 10, 2019.

Table 4-15. Clinically Indicated Suggested Doses of IV or Other Nonoral Routes of Administration for Vitamins

Vitamin	Dose for Adults
Thiamin	6 mg daily
Folate	0.6 mg daily
Ascorbic Acid	200 mg daily
Pyridoxine	6 mg daily
Vitamin K	0.15 mg daily or 5-10 mg weekly
Cyanacobalamin (B_{12})	0.1-1 mg intramuscularly or by deep subcutaneous administration at least once monthly or 0.5 mg intranasally once weekly or 1 mg sublingually once daily

IV, intravenous.
Source: Adapted with permission from ASPEN Clinical Practice Committee Nutrition Product Shortage Subcommittee. Parenteral nutrition multivitamin product shortage considerations. ASPEN website. http://www.nutritioncare.org/News/Product_Shortages/Parenteral_Nutrition_Multivitamin_Product_Shortage_Considerations/. Published 2016. Accessed November 10, 2019.

Table 4-16. Shortage Considerations for Pediatric IV Multivitamins

- Consider switching to oral or enterally administered multivitamins when oral/enteral intake is >50% of needs (excluding patients with malabsorption syndromes). The vitamin profile should be reviewed, and missing components should be supplemented, if available. Consult a pharmacist for assistance with selecting an appropriate oral multivitamin product.

- Reserve pediatric IV multivitamins for children < 2.5 kg or < 36 weeks' gestation.

- Consider use of adult IV multivitamins for children during the shortage; use 5 mL of adult multivitamins in all children > 2.5 kg or 36 weeks' gestation while saving the pediatric product for smaller neonates to conserve the supply. Supplement IV vitamin K daily (total daily dose = 200 mcg). The vitamin K content of the adult multivitamin product should be noted when supplementing with additional vitamin K.

- In the event that no pediatric IV multivitamins are available, infants < 2.5 kg or < 36 weeks' gestation should receive an adult IV multivitamin at a daily dose of 1 mL/kg up to a maximum of 2.5 mL/d.

- When using adult IV multivitamin products in neonates, be aware that these products contain propylene glycol, polysorbate, and aluminum, which may be toxic to neonates. Adult IV multivitamins may contain more aluminum than pediatric products. Clinical judgment must prevail by weighing potential vitamin deficiencies against potential propylene glycol, polysorbate, and aluminum toxicity.

- Use the full adult dose (10 mL) of adult IV multivitamins for children > 11 years of age.

- If neither pediatric nor adult IV multivitamins are available, administer individual parenteral vitamin entities in doses that are appropriate for the patient's age and weight.

  1. Thiamin, ascorbic acid, pyridoxine, folic acid, cyanocobalamin and vitamin K should be given daily.

  2. Thiamin is critical, as several deaths have resulted from thiamin deficiency when patients administered long-term PN did not receive vitamins for 3–4 wk. Patients receiving a carbohydrate load are particularly susceptible to thiamin deficiency.

  3. Unless deficiency is suspected or otherwise clinically indicated, suggested IV daily doses of vitamins are listed in Table 4-11.

IV, intravenous
Source: Adapted with permission from ASPEN Clinical Practice Committee Nutrition Product Shortage Subcommittee. Parenteral nutrition multivitamin product shortage considerations. ASPEN website. http://www.nutritioncare.org/News/Product_Shortages/Parenteral_Nutrition_Multivitamin_Product_Shortage_Considerations/. Published 2016. Accessed November 10, 2019.

Table 4-17. Clinically Indicated Suggested IV Daily Doses of Vitamins

Vitamin	Infants	Children
Thiamin	0.35–0.5 mg/kg	1.2 mg
Folic acid	0.056 mg	0.14 mg
Ascorbic acid	15–25 mg/kg	80 mg
Pyridoxine	0.15–0.2 mg/kg	1 mg
Cyancobalamin	0.0003 mg/kg	0.001 mg
Vitamin K	0.01 mg/kg	0.2 mg

Source: Adapted with permission from ASPEN Clinical Practice Committee Nutrition Product Shortage Subcommittee. Parenteral nutrition multivitamin product shortage considerations. ASPEN website. http://www.nutritioncare.org/News/Product_Shortages/Parenteral_Nutrition_Multivitamin_Product_Shortage_Considerations/. Published 2016. Accessed November 10, 2019.

Table 4-18. Shortage Considerations for L-cysteine

- Discontinue L-cysteine supplementation in PN for neonates receiving a minimum dose of 3 g/kg/d of commonly prescribed amino acid solutions. This dose of amino acids will provide a sufficient amount of sulfur amino acid substrate (methionine) for the trans-sulfuration pathway to produce adequate cysteine, thus not requiring supplementation of PN with L-cysteine. However, L-cysteine supplementation may be necessary to decrease the pH of the PN admixture to enhance calcium and phosphate solubility.

- Reduce L-cysteine supplementation in PN admixtures to 20 mg/g of amino acids provided. Common dosing of L-cysteine in PN admixtures is 30–40 mg/g of amino acids provided. However, studies have documented that as little as 20 mg/g of amino acids is adequate.

- Assess the PN admixture to determine if the daily calcium and phosphorus requirements are considered to be compatible and within solubility limits and can be attained without the addition of L-cysteine.

- When removing or reducing the dose of L-cysteine in the PN admixture, reevaluate the calcium-phosphorus solubility charts or software to ensure that a precipitate will not develop because of the increase in the pH of the PN admixture. Consider using calcium-phosphorus solubility data that do not include the presence of L-cysteine in the PN admixture.

- Consider using organic phosphate injections, if available. Organic phosphates, as compared with inorganic phosphorus products, have favorable compatibility with calcium and may be considered as a measure to provide adequate calcium and phosphate to patients with decreased risk of precipitate formation.

- Discourage using L-cysteine as an agent to reestablish vascular access device catheter patency.

PN, parenteral nutrition.
Source: Adapted with permission from ASPEN Clinical Practice Committee Nutrition Product Shortage Subcommittee. Parenteral nutrition L-cysteine product shortage considerations. ASPEN website. http://www.nutritioncare.org/News/General_News/A_S_P_E_N__Releases_New_Parenteral_Nutrition_L-Cysteine_Product_Shortage_Considerations/. Published 2015. Accessed November 10, 2019.

References

1. Mirtallo JM. Parenteral formulas. In: Rombeau JL, Rolandelli RH, eds. *Parenteral Nutrition.* 3rd ed. Philadelphia, PA: WB Saunders; 2001:118–139.

2. Singer P, Bursztein S, Kirvelä O, et al. Hypercaloric glycerol in injured patients. *Surgery.* 1992;112(3):509–514.

3. Lev-Ran A, Johnson M, Hwang DL, Askanazi J, Weissman C, Gersovitz M. Double-blind study of glycerol vs glucose in parenteral nutrition of postsurgical insulin-treated diabetic patients. *JPEN J Parenter Enteral Nutr.* 1987;11(3):271–274.

4. Fairfull-Smith RJ, Stoski D, Freeman JB. Use of glycerol in peripheral parenteral nutrition. *Surgery.* 1982;92(4):728–732.

5. Intralipid [package insert]. Uppsala, Sweden: Fresenius Kabi AB; 2015. FDA website. https://www.accessdata.fda.gov/drugsatfda_docs/label/2016/020248s020lbl.pdf. Accessed December 8, 2019.

6. Clinolipid [package insert]. Deerfield, IL: Baxter Healthcare; 2013. FDA website. https://www.accessdata.fda.gov/drugsatfda_docs/label/2013/204508s000lbl.pdf. Accessed December 8, 2019.

7. Smoflipid [package insert]. Uppsala, Sweden: Fresenius Kabi AB; 2016. FDA website. https://www.accessdata.fda.gov/drugsatfda_docs/label/2016/207648lbl.pdf. Accessed December 8, 2019.

8. Omegeven [package insert]. Graz, Austria: Fresenius Kabi; 2018. FDA website. https://www.accessdata.fda.gov/drugsatfda_docs/label/2018/0210589s000lbledt.pdf. Accessed December 8, 2019.

9. FDA information on Clinolipid 20% (Baxter). Drugs @FDA: FDA-Approved Drugs website. https://www.accessdata.fda.gov/scripts/cder/daf/index.cfm?event=overview. process&ApplNo=204508. Accessed January 14, 2020.

10. Sacks GS, Driscoll DF. Does lipid hang time make a difference? Time is of the essence. *Nutr Clin Pract.* 2002;17(5):284–290.

11. O'Grady NP, Alexander M, Dellinger EP, et al. Guidelines for the prevention of intravascular catheter-related infections. Centers for Disease Control and Prevention [erratum in *MMWR Recomm Rep.* 2002;51:711]. *MMWR Recomm Rep.* 2002;51(RR-10):1–29.

12. Pharmaceutical compounding—sterile preparations. *United States Pharmacopeia Revision Bulletin.* Rockville, MD: The United States Pharmacopeial Convention; 2007:1–61.

13. Klein S, Miles JM. Metabolic effects of long-chain and medium-chain triglycerides in humans. *JPEN J Parent Enteral Nutr.* 1994;18(5):396–397.

14. Kerner JA, Poole RL. The use of IV fat in neonates. *Nutr Clin Pract.* 2006;21(4):374–380.

15. American Academy of Pediatrics Committee on Nutrition. Use of intravenous fat emulsions in pediatric patients. *Pediatrics.* 1981;68:738–743.

16. Mayer K, Gokorsch S, Fegbeutel C, et al. Parenteral nutrition with fish oil modulates cytokine response in patients with sepsis. *Am J Respir Crit Care Med.* 2003;167(10):1321–1328.

17. Mayser P, Mayer K, Mahloudjian M, et al. A double-blind, randomized, placebo-controlled trial of n-3 versus n-6 fatty acid-based lipid infusion in atopic dermatitis. *JPEN J Parenter Enteral Nutr.* 2002;26(3):151–158.

18. Grimminger F, Führer D, Papavassilis C, et al. Influence of intravenous n-3 lipid supplementation on fatty acid profiles and lipid mediator generation in a patient with severe ulcerative colitis. *Eur J Clin Invest.* 1993;23(11):706–715.

19. Weiss G, Meyer F, Matthies B, Pross M, Koenig W, Lippert H. Immunomodulation by perioperative administration of n-3 fatty acids. *Br J Nutr.* 2002;87(suppl 1):S89–S94.

20. Goulet O, de Potter S, Antébi H, et al. Long-term efficacy and safety of a new olive-oil based intravenous fat emulsion in pediatric patients: a double-blind randomized study. *Am J Clin Nutr.* 1999;70(3):338–345.

21. Granot D, Blum S, Zbinden I, et al. Effect of ClinOleic*, an olive-oil based parenteral lipid emulsion on lymphocyte function in vitro [abstract]. *Clin Nutr.* 1996;15:9(suppl 1):3.

22. Gura KM, Duggan CP, Collier SB, et al. Reversal of parenteral nutrition-associated liver disease in two infants with short bowel syndrome using parenteral fish oil: implications for future management. *Pediatrics*. 2006;118(1):e197–e201.

23. Heird WC. Amino acids in pediatric and neonatal nutrition. *Curr Opin Clin Nutr Metab Care*. 1998;1(1):73–78.

24. ASPEN Board of Directors and The Clinical Guidelines Task Force. Guidelines for the use of parenteral and enteral nutrition in adult and pediatric patients [erratum in *JPEN J Parenter Enteral Nutr*. 2002;26(2):144]. *JPEN J Parenter Enteral Nutr*. 2002;26(1 suppl):1SA–138SA.

25. Melnick G. Value of specialty intravenous amino acids solutions. *Am J Health Syst Pharm*. 1996;53(6):671–674.

26. Schloerb PR, Skikne BS. Oral and parenteral glutamine in bone marrow transplantation: a randomized, double-blind study. *JPEN J Parenter Enteral Nutr*. 1999;23(3):117–122.

27. Ziegler TR, Benfell K, Smith RJ, et al. Safety and metabolic effects of L-glutamine administration in humans. *JPEN J Parenter Enteral Nutr*. 1990;14(4 suppl):137S–146S.

28. Greene HL, Hambidge KM, Schanler R, Tsang RC. Guidelines for the use of vitamins, trace elements, calcium, magnesium, and phosphorus in infants and children receiving total parenteral nutrition: report of the Subcommittee on Pediatric Parenteral Nutrient Requirements from the Committee on Clinical Practice Issues of the American Society for Clinical Nutrition. *Am J Clin Nutr*. 1988;48(5):1324–1342.

29. American Medical Association Department of Foods and Nutrition. Guidelines for essential trace element preparations for parenteral use. A statement by an expert panel. *JAMA*. 1979;241(19):2051–2054.

30. Kumpf VJ. Update on parenteral iron therapy. *Nutr Clin Pract*. 2003;18(4):318–326.

31. Mirtallo JM, Canada T, Johnson D, et al. Safe practices for parenteral nutrition. *JPEN J Parenter Enteral Nutr*. 2004;28(6):S39–S70.

32. Borum PR. Is L-carnitine stable in parenteral nutrition solutions prepared for preterm neonates? *Neonatal Intensive Care*. 1993;6:30–32.

33. Isaacs JW, Millikan WJ, Stackhouse J, Hersh T, Rudman D. Parenteral nutrition of adults with a 900 milliosmolar solution via peripheral veins. *Am J Clin Nutr*. 1977;30(4):552–559.

34. Fujiwara T, Kawarasaki H, Fonkalsrud EW. Reduction of postinfusion venous endothelial injury with Intralipid. *Surg Gynecol Obstet*. 1984;158(1):57–65.

35. Kochevar M, Guenter P, Holcombe B, Malone A, Mirtallo J; ASPEN Board of Directors and Task Force on Parenteral Nutrition Standardization. A.S.P.E.N. statement on parenteral nutrition standardization. *JPEN J Parenter Enteral Nutr*. 2007;31(5):441–448.

36. Waxman K, Day AT, Stellin GP, Tominaga GT, Gazzaniga AB, Bradford RR. Safety and efficacy of glycerol and amino acids in combination with lipid emulsion for peripheral parenteral nutrition support. *JPEN J Parenter Enteral Nutr*. 1992;16(4):374–378.

37. Freeman JB, Fairfull-Smith R, Rodman GH, Bernstein DM, Gazzaniga AB, Gersovitz M. Safety and efficacy of a new peripheral intravenously administered amino acid solution containing glycerol and electrolytes. *Surg Gyn Obstet*. 1983;156(5):625–631.

38. Holcombe B. Parenteral nutrition product shortages: impact on safety. *JPEN J Parenter Enteral Nutr*. 2012;36(2 suppl):44S–47S.

39. Ayers P, Adams S, Boullata J, et al. A.S.P.E.N. parenteral nutrition safety consensus recommendations. *JPEN J Parenter Enteral Nutr*. 2014;38(3):296–333.

40. Kochevar M, Guenter P, Holcombe B, Malone A, Mirtallo J; ASPEN Board of Directors and Task Force on Parenteral Nutrition Standardization. ASPEN statement on parenteral nutrition standardization. *JPEN J Parenter Enteral Nutr*. 2007;31(5):441–448.

41. ASPEN Clinical Practice Committee Nutrition Product Shortage Subcommittee. Parenteral nutrition amino acids product shortage considerations. ASPEN website. http://www.nutritioncare.org/News/General_News/Parenteral_Nutrition_Amino_Acids_Product_Shortage_Considerations/. Published 2016. Accessed November 10, 2019.

42. ASPEN Clinical Practice Committee Nutrition Product Shortage Subcommittee. Parenteral nutrition electrolyte and mineral product shortage considerations. http://www. nutritioncare.org/News/General_News/Parenteral_Nutrition_Electrolyte_and_Mineral_ Product_Shortage_Considerations/. Published 2015. Accessed November 10, 2019.

43. ASPEN Clinical Practice Committee Nutrition Product Shortage Subcommittee. Parenteral nutrition trace element product shortage considerations. ASPEN website. http://www.nutritioncare.org/News/General_News/Parenteral_Nutrition_Trace_ Element_Product_Shortage_Considerations/. Published 2016. Accessed November 10, 2019.

44. ASPEN Clinical Practice Committee Nutrition Product Shortage Subcommittee. Parenteral nutrition lipid injectable emulsion product shortage considerations. ASPEN website. http://www.nutritioncare.org/News/General_News/2017_Parenteral_Nutrition_ Lipid_Injectable_Emulsion_Product_Shortage_Considerations/. Published 2017. Accessed November 10, 2019.

45. ASPEN Clinical Practice Committee Nutrition Product Shortage Subcommittee. Parenteral nutrition multivitamin product shortage considerations. ASPEN website. http://www.nutritioncare.org/News/Product_Shortages/Parenteral_Nutrition_ Multivitamin_Product_Shortage_Considerations/. Published 2016. Accessed November 10, 2019.

46. ASPEN Clinical Practice Committee Nutrition Product Shortage Subcommittee. Parenteral nutrition L-cysteine product shortage considerations. ASPEN website. http:// www.nutritioncare.org/News/General_News/A_S_P_E_N__Releases_New_Parenteral_ Nutrition_L-Cysteine_Product_Shortage_Considerations/. Published 2015. Accessed November 10, 2019.

47. Vanek VW, Borum P, Buchman A, et al. A.S.P.E.N. position paper: recommendations for changes in commercially available parenteral multivitamin and multi-trace element products. *Nutr Clin Pract.* 2012;27(4):440–491.

How to Prescribe Parenteral Nutrition Therapy

Introduction

Parenteral nutrition (PN) is a complex prescription therapy associated with significant adverse effects. Deaths have occurred when safe practice guidelines were not followed.[1] Appropriate and safe prescribing and ordering of PN is a critical first step and an essential component of the PN use process. The safe prescribing of PN requires a thorough knowledge of protein and energy requirements, macronutrients, micronutrients, fluid homeostasis, and acid-base balance. The prescriber should be well versed in the appropriate indications for PN and basics in sterility and infection control, as well as vascular access devices (VADs; peripheral and central) and their associated complications.

Safe prescribing of PN begins with PN-specific interdisciplinary education and institutional policies focused on writing clear PN orders. Furthermore, clear communication among physicians, nurse practitioners, physician assistants, dietitians, pharmacists, and other nurses involved in this process is critical.

Healthcare organizations should use a standardized process for PN management, and this process should include clinicians with expertise in the area of nutrition support, preferably from multiple disciplines.[2-4] This process includes the following:

- Developing written policies and procedures for all aspects of PN therapy in the manner described in the American Society for Parenteral and Enteral Nutrition's (ASPEN's) guidelines and consensus documents; that is, *Safe Practices for Parenteral Nutrition and the ASPEN Parenteral Nutrition Safety Consensus Recommendations*[1,2]

- Developing a comprehensive PN education program and competency assessment and assessing competency at least annually for healthcare professionals who are involved in the care of patients receiving PN therapy.[5]

- Developing a written policy addressing credentials, training, and competency certifications required of clinicians who prescribe PN[5] (see chapter 9 on PN competencies).

Prior to ordering PN therapy, the patient and caregivers should be informed of the risks and benefits associated with PN. The primary healthcare team, in collaboration with nutrition support professionals, should evaluate, clearly define, and accurately document the patient's medical problems and the indications for PN.[2] The patient should have an appropriate indication for PN therapy based on published guidelines and evidence for the use of PN, which needs to be documented in the medical record.[1] Furthermore, the therapeutic goals of PN therapy must be specified and documented.[2] The therapeutic goals should include the following:

- Energy and protein goals appropriate for the patient's condition and based on published evidence and guidelines. (General considerations for nutrient requirements are addressed later in this chapter.)

- Parameters and frequency of monitoring to assess efficacy, detect and prevent complications, evaluate changes, and document outcomes.[1] Appropriate monitoring parameters for PN should include fluid requirements, serum electrolyte concentrations, serum glucose concentrations, hepatic function, renal function, serum triglyceride concentrations, and signs or symptoms of VAD complications.[1]

Therapeutic goals should also include PN therapy end points, response to treatment, and treatment failure.

PN Order Format

PN needs to be prescribed using a standardized PN order format.[1,2,4] Standardized electronic PN orders (eg, a computerized prescriber order entry [CPOE] system) should be used to prescribe PN for all patients.[1,2,6–8] Handwritten orders should be avoided because of potential for error. Verbal and telephone orders for PN should also be avoided. Clinical decision support should be available within electronic PN orders to alert and prevent prescribers from ordering doses of macronutrients, micronutrients, and/or nonnutrient medications that exceed recommended/safe clinical limits or that exceed limits of compatibility/stability (eg, hard limits when maximum concentrations have been exceeded).[1,2,6,7] When a CPOE system is not available, PN should be prescribed using a standardized order template as an editable electronic document to avoid handwritten orders.

PN order templates should be designed so they are clear and easily understood by all healthcare professionals involved in the care of patients receiving PN.[1] Table 5-1 lists components to be included on the PN order. All PN order templates should include the required components listed in the sequence in Table 5-1. This sequence should match the PN labels as well (see chapter 6 for PN labeling and Figures 5-1 and 5-2 for PN order templates).

Table 5-1. Required Components for PN Orders and Preferred Sequence

Components for the PN Order

Patient Information	Patient identifiers (patient name, medical record number or other unique identifiers, birth date/age, patient location)
	Patient location (home address for home PN patients)
	Allergies and reactions • Height and dosing weight (metric) • Diagnosis(es)/indication(s) for PN • VAD/location
	Administration date/time
PN ingredients (should match PN label)	• Amino acids • Dextrose • ILE • Sodium phosphate • Sodium chloride • Sodium acetate • Potassium phosphate • Potassium chloride • Potassium acetate • Magnesium sulfate or magnesium chloride • Calcium gluconate • Multivitamins • Trace elements • Additives (eg, cysteine, regular insulin) as clinically appropriate and compatible
PN instructions	Total volume, infusion rate, start and stop times, cycle information
	Prescriber and contact information

ILE, lipid injectable emulsion; PN, parenteral nutrition; VAD, vascular access device.
Source: Adapted with permission from Ayers P, Adams S, Boullata J, et al; ASPEN. A.S.P.E.N. parenteral nutrition safety consensus recommendations. *JPEN J Parenter Enteral Nutr.* 2014:38(3):296–333.

Figure 5-1. Parenteral Nutrition Order Template: Adult Patient

Patient Information

PATIENT NAME   **MEDICAL RECORD #**   **BIRTH DATE/AGE**

HEIGHT (CM)   **DOSING WEIGHT (KG)**   **DIAGNOSIS(ES)/INDICATION(S) FOR PN:**

VAD/CVC TYPE   **LOCATION**

ADMINISTRATION DATE/TIME

Base Formula	Amount (kg/d)	
Amino acids		g
Dextrose		g
ILE		g

Electrolytes	Amount (kg/d)	
Sodium phosphate		mmol
Sodium chloride		mEq
Sodium acetate		mEq
Potassium phosphate		mmol
Potassium chloride		mEq
Potassium acetate		mEq
Magnesium sulfate		mEq
Calcium gluconate		mEq

Vitamins, trace elements, additives	Amount (kg/d)	
Multicomponent vitamins		mL
Multicomponent trace elements		mL
Other additives (eg, cysteine, regular insulin) as clinically appropriate and compatible:		

PN Instructions

Total Volume: _____ mL, Infusion rate: _____ mL/h, Start and stop times: _____

Cycle information: _____

Prescriber and contact information: _____

CVC, central venous catheter; Ht, height; ILE, lipid injectable emulsion; PN, parenteral nutrition; Wt, weight.
Source: Adapted with permission from Ayers P, Adams S, Boullata J, et al; ASPEN. A.S.P.E.N. parenteral nutrition safety consensus recommendations. *JPEN J Parenter Enteral Nutr.* 2014:38(3):296–333.

Figure 5-2. Parenteral Nutrition Order Template: Pediatric/ Neonatal Patient

Patient Information

PATIENT NAME   **MEDICAL RECORD #**   **BIRTH DATE/AGE**

HEIGHT (CM)   **DOSING WEIGHT (KG)**   **DIAGNOSIS(ES)/INDICATION(S) FOR PN:**

VAD/CVC TYPE   **LOCATION**

ADMINISTRATION DATE/TIME

Base Formula	Amount (kg/d)	
Amino acids	_____	g
Dextrose	_____	g
ILE	_____	g

Electrolytes	Amount (kg/d)	
Sodium phosphate	_____	mmol
Sodium chloride	_____	mEq
Sodium acetate	_____	mEq
Potassium phosphate	_____	mmol
Potassium chloride	_____	mEq
Potassium acetate	_____	mEq
Magnesium sulfate	_____	mEq
Calcium gluconate	_____	mEq

Vitamins, trace elements, additives	Amount (kg/d)	
Multicomponent vitamins	_____	mL
Multicomponent trace elements	_____	mL
Other additives (eg, cysteine, regular insulin) as clinically appropriate and compatible:		

CVC, central venous catheter; Ht, height; ILE, lipid injectable emulsion; PN, parenteral nutrition; Wt, weight.
Source: Adapted with permission from Ayers P, Adams S, Boullata J, et al; ASPEN. A.S.P.E.N. parenteral nutrition safety consensus recommendations. *JPEN J Parenter Enteral Nutr.* 2014:38(3):296–333.

All PN ingredients should be ordered in amounts per day (eg, for adult patients) or amounts per kilogram per day (eg, pediatric and neonatal patients) rather than in amounts per liter, by percent concentration, or by volume.[1,2] Amount per day refers to macronutrients in grams per day and micronutrients in milliequivalents, millimoles, milligrams, or micrograms per day. Electrolytes should be ordered as the complete salt form rather than as the individual ion.[1,2] Each individual macronutrient and micronutrient ordered should be listed with its corresponding dose.[1,2] If available, the total ion amounts and concentrations may be reported or displayed to the prescriber within the PN order.

The PN order template should contain the full generic name for each ingredient.[1,2,5] Proprietary names should only be used if multiple products exist and/or when the proprietary name may assist in identifying unique properties of the specific dosage form (eg, inherent electrolytes in amino acid formulations, fatty acids in lipid injectable emulsion [ILE]).[1,5] Any abbreviations should follow The Joint Commission standards on abbreviations.[5,9] Abbreviations on the Institute for Safe Medication Practices list of error-prone abbreviations, symbols, and dose designations should not be used.[10]

Prescribing a PN formulation that includes nonnutrient medications should be avoided. When no other reasonable alternatives exist, nonnutrient medications should only be included on the PN order if data support compatibility/stability.[1,2] PN orders should be prescribed with a time limitation to allow for appropriate patient evaluation at predetermined intervals based on clinical status and required level of care.[1,2,11,12]

The PN order template in CPOE systems should display current patient monitoring values and their date and time of entry to include parameters such as laboratory values, temperature, weight, and so forth. The PN order should include related orders for routine care, laboratory tests, and relevant monitoring parameters.[1,2] Recommendations for frequency of laboratory monitoring are as follows:

- Patients who are new to PN should be monitored daily until stable (more frequently if clinically significant metabolic abnormalities are found or patient is at risk for refeeding syndrome).[2]

- Patients in an unstable clinical condition (eg, acutely ill, critically ill, recovering from critical illness, recent surgery) should be monitored daily until stable (more frequently if clinically significant abnormalities are observed).[2]

- Stable patients in the hospital with no required changes in formulation for 1 week should be monitored every 2–7 days.[2]

- Stable patients in a hospital, in long-term care, or in a home setting with no changes in formulation for >1 week should be monitored every 1–4 weeks or longer for select clinically stable patients.[2]

Institutions should create a home PN order template/format that provides a safe plan for multiple days of therapy. The prescription for home PN therapy should be written in a format that specifically reflects trends in laboratory values and previous days of PN therapy.

Using a checklist when ordering PN will assure that all elements of the PN order are included and optimize communication between all members of the healthcare team. See Figure 5-3 for an example of a PN prescribing checklist.

Figure 5-3.

Prescribing PN **CHECKLIST**

The American Society for Parenteral and Enteral Nutrition (A.S.P.E.N.) champions the best evidence-based practices that support parenteral nutrition (PN) therapy in varying age populations and disease states. The appropriate use of this complex therapy aims to maximize clinical benefit while minimizing the potential risks for adverse events.

The purpose of this checklist is to promote safe practices by prescribers in developing optimal PN prescriptions using the best practices available.

☐ **Inform patient and caregivers of the risks and benefits associated with PN.**

☐ **Evaluate, clearly define, and accurately document the patient's medical problem(s) and appropriate indication(s) for PN based on published evidence.**

☐ **Specify and document PN therapeutic goals and monitoring parameters including:**
  ○ Energy and protein goals
  ○ Monitoring parameters and frequency of monitoring
   • Fluid requirements
   • Serum electrolytes
   • Serum glucose
   • Hepatic function
   • Renal function
   • Serum triglycerides
   • Assess vascular access
  ○ PN therapy end points, response to treatment, and treatment failure.

☐ **Prescribe PN in a medication safety zone to minimize errors.**

☐ **Use a standardized PN order format including a standardized sequence of PN components.**
  ○ PN order elements:
   • Patient named or other identifier
   • Birth date and/or age
   • Allergies and associated reactions
   • Height and dosing weight (metric units)
   • Diagnosis/diagnoses
   • Indication(s) for PN
   • Prescriber contact information
   • Date and time order submitted
   • Administration date and time
   • Volume and infusion rate
   • Infusion schedule (continuous or cyclic)
   • Type of formulation (dextrose/amino acids with separate infusion of IVFE or total nutrient admixture)
  ○ PN components:
   • Adults – ordered as amounts/day
   • Pediatrics - ordered as amounts/kg/day
   • Neonates - ordered as amounts/kg/day
   • A dose for each macronutrient
   • A dose for each electrolyte ordered as a complete salt form
   • A dose for multivitamins
   • A dose for individual vitamins, if ordered
   • A dose for multi-trace elements
   • A dose for individual trace elements, if ordered
   • A dose for insulin, if ordered
   • A dose for non-nutrient medications, if ordered

☐ **Use CPOE to prescribe PN**

☐ **Avoid handwritten orders**

☐ **Avoid verbal and telephone orders**

☐ **When a CPOE system is not available, PN should be prescribed using a standardized order template as an editable electronic document in order to avoid handwritten orders.**

☐ **Prescribe home/alternative site PN therapy using a home/alternative site PN-specific order/ template that allows for multiple days of therapy and reflects trends in laboratory values.**

CHAPTER 5

How to Prescribe Parenteral Nutrition Therapy

CPOE, computerized prescriber order entry; PN, parenteral nutrition.
Source: Reprinted with permission from ASPEN. Parenteral nutrition safety consensus recommendations and clinical guidelines. ASPEN website. http://www.nutritioncare.org/Guidelines_and_Clinical_Resources/ Toolkits/Parenteral_Nutrition_Safety_Toolkit/Parenteral_Nutrition_Safety_Consensus_Recommendations_ and_Clinical_Guidelines/. Accessed January 21, 2020.

General Considerations for Nutrient Requirements

Adult Patients

The usual goals for protein, carbohydrate, fat, and fluid intake for adult patients receiving PN are presented in Table 5-2.[1,13] Guidelines for mineral and electrolyte intake for adult patients are presented in Table 5-3.[1,14-16] Guidelines for vitamins and trace elements for adult patients may be found in chapter 4. Electrolytes may be manipulated to avoid electrolyte and acid-base imbalances. Although it is inappropriate to use PN to manage short-term fluid and electrolyte shifts, the fluid, mineral, and electrolyte content of PN is frequently individualized. Consideration is given to the patient's existing deficits, dry weight, ongoing losses, and changes in organ function or drug therapy. Generally, the patient should have satisfactory hydration, electrolyte, and acid-base status prior to initiating PN. Individualized PN may help balance hydration, electrolytes, and acid-base status. However, to best achieve nutrition goals with PN, fluid and metabolic abnormalities should be corrected as much as possible before PN initiation.

The initial PN formulation for adults is based on the ability to tolerate volume and macronutrients. Because protein intake in an adult is associated with minimal metabolic adverse effects, protein intake of 1–1.5 g/kg/d can be provided on day 1. The initial maximum carbohydrate given in an adult is usually 150–200 g/d. For adult patients with diabetes mellitus or hyperglycemia of stress, 100–150 g of dextrose per day can be administered initially.[17] For many adult patients, PN may be increased such that energy and protein goals are achieved within 72–96 hours. The dextrose content of the PN can be increased if the patient has capillary blood glucose values consistently ≤180 mg/dL. The ILE in the PN can be added or increased if the patient has serum triglycerides ≤400 mg/dL.

Table 5-2. Suggested Nutrient Intake for Adult Patients Receiving PN[a,1,13]

PN Component	Patients With Critical Illness	Stable Patients
Protein	1.5–2 g/kg/d	0.8–1 g/kg/d
Carbohydrate	≤4 mg/kg/min	4–5 mg/kg/min
ILE	≤1 g/kg/d	1 g/kg/d
Total energy	25–30 kcal/kg/d	20–30 kcal/kg/d[b]
Fluid	Minimum needed to deliver adequate macronutrients	30–40 mL/kg/d[c]

ILE, lipid injectable emulsion; PN, parenteral nutrition.
[a]Estimated dry weight is used as the basis of calculations.
[b]Varies according to activity levels.
[c]May vary if the patient has ongoing fluid losses.

Table 5-3. Daily Electrolyte Guidelines for Adult PN Formulations[14–16]

Nutrient	Standard Daily Requirementa	Factors That Increase Needs	Dosage Form
Calcium	10–15 mEq	High protein intake	Calcium gluconate
Magnesium	8–20 mEq	GI losses, drugs, refeeding	Magnesium sulfate
Phosphorus	20–40 mmol	High dextrose intake, refeeding	Sodium phosphate, potassium phosphate
Sodium	1–2 mEq/kg[a]	Diarrhea, vomiting, NG suction, GI losses	Sodium phosphate, sodium chloride, sodium acetate
Potassium	1–2 mEq/kg[b]	Diarrhea, vomiting, NG suction, medications, refeeding, GI losses	Potassium phosphate, potassium chloride, potassium acetate
Acetate	As needed to maintain acid-base balance	Renal insufficiency, metabolic acidosis, GI losses of bicarbonate	Sodium acetate, potassium acetate
Chloride	As needed to maintain acid-base balance	Metabolic alkalosis, volume depletion	Sodium chloride, potassium chloride

GI, gastrointestinal; NG, nasogastric.
[a]Standard intake ranges based on generally healthy people with normal losses.
[b]Multiple salts of these electrolytes may be provided for a total of 1–2 mEq/kg.

Pediatric and Neonatal Patients

The usual goals for energy, protein,[5,18,19] and fluid requirements[20,21] for pediatric patients receiving PN are presented in Tables 5-4, 5-5, and 5-6, and guidelines for electrolyte and mineral requirements[14-16] are presented in Table 5-7. Recommendations for vitamin dosages[22] are provided in Table 5-8 for pediatric PN formulations, with further information about specific vitamin and trace elements for pediatric and neonatal patients found in chapter 4.

Table 5-4. Daily Energy Requirements for Pediatric Patients[a,5,18,19]

Age	Total Daily Energy Requirements (kcal/kg)
Preterm neonate	90–120
<6 mo	85–105
6–12 mo	80–100
1–7 y	75–90
7–12 y	50–75
12–18 y	30–50

[a]Assumes normal age-related organ function and normal losses.

Table 5-5. Daily Protein Requirements for Pediatric Patients[a,5,18,19]

Age	Daily Protein Requirements (g/kg/d)
Preterm neonate	3–4
Infants	2–3
Children (>10 kg or 1–10 y of age)	1–2
Adolescents (11–17 y of age)	0.8–1.5

[a]Assumes normal age-related organ function and normal losses.

Table 5-6. Daily Fluid Requirements for Pediatric Patients[a,20,21]

Body Weight	Fluid Requirements (mL/kg)
<1-1.5 kg	150
1.5-2.5 kg	120
First 10 kg	100
Second 10 kg	50
Each additional kilogram	20

[a]Assumes normal age-related organ function and normal losses.

Table 5-7. Daily Electrolyte and Mineral Requirements for Pediatric Patients[a,14-16]

Electrolyte	Preterm Neonates	Infants/Children	Adolescents and children > 50 kg
Sodium	2-5 mEq/kg	2-5 mEq/kg	1-2 mEq/kg
Potassium	2-4 mEq/kg	2-4 mEq/kg	1-2 mEq/kg
Calcium	2-4 mEq/kg	0.5-4 mEq/kg	10-20 mEq/d
Phosphorus	1-2 mmol/kg	0.5-2 mmol/kg	10-40 mmol/d
Magnesium	0.3-0.5 mEq/kg	0.3-0.5 mEq/kg	10-30 mEq/d
Acetate	As needed to maintain acid-base balance	As needed to maintain acid-base balance	As needed to maintain acid-base balance
Chloride	As needed to maintain acid-base balance	As needed to maintain acid-base balance	As needed to maintain acid-base balance

[a]Assumes normal age-related organ function.

Table 5-8. Daily Dose Recommendations for Pediatric Multivitamins[a,18,22]

Manufacturer		AMA-NAG	
Weight (kg)	Dose	Weight (kg)	Dose
<1	1.5 mL	<2.5	2 mL/kg
1–3	3.25 mL	>2.5	5 mL
>3	5 mL		

AMA-NAG, American Medical Association Nutrition Advisory Group.

[a]Assumes normal age-related organ function. Pediatric multivitamin formulation (5 mL): A, 2300 United States Pharamcopeia units; D, 400 United States Pharamcopeia units; E, 7 United States Pharamcopeia units; K, 200 mcg; ascorbic acid, 80 mg; thiamin, 1.2 mg; riboflavin, 1.4 mg; niacin, 17 mg; pantothenic acid, 5 mg; pyridoxine, 1 mg; cyanocobalamin, 1 mcg; biotin, 20 mcg; folic acid, 140 mcg.

The initiation rate of PN for neonatal and pediatric patients will often replace maintenance intravenous fluids, thereby meeting maintenance fluid requirements. Generally, the time to reach energy and protein goals with PN is inversely related to age. For example, 3–5 days of PN therapy (advanced incrementally each day) is generally required for neonatal patients before nutrition goals are reached, whereas for children and adolescents, PN goals can often be met in 48–72 hours. Daily protein requirements are inversely related to developmental age and weight. In preterm neonates, protein requirements exceed 2.5 g/kg/d, whereas requirements in healthy individuals decline to about 1.5–2 g/kg/d around 1 year of age. By adolescence, the requirements approach adult values, generally ranging from 0.8–1.5 g/kg/d. In the early years of PN therapy, it was common practice for clinicians to initiate protein in neonates at lower doses that would gradually be advanced to goal over several days. This practice has largely been abandoned because of the lack of evidence to support it and the benefits documented with early initiation of amino acids in premature infants (ie, ≥2–2.5 g/kg/d within a few hours after birth).[23,24]

Dextrose infusions are generally initiated at doses that approximate endogenous glucose production rates (about 6–8 mg/kg/min for neonates and infants) and are increased gradually in daily increments until energy goals are achieved or the maximum of 12–14 mg/kg/min is reached (about 20 g/kg/d).[25] The upper limit of carbohydrate intake appears to peak between the ages of 1 and 3 years and gradually decreases with age, approaching adult values (4–5 mg/kg/min or 7 g/kg/d) during adolescence (8–10 mg/kg/min or 12–14 g/kg/d).[26] When ILE is administered to supplement nonprotein energy, dextrose intake at or below the upper limit is generally sufficient for adequate weight gain.

ILE provides a concentrated source of energy and prevents essential fatty acid deficiency (EFAD). Preterm neonates are especially prone to developing EFAD because of low body fat stores. For neonates receiving PN, ILE should be initiated within 3 days of birth. It is usually started at doses of 1.5–2 g/kg/d and advanced daily (in increments of 0.5–1 g/kg/d) to a goal dose of 3 g/kg/d. For term neonates, infants, and children, ILE is commonly initiated at 1.5–2 g/kg/d and advanced daily to a goal of 2–3 g/kg/d for children and generally 2 g/kg/d for adolescents.[27,28]

After a review of organ function, medication profile, and serum concentrations, electrolytes are adjusted according to the following general guidelines:

1. Because magnesium, phosphorus, and potassium needs increase with anabolism and are carbohydrate dependent, repletion levels of these minerals may be needed for the first few days of PN. However, neonates starting PN within 24 hours after birth should receive only calcium for the first day.

2. Potassium, magnesium, and phosphorus administration is adjusted according to changes in the serum concentrations, acid-base balance, drug therapy, and the use of renal replacement or dialysis therapy.

Elevated serum or capillary glucose concentrations or fluid volume intolerance may preclude an increase in dextrose intake or PN volume, respectively. If fluid restriction is necessary, the required amounts of protein and energy substrate are concentrated within the volume tolerated.

Sample Calculations

Figure 5-4 illustrates one method of calculating the appropriate amounts of dextrose, amino acids, and ILE for manual preparation of a PN admixture (ie, in an institution that does not use an automated compounding device and does not prepare total nutrient admixtures). Figure 5-5 depicts the calculations for a fluid-restricted PN formulation (ie, 1.5 L/d) with the same provision of energy and protein. The calculations are based on the use of commercially available products. Figure 5-6 illustrates calculations for a pediatric PN formulation.

Figure 5-4. Calculation of PN Formulation

Calculations

Energy: 30 kcal/kg/d × 80 kg = 2400 total kcal/d.

Protein: 1.5 g/kg/d × 80 kg = 120 g/d.

ILE range (20%–30% of total kcal/d): 2400 kcal/d × 0.2 = 480 kcal/d to 2400 kcal/d × 0.3 = 720 kcal/d.

Fluid: 30–40 mL/kg/d × 80 kg = 2400–3200 mL/d.

Using amounts amenable to manual compounding

ILE: 250 mL of ILE 20% × 2 kcal/mL = 500 ILE kcal.

Therefore, % goal energy as ILE = 500 kcal ÷ 2400 kcal = 21%.

Energy to be supplied as dextrose and protein = 2400 kcal − 500 kcal = 1900 kcal/d.

Energy to be supplied by protein (amino acids) = 120 g/d × 4 kcal/g = 480 kcal/d.

Therefore, energy to be supplied by dextrose to reach goal = 1900 kcal − 480 kcal = 1420 kcal/d.

This represents 1420 kcal ÷ 3.4 kcal/g = 418 g dextrose.

Choosing amino acids 8.5% for compounding,

8.5 g/100 mL = 120 g/x mL; solving for x yields 1411 mL of amino acids 8.5%; round off to 1400 mL, which contains 119 g protein.

Therefore, 119 g protein × 4 kcal/g = 476 kcal from protein.

Choosing dextrose 30% for compounding,

30 g/100 mL = 418 g/x mL; solving for x yields 1393 mL of dextrose 30%; round off to 1400 mL, which contains 420 g dextrose.

Therefore, 420 g dextrose × 3.4 kcal/g = 1428 kcal from dextrose.

Therefore, total energy from regimen of 1400 mL of dextrose 30% + 1400 mL of amino acids 8.5% + ILE 20% 250 mL = 1428 + 476 + 500 = 2404 kcal/d.

Determining administration rate

Amino acid/dextrose: 1400 mL amino acid + 1400 mL dextrose = 2800 mL/d. Add 30 mL/L to approximate the volume of additives: 30 mL/L × 2.8 L/d = 84 mL/d from additives.

2800 mL + 84 mL = 2884 mL/d

2884 mL/d per 24 h/d = 120 mL/h for dextrose/amino acid formulation.

ILE: 250 mL/d = 21 mL/h over approximately 12 h if administered separately.

ILE, lipid injectable emulsion; PN, parenteral nutrition.

Figure 5-5. Calculation for Fluid-Restricted PN Formulation

Scenario 1:

Stock solutions used by the pharmacy for compounding PN are amino acids 10%, dextrose 70%, and ILE 20%. PN formulations are manually compounded (without an ACD) as 2-in-1 formulations.

CALCULATIONS

Using amounts amenable to manual compounding:

Amino acids 10%: 1000 mL yields 100 g; 100 g × 4 kcal/g yields 400 kcal/d.
Dextrose 70%: 250 mL yields 175 g; 175 g × 3.4 kcal/g yields 595 kcal/d.
ILE 20%: 250 mL × 2 kcal/mL yields 500 kcal/d; the ILE is infused separately.

Therefore, 400 + 595 + 500 = 1495 kcal/d in 1500 mL/d.

Scenario 2:

Stock solutions used by the pharmacy for compounding PN are amino acids 20%, dextrose 70%, and ILE 30%. The pharmacy compounds TNA solutions with an ACD.

CALCULATIONS

Amino acids 20%: 20 g/100 mL = 120 g/x mL; solving for x yields amino acids 20% 600 mL.

120 g amino acids × 4 kcal/g = 480 kcal/d from amino acids.

ILE provides 20%–30% of total energy as ILE:

2400 kcal/d × 0.2 to 0.3 = 480–720 kcal/d.

Because the PN admixture volume is restricted to 1.5 L/d, provide 30% of energy or 720 kcal/d with ILE 30%, which is more energy dense (3 kcal/mL) than dextrose 70% (2.38 kcal/mL).

ILE 30% provides 3 kcal/mL; therefore, 720 kcal/d ÷ 3 kcal/mL = 240 mL.

Dextrose: energy needed from dextrose = 2400 kcal − 480 kcal from amino acids − 720 kcal from ILE = 1200 kcal/d.

1200 kcal ÷ 3.4 kcal/g = 353 g dextrose.

Dextrose 70% provides 70 g/100 mL = 353 g/0.7 = 504 mL.

Thus, the volume for the macronutrients is amino acids 20% (600 mL) + ILE 30% (240 mL) + dextrose 70% (504 mL) = 1344 mL/d. Additives including electrolytes, parenteral multivitamins, and trace elements will provide an additional 100–120 mL/d depending on dosages used. A final volume of 1500 mL/d or less can be achieved.

ACD, automated compounding device; ILE, lipid injectable emulsion; PN, parenteral nutrition; TNA, total nutrient admixture.

Figure 5-6. Calculation of Pediatric Parenteral Nutrition Formulation

Pediatric PN Calculations

Patient Specifics: neonate, 38 weeks' gestation, 3.4 kg, now day of life 3
Status after repair of duodenal atresia with end to end anastomosis
Central venous line placed in surgery
Currently receiving dextrose 5%, NaCl 0.22% with KCl 20 mEq/L
Serum laboratory values are within normal limits

Step 1: Determine PN Infusion Rate and Total Daily Volume

PN volume is based on maintenance fluid requirements: 100 mL/kg/d × 3.4 kg = 340 mL/d.

PN infusion rate = 340 mL/d divided by 24 h/d = 14.2 mL/h (consider rounding this to 14 mL/h to avoid potential infusion pump programming errors associated with numbers with decimals).

Step 2: Determine the Daily Amino Acid Dose and Energy Provided

Use pediatric amino acid product because patient is a neonate.
Daily amino acid dose = 2.5 g/kg/d × 3.4 kg = 8.5 g/d.

Energy provided by amino acids (protein) = 8.5 g × 4 kcal/g = 34 kcal/3.4 kg = 10 kcal/kg/d.

Step 3: Determine the Corresponding Dose of L-cysteine

L-cysteine dose is based on amino acid dose (40 mg L-cysteine per gram of amino acid) =
40 mg/g × 8.5 g = 340 mg L-cysteine.

Step 4: Determine the Daily Dextrose Concentration and Energy Provided

Begin with dextrose intake equivalent to dextrose10%, as the neonate is already receiving dextrose 5%, and serum laboratory values are within normal limits.

Dextrose 10% = 10 g dextrose/100, 100 mL × 340 mL = 34 g/d dextrose.

Energy provided by dextrose = 34 g × 3.4 kcal/g = 115.6 kcal/3.4 kg = 34 kcal/kg/d.

Step 5: Determine the Electrolyte and Mineral Content

Calcium: 2.5 mEq/kg = 8.5 mEq calcium gluconate.

Phosphorus: 1 mmol/kg (as sodium or potassium phosphate) = 3.4 mmol phosphorus.

Then determine the amount of sodium or phosphate provided by the phosphate salt:

1 mmol sodium phosphate provides 1 mmol phosphate and 1.33 mEq sodium.
1 mmol potassium phosphate provides 1 mmol phosphate and 0.1.47 mEq.

Potassium: If you give the phosphorous as sodium phosphate, the amount of sodium provided is 4.5 mEq (1 mmol/kg × 3.4 kg =3.4 mmol phosphate × 1.33 = 4.5 mEq sodium).

Magnesium: 0.4 mEq/kg × 3.4 kg = 1.4 mEq magnesium sulfate.

Sodium: Currently receiving IVF with NaCl 0.22%, which has a sodium content of sodium 38.5 mEq/L. The IVF infuses at 14.2 mL/h = 340 mL/d or 0.34 L/d.

The sodium provided by this IVF = 38.5 mEq/L × 0.34 L = 13 mEq sodium.

In determining the amount of sodium to add to the PN, the sodium from the sodium phosphate (4.5 mEq) must be considered. Total sodium 13 mEq less 4.5 mEq sodium from sodium phosphate = 8.5 mEq sodium to be given as chloride and/or acetate salts. Because this is a term neonate with normal serum laboratory values, initiate PN with the remainder of sodium anion as chloride and plan to adjust PN (ie, add acetate) as needed basis to maintain acid-base balance.

Potassium: Currently receiving IVF with KCl 20 mEq/L. To determine the amount of potassium provided: 20 mEq/L × 0.34 L = 6.8 mEq potassium.

All potassium will be given as the chloride salt because phosphorus and acetate needs have already been addressed with sodium.

Step 6: Determine the Multivitamin and Trace Element Content

Multivitamin dose: 5 mL/d based on weight of 3.4 kg (per manufacturer labeling and AMA-NAG guidelines; see Table 5-8).

Trace elements: give with a multiple trace element product or via individualized trace element products (see chapter 4 for more specific information).

Step 7: Determine ILE Dose, Volume, Rate, and Calories Provided

Begin with 1 g/kg/d × 3.4 kg = 3.4 g/d.
Using ILE 20% = 20 g per 100 mL; 2 kcal/mL.
3.4 g divided by 0.2 (100 mL/20 g) = ILE 20% 17 mL/d.

ILE infusion rate = 17 mL divided by 24 h = 0.7 mL/h.

Energy provided by ILE = 0.7 mL/h × 24 h/d = 16.8 mL × 2 kcal/mL = 33.6 kcal/3.4 kg = 10 kcal/kg/d.

Step 8: Summarize Final PN and ILE Regimen and Energy Provided

PN to infuse at 14.2 mL/h = 340.8 mL/d.
ILE to infuse at 0.7 mL/h = 16.8 mL/d.
Total volume/d = 357.6 mL/3.4 kg = 105 mL/kg/d.

Energy provided:

Protein   10 kcal/kg/d
Dextrose   34 kcal/kg/d
ILE   10 kcal/kg/d

Energy provided on day 1 PN/ILE = 54 kcal/kg/d.

AMA-NAG, American Medical Association Nutrition Advisory Group; IVF, intravenous fluid; ILE, lipid injectable emulsion; PN, parenteral nutrition.

References

1. Mirtallo J, Canada T, Johnson D, et al; ASPEN Board of Directors and Task Force for the Revision of Safe Practices for Parenteral Nutrition. Safe practices for parenteral nutrition [erratum in *JPEN J Parenter Enteral Nutr.* 2006;30(2):177]. *JPEN J Parenter Enteral Nutr.* 2004;28(6):S39–S70.

2. Ayers P, Adams S, Boullata J, et al; ASPEN. A.S.P.E.N. parenteral nutrition safety consensus recommendations. *JPEN J Parenter Enteral Nutr.* 2014;38(3):296–333.

3. Kochevar M, Guenter P, Holcombe B, Malone A, Mirtallo J; ASPEN Board of Directors and Task Force on Parenteral Nutrition Standardization. A.S.P.E.N. statement on parenteral nutrition standardization. *JPEN J Parenter Enteral Nutr.* 2007;31(5):441–448.

4. MacKay M, Anderson C, Boehme S, Cash J, Zobell J. Frequency and Severity of Parenteral Nutrition Medication Errors at a Large Children's Hospital After Implementation of Electronic Ordering and Compounding. *NCP Nutr Clin Pract.* 2016 Apr;31(2):195-206. doi: 10.1177/0884533615591606.

5. Jacobson JO, Polovich M, Gilmore TR, et al. Revisions to the 2009 American Society of Clinical Oncology/Oncology Nursing Society chemotherapy administration safety standards: expanding the scope to include inpatient settings. *Oncol Nurs Forum.* 2012;39(1):31–38.

6. Maat B, Rademaker Carin MA, Oostveen MI, Krediet TG, Egberts TC, Bollen CW. The effect of a computerized prescribing and calculating system on hypo- and hyperglycemias and on prescribing time efficiency in neonatal intensive care patients. *JPEN J Parenter Enteral Nutr.* 2013;37(1):85–91.

7. Shamliyan TA, Duval S, Du J, Kane RL. Just what the doctor ordered: review of the evidence of the impact of computerized physician order entry on medication errors. *Health Serv Res.* 2008;43(1 pt. 1):32–53.

8. Brown CL, Garrison NA, Hutchinson AA. Error reduction when prescribing neonatal parenteral nutrition. *Am J Perinatol.* 2007;24(7):417–427.

9. The Joint Commission. *Comprehensive Accreditation Manual for Hospitals: The Official Handbook.* Oak Brook, IL: Joint Commission Resources; 2013.

10. Institute for Safe Medication Practices. List of error-prone abbreviations, symbols, and dose designations. ISMP website. http://www.ismp.org/tools/errorproneabbreviations. pdf. Accessed September 21, 2012.

11. de Vries TPGM, Henning RH, Hogerzeil HV, Fresle DA; World Health Organization. *Guide to Good Prescribing: A Practical Manual.* Geneva, Switzerland: World Health Organization Action Programme on Essential Drugs; 1994. http://apps.who.int/medicinedocs/pdf/whozip23e/whozip23e.pdf. Accessed May 20, 2012.

12. Pollock M, Bazaldua O, Dobie A. Appropriate prescribing of medications: an eight-step approach. *Am Fam Physician.* 2007;75(2):231–236, 239–240.

13. McClave SA[1], Taylor BE[2], Martindale RG[3], Warren MM[4], Johnson DR[5], Braunschweig C[6], McCarthy MS[7], Davanos E[8], Rice TW[9], Cresci GA[10], Gervasio JM[11], Sacks GS[12], Roberts PR[13], Compher C[14]; Society of Critical Care Medicine; ASPEN. Guidelines for the Provision and Assessment of Nutrition Support Therapy in the Adult Critically Ill Patient: Society of Critical Care Medicine (SCCM) and American Society for Parenteral and Enteral Nutrition (A.S.P.E.N.). *JPEN J Parenter Enteral Nutr.* 2016 Feb;40(2):159-211. doi: 10.1177/0148607115621863.

14. Derenski K, Catlin J, Allen L. Parenteral nutrition basics for the clinician caring for the adult patient. *Nutrition in Clinical Practice.* 2016;31(5):578-595.

15. Institute of Medicine. Minerals. In: *Recommended Dietary Allowances.* 10th ed. Washington, DC: National Academy Press; 1989:174–194.

16. Baumgartner TG. *Clinical Guide to Parenteral Micronutrition.* 3rd ed. Deerfield, IL: Fujisawa USA; 1997.

17. Rudman D, Millikan WJ, Richardson TJ, Bixler TJ 2nd, Stackhouse J, McGarrity WC. Elemental balances during intravenous hyperalimentation of underweight adult subjects. *J Clin Invest.* 1975:55(1):94–104.

18. ASPEN Board of Directors and the Clinical Guidelines Task Force. Guidelines for the use of parenteral and enteral nutrition in adult and pediatric patients [erratum in *JPEN J Parenter Enteral Nutr*. 2002;26(2):144]. *JPEN J Parenter Enteral Nutr*. 2002;26(1 suppl):1SA–138SA.

19. American Medical Association Department of Foods and Nutrition. Multivitamin preparations for parenteral use: a statement by the Nutrition Advisory Group. *JPEN J Parenter Enteral Nutr*. 1979:3(4):258–262.

20. American Medical Association Department of Foods and Nutrition. Guidelines for essential trace element preparations for parenteral use: a statement by an expert panel. *JAMA*. 1979;241(19):2051–2054.

21. Food and Nutrition Board, National Academy of Sciences, Institute of Medicine. *Recommended Dietary Allowances*. 10th ed. Washington, DC: National Academy Press; 1989.

22. Gallagher-Allred C. Fluid and electrolyte requirements. In: Krey SH, Murrar RL, eds. *Dynamics of Nutrition Support*. Norwalk, CT: Appleton-Century-Crofts; 1986:249–275.

23. Vanek VW, Borum P, Buchman A, et al; Novel Nutrient Task Force, Parenteral Multi-Vitamin and Multi–Trace Element Working Group; ASPEN Board of Directors. A.S.P.E.N. position paper: recommendations for changes in commercially available parenteral multivitamin and multi-trace element products. *NCP Nutr Clin Pract*. 2012;27(4):440–491.

24. Denne SC, Poindexter BB. Evidence supporting early nutritional support with parenteral amino acid infusion. *Semin Perinatol*. 2007;31(2):56–60.

25. Shulman RJ, Phillips S. Parenteral nutrition in infants and children. *J Pediatr Gastroenterol Nutr*. 2003;36(5):587–607.

26. McMahon M, Manji N, Driscoll DF, Bistrian BR. Parenteral nutrition in patients with diabetes mellitus: theoretical and practical considerations. *JPEN J Parenter Enteral Nutr*. 1989;13(5):545–553.

27. Kalhan SC, Kiliç I. Carbohydrate as nutrient in the infant and child: range of acceptable intake. *Eur J Clin Nutr*. 1999;53(suppl 1):S94–S100.

28. Ben XM. Nutritional management of newborn infants: practical guidelines. *World J Gastroenterol*. 2008;14(40):6133–6139.

29. Ibrahim HM, Jeroudi MA, Baier RJ, Dhanireddy R, Krouskop RW. Aggressive early total parenteral nutrition in low-birth-weight infants. *J Perinatol*. 2004;24(8):482–486.

CHAPTER 6

Review and Verification of Parenteral Nutrition Orders, Preparing Parenteral Nutrition Formulations, and Labeling

Introduction

This chapter describes the steps of the parenteral nutrition (PN) process that occur once PN is prescribed and the order is transmitted to the pharmacy. These steps include review and verification of the PN order, compounding/preparing the PN formulation, and labeling the PN admixture.

PN orders should be prescribed, transmitted to the pharmacy, reviewed and verified, and compounded when supported by properly trained and competent personnel who regularly perform this task. This process usually takes place during the daytime hours.[1]

PN Order Review and Verification

Before any PN order is compounded, it is reviewed and verified by a knowledgeable pharmacist for safety, efficacy, and appropriateness. The verification process ensures that the order is clear, complete, and timely and that an appropriate vascular access is in place for new patients beginning PN.[1-3] This is the opportunity to identify and correct the many errors in PN prescribing.[4]

117

The review process includes both a clinical review and a pharmaceutical review. Unfortunately, the pharmacist review did not exist in many organizations, with 23% dedicating no full-time staff to this critical step, according to a national survey.[5] The clinical review evaluates each macronutrient, each micronutrient, and any nonnutrient medication to confirm that each dose meets the patient's needs based on indication, body weight, organ function, current laboratory values, and other medications and is consistent with the most recent care plan.

The pharmaceutical review is conducted to assess the compatibility of the prescribed PN components and the expected stability of the formulation.[1,2] This review will ensure that each component is compatible with every other component at the prescribed doses and volumes, and that the final admixture remains stable through the end of infusion. A specific example is provided within the PN preparation section, but components should be evaluated during the distinct safety step of PN order review prior to preparation. An independent double-check will be required if there was any transcription or calculation that took place during review.

Using a checklist to standardize the review and verification processes ensures that all elements are included and that the order is complete and has been evaluated for safety (see Figure 6-1: "PN Order Review and Verification Checklist"). Identification of missing elements, errors, or safety concerns requires follow-up with the prescriber and clarification of the order.[1] Any interventions to clarify or correct the PN order can be documented for future compilation and evaluation.

PN Preparation

Admixtures: Dextrose/Amino Acids vs Total Nutrient Admixtures

PN formulations may be prepared for administration in one of 2 types. The 2-in-1 formulation incorporates 2 macronutrients (dextrose and amino acids) in a single base solution along with the prescribed micronutrients (electrolytes, vitamins, and trace elements) in 1 or multiple containers each day. Lipid injectable emulsion (ILE) is administered separately as a piggyback infusion.

Figure 6-1.

PN Order Review and Verification
CHECKLIST

The **American Society for Parenteral and Enteral Nutrition** (A.S.P.E.N.) champions the best evidence-based practices that support parenteral nutrition therapy in varying age populations and disease states. The appropriate use of this complex therapy aims to maximize clinical benefit while minimizing the potential risks for adverse events.

The **purpose of this checklist** is to promote safe practices by pharmacists and other clinicians in the PN order review and verification process.

☐ **Verify PN order elements for:**
- ☐ Patient name- or other identifier
- ☐ Birth date and/or age
- ☐ Allergies and associated reactions
- ☐ Height and dosing weight (metric units)
- ☐ Diagnosis/diagnoses
- ☐ Indication(s) for PN
- ☐ Administration route/ vascular access device (peripheral vs central)
- ☐ Prescriber contact information
- ☐ Date and time order submitted
- ☐ Administration date and time
- ☐ Volume and infusion rate
- ☐ Infusion schedule (continuous or cyclic)
- ☐ Type of formulation (dextrose/amino acids with separate infusion of IVFE or total nutrient admixture)

☐ **Verify PN ingredients for:**
- ☐ Adults - amounts/day
- ☐ Pediatrics - amounts/kg/day
- ☐ Neonates - amounts/kg/day
- ☐ Electrolytes as complete salt form
- ☐ A dose for each macronutrient
- ☐ A dose for each electrolyte
- ☐ A dose for multivitamins
- ☐ A dose for individual vitamins, if ordered
- ☐ A dose for multi-trace elements
- ☐ A dose for individual trace elements, if ordered
- ☐ A dose for insulin, if ordered
- ☐ A dose for non-nutrient medications, if ordered

☐ **Perform clinical review of PN order for:**
- ☐ Indication consistent with published guidelines
- ☐ Appropriate dose of each additive
- ☐ Appropriate osmolarity for route of administration (peripheral vs. central)

☐ **Compare order to previous day's order to assess component doses for substantial changes**

☐ **Perform PN order safety review for:**
- ☐ Compatibility of ingredients
- ☐ Stability of formulation

☐ **Perform independent double-check for:**
- ☐ Transcribed order data prior to compounding
- ☐ Calculations or conversion of units of measure

In contrast, the total nutrient admixture (TNA) system, also referred to as a 3-in-1 or all-in-one admixture, incorporates dextrose, amino acids, and ILE along with the other prescribed micronutrients together in a single container for administration. Specific advantages and disadvantages associated with the use of each PN formulation system are outlined in Table 6-1.

Table 6-1. Advantages and Disadvantages of the TNA System

Advantages and Disadvantages of the Total Nutrient Admixture System

Advantages:
- All components are aseptically compounded by the pharmacy.
- Preparation is more efficient for pharmacy personnel, especially when it is automated.
- Administering TNA involves less manipulation than administering 2-in-1 formulations plus separate ILE, and there is therefore less risk of contamination of the system during administration.
- If contamination does occur, the bacterial growth is more inhibited or slower with TNA than with separate ILE, although there is no clinical difference in infectious complications between 2-in-1 vs 3-in-1 formulations.

- TNA may be more cost-effective overall in certain settings:
  - It requires less nursing time because it is administered via a single container per day and there is no piggyback ILE to administer.
  - The supply and equipment expenses are lower with TNA because only 1 infusion pump and IV tubing are needed.
- In home care settings, TNA is more convenient to store, involves fewer supplies, and is easier to administer.
- In some situations, dextrose and venous access tolerance may be better with TNA than with 2-in-1 formulations.
- TNA may have possible applications in fluid-restricted patients because ILE 30% is restricted to use in TNA.
- Fat clearance may be better when ILE is administered over more than 12 hours.

Disadvantages:
- Larger particle size of admixed ILE precludes use of 0.22-μm (bacteria-eliminating) filter and requires the larger pore size filter of 1.2 μm.
- Admixed ILE is less stable and more prone to separation of lipid components.
- TNA formulations are more sensitive to destabilization with greater divalent and monovalent electrolyte concentrations.
- TNA formulations are more sensitive to destabilization with low concentrations of dextrose and amino acids.
- TNA formulation may be unstable when the final concentration of ILE is low.
- Compatibility and solubility of calcium gluconate and sodium/potassium phosphate are less in TNA formulations than in 2-in-1 formulations.
- Lower pH amino acid formulations may destabilize the ILE portion of admixture.
- It is difficult to visualize precipitate or particulate material in the opaque admixture.
- Certain medications are incompatible with the ILE portion of TNA.
- The risk for catheter occlusion is greater and the catheter lifespan is shorter with daily ILE.

- TNA is less stable over time than dextrose–amino acid PN formulations with separate ILE.

ILE, lipid injectable emulsion; IV, intravenous; PN, parenteral nutrition; TNA, total nutrient admixture.
Source: Reprinted with permission from Patel R. Parenteral nutrition formulations In: Mueller CM, ed. *The ASPEN Adult Nutrition Support Core Curriculum.* 3rd ed. Silver Spring, MD: American Society for Parenteral and Enteral Nutrition; 2017.

National Standards for Compounded Sterile Preparations: PN Compounding

Compounding an accurate formulation free of microbial and particulate matter is essential to ensuring the safe administration of PN. The United States Pharmacopeia (USP) is a private, nonprofit organization recognized by the federal government as the official group responsible for setting national standards for drug purity and safety. USP General Chapter <797> *Pharmaceutical Compounding—Sterile Preparations* is an official monograph enforceable by regulatory agencies concerning the procedures and requirements for the pharmaceutical compounding of sterile products.[6] Chapter <797> is currently under revision at the time of this publication, with expected updates having been put on hold. The most current Chapter <797> identifies 3 different risk levels (low, medium, and high) for each compounded sterile product (CSP) based on the potential for microbial contamination. Risk level assessment is important because storage and expiration limits of CSPs are assigned based on risk level. *Beyond-use dating* is the terminology for what was formerly referred to as expiration dating. The beyond-use dating of individual CSPs cannot exceed the limits delineated in Chapter <797> unless formal sterility testing is performed.

Levels of risk assessment and beyond-use dating guidelines for CSPs based on risk level are outlined in Table 6-2; these represent maximum beyond-use dating. For example, a pharmacy-prepared PN formulation stored at room temperature (20°C–25°C) cannot be used after 30 hours, whereas a PN formulation stored under refrigeration has a beyond-use date of up to 9 days after preparation. This is based solely on sterility concerns, without taking into account compatibility or stability, which could be shorten the beyond-use date. Therefore, certain PN formulations, particularly those mixed as a TNAs and those with maximum calcium and phosphate concentrations, may have shorter beyond-use dating because of stability and/or compatibility issues.

Healthcare organizations that do not possess the technological resources or staffing to prepare PN admixtures according to USP Chapter <797> should consider outsourcing PN production to a sterile compounding facility.[7]

Table 6-2. Risk Level Classification and Beyond-Use Dating Guidelines for Compounded Sterile Preparations[a]

| | | Beyond-Use Dating | |
| | | Room, 20°C–25°C | Refrigeration, 2°C–8°C |
Risk Level	Examples		
Low	Reconstitution of a single dose vial of lyophilized powder with a sterile diluent for transfer into another container; eg, pediatric parenteral multivitamins	48 h	14 d
Medium	Mixing of multiple manufactured additives for transfer into a large-volume parenteral solution; eg, PN formulations	30 h	9 d
High	Preparation of nonsterile powder for intravenous infusion; eg, extemporaneously compounded L-glutamine for supplementation in PN formulation	24 h	3 d

Source: Reprinted with permission from Barber JR, Sacks GS. Parenteral nutrition formulations. In: Mueller CM, ed. *The ASPEN Adult Nutrition Support Core Curriculum.* 3rd ed. Silver Spring, MD: ASPEN; 2017.
[a]Chapter <797> is currently under review/revision.

Compounding Methods

PN formulations may be compounded manually or with the use of automated compounding devices (ACDs). With manual compounding, the base formulation (ie, dextrose, amino acids, and sterile water for injection) may be aseptically mixed by hand or, more typically, by gravity through the use of a gravimetric compounder. After the base formulation has been made, all additional additives are drawn up in individual syringes prior to being added to the PN formulation. Verification of manual additives requires inspection of the actual vials and syringes that contain the additives before admixing. Proxy methods of verification such as the syringe pull-back method of verification should not be used in the preparation of PN formulations.[1] When the manual compounding method is used, the process should be standardized to promote safety and efficacy. A checklist should be incorporated into the manual process.[1]

ACDs originally were developed to assist with streamlining the manufacturing sequence for PN admixtures. The main advantage of ACDs is enhanced accuracy of the dosage form. Instead of trying to compound easily measured volumes (eg, 250- or 500-mL increments for amino acids or dextrose), any volume (generally >10 mL) of a formulation can be programmed for pumping from large stock containers by the ACD. Not only can PN formulations be more easily tailored to meet patient-specific needs, but the technology should improve accuracy, enforce the proper compounding sequence, and reduce opportunities for human-touch contamination.[1] All features of the ACD should be incorporated into the compounding process to optimize safety. During the initial setup, the vendor-validated process and the setup should be performed by 2 staff members using an independent double-check process. All additives and base solutions shall be verbally affirmed during the setup. Barcode technology should be used to verify products during the setup and replacement of ingredients. Tubing should be traced from the source container to the port where it attaches to the ACD.[1] When an ACD is used, manual compounding should be restricted to PN component volumes that the ACD cannot accurately deliver. Manual compounding may also be used if there is an interaction between the PN component and a component on the ACD, or between 2 PN components that cannot be mitigated by sequencing the addition of the ingredients. Such potential incompatibilities should be recognized during the PN order review step. Furthermore, limits or alerts can be placed on the doses of each PN component and automated in the ACD database. A soft limit is an alert to an unusual dose and requires more evaluation. Hard (catastrophic) limits refer to alerts that indicate a component is outside the determined safe range and should not be exceeded. Clinical limits vary by the patient population (ie, neonates, pediatrics, adults). These built-in alerts and any other changes made to the ACD database should be restricted to a limited number of pharmacy staff and any changes.[1]

For institutions compounding more than a few PN formulations per day, ACDs are associated with decreased pharmacy labor and supply costs. Ultimately, ACDs enable clinicians to administer safer and more precise PN formulations to patients.

Quality Control

At least 3 verification processes should occur in the pharmacy during the preparation process: (1) after the initial order entry, whether with a manual or electronic interface, of PN into the ACD, (2) before manually injecting additives into the PN, and (3) once the PN has been compounded.

Chapter <797> also describes the procedures for ensuring the accuracy and precision of the compounding process.[6] See Table 6-3 for a review of these quality procedures.[8,9]

Standardized Commercial PN Products: Multichamber-Bags

In addition to manual or automated methods for compounding PN formulation from the individual components as already discussed, there are several standardized commercially available PN products (see chapter 4 and chapter 12 for additional information on these products).[9] These multichamber products require manipulation of the container to mix the separated macronutrient components together. The products serve as a starting point for compounding in the pharmacy. Following activation and mixing of the chamber contents, addition of prescribed micronutrients is performed manually in the pharmacy prior to labeling and dispensing.

Table 6-3. Quality Assurance Procedures for the Compounding Process

Criteria	Definition
Accuracy	
Volumetric	Assess the accuracy of the compounder to deliver both small and large volumes of additives.
Gravimetric	Assess the accuracy of the compounder to deliver the appropriate amounts of the additives. Weight-based delivery of PN additives is the principal method by which automated compounders prepare PN formulations. In general, as a final check, the PN formulation is weighed and is expected to be within an acceptable margin of error. Compounders can evaluate weight of total contents as well as weight of individual additives. Evaluating weight of total contents and individual additives is preferred when using additives with a narrow margin of safety, such as potassium.
Chemical	If clinical laboratories (designed for biological samples) assess the accuracy of the final admixture (ie, dextrose and/or electrolyte content), they must use USP-approved measurements and ranges. Assays should be within USP-defined ranges (ie, no less than 95% and no more than 105%) of the labeled amount of the exact compound to be analyzed (eg, anhydrous dextrose, not dextrose monohydrate).
Refractometry	A measure of the final additive concentration. Dextrose concentration is frequently assessed by this technique. Refractometry measures a physical characteristic of dextrose (eg, refractive index), so it is an *indirect* determinant of dextrose concentration and subject to interference by other components, as well as to variation in technique from one operator to another and in subsequent interpretation of the final results. This method is limited to PN preparations that do not contain ILE.
Precision	
	Daily records are kept to document variations in the accuracy measures above. Records are analyzed at least weekly to avoid cumulative errors over time.
Finished Product Release Checks	
Visual inspection	Solutions visually examined for particulates/foreign matter and integrity of the system (cloudiness, leakage).
Pharmacy double-check	Pharmacist to check finished product, including labeling, to confirm accuracy. Pharmacist should double-check all additive vials and syringes, their volumes, and their quantities to confirm that the ingredients measured match the written order prior to dispensing the final preparation. A pharmacist other than the compounding personnel is preferred for this inspection process.

ILE, lipid injectable emulsion; PN, parenteral nutrition; USP, United States Pharmacopeia.

PN Compounding Additive Sequence

Finally, the sequence in which the components of a PN formulation are combined can affect compatibility and the overall stability of the final product. The additive sequence in compounding must be optimized and validated as a safe and efficacious method.[8] The order of admixing is determined by the method used (eg, automated vs manual compounding) and has been outlined in Table 6-4. This general recommendation assumes that the appropriateness of dose and form of each individual component was already determined during the review process.

Table 6-4. Order of Admixing a PN Formulation

Method	Procedure
Automated compounding	Procedure depends on the ACD. Obtain assistance in optimizing the compounding and additive sequence through consultation with the manufacturer of macronutrients being used as well as the manufacturer of the ACD (brand-specific issues might influence the compatibility of the final formulation).
Manual compounding	The steps below should be followed in the order presented (step 1 first and step 9 last) to optimize the stability of the PN formulation. 1. Combine dextrose, amino acids, and sterile water for injection. 2. Add phosphate. 3. Add sodium, potassium, and magnesium (in any order). 4. Add trace minerals. 5. Agitate the solution well. 6. Add calcium (or a calcium-containing multielectrolyte solution) and agitate the solution well again. 7. Observe the solution for precipitates or contaminants (eg, rubber cores). If either is present, discard the solution. If a precipitate is present, review the quantities of additives for incompatibilities (especially calcium and phosphorus) and adjust nutrient doses as needed to achieve compatibility. 8. If a TNA is being admixed, add the ILE next, gently agitate, and observe for signs of the emulsion cracking. 9. Add vitamins last, as close to the time of administration of the PN admixture as possible. For home PN patients, the patient or caregiver should add vitamins just prior to infusion. Note: When a TNA is admixed, dextrose and ILE should never be added directly to one another. The low pH of dextrose solutions will disrupt the ILE.

ACD, automated compounding device; ILE, lipid injectable emulsion; PN, parenteral nutrition; TNA, total nutrient admixture.

A PN compounding checklist is a useful tool to enhance the safety and to ensure that all elements of compounding PN formulations are complete (see Figure 6-2).

Figure 6-2.

PN Compounding **CHECKLIST**

The **American Society for Parenteral and Enteral Nutrition** (A.S.P.E.N.) champions the best evidence-based practices that support parenteral nutrition (PN) therapy in varying age populations and disease states. The appropriate use of this complex therapy aims to maximize clinical benefit while minimizing the potential risks for adverse events.

The **purpose of this checklist** is to promote safe practices by pharmacy staff to prepare optimal PN formulations.

Automated Compounding Device (ACD) Setup
- ☐ Use vendor-validated setup for ACD
- ☐ Initial - ACD setup performed using 2 staff members:
  - ○ Use independent double-check process
  - ○ Use printed check
  - ○ Verbally affirm all additives and base solutions including
    - • name
    - • concentration
    - • container size
- ☐ Use barcode technology to verify products during setup and replacement of ingredients
- ☐ Trace tubing from the source container to port where attached to ACD during initial setup and with each change in the source container
- ☐ Pharmacist verifies all empty containers when multiple containers of a single additive are used
- ☐ Use ACD to deliver all ingredients

Manual compounding
- ☐ Use manual compounding when
  - ○ The volume of PN component to be mixed is less than the ACD can accurately deliver
  - ○ There is an interaction between a PN component and a component of the ACD (e.g., insulin and tubing)

- ○ There is a chemical reaction between PN components that cannot be mitigated by sequencing the addition of ingredients
- ○ There is a shortage of a specific PN components and manual compounding is part of a conservation measure
- ☐ Verify and inspect manual additive vials and syringes with the additive prior to adding to PN (Do not use proxy methods of verification such as syringe pull-back method)
- ☐ Use check list or sign-off sheet for manual additives

Standardized, Commercial - Parenteral Nutrition Products
- ☐ Open seal/remove bar between the chambers, mix components, and add other components prior to dispensing from pharmacy.

Review and verify PN order
- ☐ After initial order entry
- ☐ Prior to injecting manual additives
- ☐ After compounding

Prior to dispensing PN
- ☐ Review and compare PN order, label on PN product and compounding label prior to dispensing
- ☐ Visually inspect PN

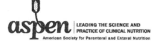

LEADING THE SCIENCE AND PRACTICE OF CLINICAL NUTRITION
American Society for Parenteral and Enteral Nutrition

For full recommendations, rationale, and references, go to Ayers P, Adams S, Boullata J, Gervasio J, Holcombe B, Kraft M, et al. A.S.P.E.N. Parenteral Nutrition Safety Consensus Recommendations. *JPEN J Parenter Enteral Nutr.* 2014;38:296-333.

www.nutritioncare.org/pnsafety

www.nutritioncare.org

ACD, automated compounding device; PN, parenteral nutrition.
Source: Reprinted with permission from ASPEN. Parenteral nutrition safety consensus recommendations and clinical guidelines. ASPEN website. http://www.nutritioncare.org/Guidelines_and_Clinical_Resources/Toolkits/Parenteral_Nutrition_Safety_Toolkit/Parenteral_Nutrition_Safety_Consensus_Recommendations_and_Clinical_Guidelines/. Accessed January 24, 2020.

Stability and Compatibility of PN Formulations

Although stability and compatibility are often used interchangeably in some medical literature, a distinction exists between them, especially in reference to PN. Stability refers to maintaining chemical integrity and pharmacologic activity of each component of the final admixture, or of the dosage form (ie, TNA emulsion), until the end of infusion. Compatibility refers to lack of interaction between each PN component with every other PN component, at the prescribed dose and volume, until the end of the infusion.

Stability of TNAs

The ILE consists of an interior oil phase dispersed in an external water phase. Polar and nonpolar regions on the same fat droplet are responsible for maintaining stability. The polar regions create a negative charge, or Zeta potential, on the surface of the fat droplet that promotes repulsion between neighboring lipid particles of the same charge.[10,11] When the surface charge becomes less negative, fat droplets begin to aggregate into larger fat globules (>1 μm in diameter), and the emulsion becomes unstable. Clinically, the ILE becomes unsafe for administration at this point because fat globules may obstruct the microvasculature and lodge in the pulmonary vasculature, compromising respiratory function.

Factors that may alter the electrical charge on the fat droplet surface include reductions in pH and addition of electrolyte salts. A pH in the range of 6–9 is most favorable for ILE stability, whereas additives that lower or increase it may irreversibly destabilize or "crack" the emulsion.[11] When a cracked ILE occurs, the oil phase separates from the water phase, initially creating subtle changes in the uniformly white appearance of the emulsion, which may progress to yellow oil streaks throughout the bag or development of an amber oil layer at the top of the admixture bag. A TNA with this appearance is unsafe for use. Low pH is especially damaging because, in addition to effects on electrical charge, the egg phospholipids emulsifier begins to degrade.

The single most critical factor influencing the pH of a PN formulation is the crystalline amino acids solution used for compounding. The final pH of a PN formulation is generally very near that of the amino acids solution unless the buffering capacity of the amino acids has been overwhelmed by other PN components. Therefore, the selection of amino acid product, the contents of which vary by manufacturer, is critical to overall emulsion stability.

Use of these amino acid formulations can be particularly problematic for outpatient use and use elsewhere when PN is made several days in advance of use; in addition, other factors influencing TNA stability are marginal for ILE stability. Addition of L-cysteine hydrochloride, as is routine with neonatal PN formulations and some pediatric PN formulations, renders the final admixture pH to be <5, promoting ILE destabilization. However, some prescribers may request the use of pediatric amino acid products in adult PN patients because the pediatric amino acid products are the only products with taurine.

A concentrated dextrose solution should not be added directly to an ILE because of its acidic pH; rather, dextrose should be combined with the amino acid solution first during the compounding process. The amino acid solution serves as a buffer, and low final concentrations of amino acids (<4% depending on other factors) may not provide adequate buffer capacity to prevent destabilization of a TNA.[12] Low ILE concentrations, especially <2%, may also result in an unstable TNA.[13] When compounding PN for 3–7 days in advance of use, final ILE concentrations may need to be higher for a stable TNA, especially if other components contribute to destabilization.

Stability studies should be reviewed carefully to ensure that the assigned beyond-use dating is reasonable for the final concentrations of base components and the combination of additives in the PN formulation. Manufacturers' data often list a range of amino acids, dextrose, and ILE concentrations that have been evaluated for TNA stability, but less commonly are the specific combinations of base components, electrolytes, vitamins, and trace elements present in the PN formulations reported. Although this information provides some guidance to stability limits, it does not provide adequate practice guidelines. For instance, a range of final concentrations for each base component (amino acids, dextrose, and ILE) are typically listed. If, for example, amino acids 1%, dextrose 10%, and ILE 1% are each listed as within the range tested, there is no indication that this particular combination was tested. Although a final concentration of ILE 1% may be stable with amino acids ≥5%, this ILE concentration is not likely to be compatible with a final amino acids 1% concentration, but this is not stated.

Home care practitioners must be particularly vigilant in assessing appropriate combinations of final concentrations and the beyond-use dating assigned. A PN formulation may be stable when used within 30 hours of compounding (in hospital) but begin to destabilize before use when assigned a longer beyond-use date.

Excess numbers of cations, especially divalent cations such as calcium (Ca^{2+}) or magnesium (Mg^{2+}), can reduce or neutralize the negative surface charge exerted by the emulsifier, thereby removing the repulsive force and allowing fat particles to combine.[10] Trivalent cations, such as iron dextran (Fe^{3+}), have even greater destabilizing effects. There is no dose or form of iron that can be added to any TNA because of instability. As with base components, home care providers must be especially alert for inappropriate concentrations of electrolytes because the process of coalescence is not immediate and formulations that are stable for 30 hours may not be stable for longer periods of time.

Calcium and Phosphate Solubility

The development of microprecipitates within PN formulations can occur as a result of incompatible combinations. Calcium-phosphate solubility is a major compatibility concern with PN formulations. For patient safety, all healthcare professionals who prescribe PN formulations that deviate from preestablished standards should be familiar with limitations for addition of calcium and phosphate. This allows the pharmacist responsible for the PN compounding to serve as a *tertiary* check for calcium phosphate solubility rather than as a single evaluator. In the review process by the clinical pharmacist, the compatibility of calcium and phosphate should be evaluated by the separate safety step of order review, before reaching the preparation step.

Several factors can influence the calcium and phosphate solubility in a PN formulations. See Table 6-5 for these factors.[14]

Table 6-5. Factors That Influence Calcium and Phosphorus Compatibility in PN Formulations

Increased risk of calcium phosphate precipitation:
- Increased calcium concentration
- Increased phosphate concentration (including amino acids with phosphorus content)
- Calcium chloride salt use (vs calcium gluconate)
- Increased temperature of PN admixture

Increased calcium phosphate solubility:
- Increased amino acid concentration
- Increased dextrose concentration
- Lower pH of the PN admixture

PN, parenteral nutrition.
Source: Reprinted with permission from Patel R. Parenteral nutrition formulations. In: Mueller CM, ed. *The ASPEN Adult Nutrition Support Core Curriculum.* 3rd ed. Silver Spring, MD: ASPEN; 2017.

The pH of the final PN formulation plays a major role in dictating the solubility of calcium and phosphate. A low pH favors the presence of monobasic calcium phosphate, a relatively soluble salt-form of calcium. Increasing the pH results in a greater availability of dibasic phosphate to bind with free calcium ions and precipitate. Thus, lowering the pH of the PN admixture lowers the likelihood that calcium and phosphate will precipitate. This concept has been used extensively in compounding pediatric PN formulations.[15] For example, relatively large doses of calcium and phosphate are routinely required in neonatal PN formulations to optimize bone formation.[12] Although pediatric amino acid products are formulated at a lower pH, L-cysteine hydrochloride can be added to further decrease pH and thereby increase calcium phosphate solubility.[16] Because L-cysteine is considered a semi-essential amino acid in premature infants, its addition to pediatric formulations serves a dual purpose. Yet an acidic pH creates an unfavorable environment for ILE, possibly destabilizing the final emulsion. As a result, TNAs are discouraged for use in the neonatal and pediatric population, in whom lowering the pH is an effective technique for increasing calcium phosphate solubility.

The concentration or amounts of calcium and phosphate ions are directly related to the risk of precipitation.[14] A variety of resources are available to assist clinicians in determining appropriate calcium and phosphate concentrations to avoid precipitation. Product-specific solubility curves have been published that depict solubility limits for calcium and phosphate salts.[15,16] Unfortunately, most of these curves were developed using fixed concentrations of amino acids, dextrose, calcium, and phosphate and often omitted other components that might influence calcium phosphate solubility. Additionally, these curves rarely evaluated the higher amino acid concentrations as used currently. This makes applying such curves for determining solubility characteristics of patient-specific formulations difficult. When ACDs are used in the admixture process, the manufacturer's software may be helpful in predicting calcium and phosphate solubility for a given formulation.

The salt form of calcium added to the PN formulation can have a dramatic impact on the risk of precipitation. Calcium gluconate and calcium gluceptate are generally less dissociated salt forms of calcium than the chloride salts.[17] As a result, the amount of free calcium available to form insoluble complexes with phosphate is reduced. Solubility curves for calcium phosphate are specific to the calcium salt and cannot be interchanged; most solubility curves are for calcium gluconate. High localized phosphate or calcium concentrations can occur if the final container is not sufficiently agitated or the contents are not sufficiently dispersed during the compounding process.

Aluminum Contamination

On July 26, 2004, federal regulations regarding labeling of aluminum content in large-volume parenteral (LVP) solutions, pharmacy bulk packaging (PBP), and small-volume parenteral (SVP) solutions became effective.[18] Despite significant aluminum content in albumin, blood products, and certain medications, only products regulated by the Endocrine and Metabolic Products Division of the US Food and Drug Administration (FDA), including products used in compounding PN formulations, are governed by the regulation.

The maximum aluminum load permitted in LVPs, including dextrose solutions, amino acid solutions with and without electrolytes, and premade PN solutions, is 25 mcg/L. Labels on PBP and SVPs must include the statement "not more than 25 mcg/L of aluminum" or provide the aluminum content in micrograms per liter at product expiration. Thus, the label contains the potential *maximum* aluminum content, not the actual amount of aluminum at the time of use. Aluminum content increases over time and is influenced by the container material and closures. Products with an affinity for aluminum can leach aluminum from glass containers and elastomeric closures, causing a significant rise in aluminum contamination over the shelf life of the product. Specific amino acids, calcium salts, and phosphate salts have a high affinity for aluminum; therefore, storage of these products in plastic containers typically results in significantly less aluminum content at expiry than storage in glass containers.[19,20] Raw product contamination with aluminum also contributes to the aluminum load and may be responsible for some of the significant variability in aluminum content between different salt forms of products, such as calcium gluconate and calcium chloride.

Aluminum is widespread in the environment; however, under normal circumstances, <1% of ingested aluminum is absorbed from the gastrointestinal tract.[20,21] The lungs also serve as an effective barrier. Unfortunately, the body has no effective barriers to aluminum contaminants in parenteral products and must rely on excretion to prevent toxicity. The kidneys are the primary route for elimination of aluminum and remove unbound aluminum from the blood. However, 95% of the aluminum is bound to protein, primarily transferrin, and cannot be excreted; thus, elimination occurs slowly as equilibrium between bound and unbound aluminum maintains about 5% of the aluminum available for filtration via the kidneys.[21,22] Eventually about 60% of infused aluminum is eliminated in patients with adequate renal function.[21] The remaining aluminum is deposited in tissues, including brain, bones, liver, and lungs.

Adult patients at risk of aluminum toxicity include those with significant renal dysfunction, high intake of parenteral products including PN, or iron deficiency.[18,21] These patients have either impaired excretion and/or excessive exposure, such that aluminum accumulation is likely to occur. Progressive encephalopathy, patchy osteomalacia, reduced parathyroid hormone secretion, and microcytic anemia resistant to erythropoietin (plus iron) have been associated with aluminum toxicity. The final FDA ruling regarding labeling of aluminum content selected 4–5 mcg/kg/d as the upper limit of acceptable aluminum exposure and requires a warning statement in the manufacturer's product information to this effect.[18] There is no mandate for calculation of potential aluminum load or for inclusion of this information on compounded PN in the FDA ruling; however, minimizing aluminum exposure is an important clinical consideration for patients at risk of toxicity.

Labeling PN Formulations

The pharmacy-generated label is a critical tool used to compare the PN ingredients and administration information against the PN order. The label should reflect the PN order in terminology, sequence of ingredients, and units of measure (see chapter 4). It is not acceptable to label the PN using the volume of the original percentage concentration added, the final percentage concentration after admixture, or the amount per liter. Additives, especially electrolytes, should be labeled in the amount (millimoles, milliequivalents) per day — or per kilogram per day in pediatrics.[1,2] Standardized pharmacy labels for PN formulations provide information in a clear, uniform, and organized manner and improve the verification processes for pharmacists.[8]

Additionally, the label is compared with the PN order for accuracy and to verify the beyond-use date prior to administration and serves as a final check for those administering the PN, including nurses or patients and caregivers.[1] Listing ingredients in a uniform sequence and units of measure removes the need for calculations and reduces the risk of misinterpretation, especially when patients are transferred from 1 healthcare environment to another. The ASPEN published report, "Safe Practices for Parenteral Nutrition,"[8] recommends pharmacist-to-pharmacist communication when a patient transfers between healthcare environments, to ensure the accurate transfer of the PN prescription.

The PN label should match the PN order as described in chapter 5 (see Figures 5-1 and 5-2). Standardized PN labels for adults and neonatal/pediatric patients are shown in Figures 6-3 and 6-4. Some key elements for labeling are listed in Table 6-6.

Table 6-6. Key Elements When Labeling PN

Amounts	PN ingredients should be listed in amounts per day (adult patients) and amounts per kilogram per day (neonates and pediatric patients) rather than in amounts per liter, percent concentration, or volume. "Amount per day" refers to macronutrients in grams per day and micronutrients in milliequivalents, millimoles, micrograms, or milligrams per day.
Electrolytes	Electrolytes are listed as the complete salt form rather than the individual ions.
ILEs	If an ILE is not included in the PN admixture but is administered as a separate infusion (intravenous piggyback) from a dextrose/amino acid admixture, then a separate label for ILE should be used (see Figures 6-5 and 6-6).
Dosing weight	The dosing weight (the weight used to calculate nutrient doses) is required on the label.
Route of administration	The route of administration (central vs peripheral) should be specified.
Volume overfill	The volume of overfill is included on the label.
Date/time	Administration date and time and beyond-use date and time are included on the label.
Infusion	Infusion duration and rates are to be expressed on the label.

ILE, lipid injectable emulsion; PN, parenteral nutrition.

Labels for PN preparations administered at home or alternative sites should have the same format as those used in acute care but also be consistent with USP General Chapter <17>.[23] This USP chapter offers direction on organizing the label in a patient-centered manner that optimizes the clarity of information on the label. Additionally, the labels for home PN should include a list of patient and caregiver additives, and these additives should be easily identified and differentiated from the other PN components. Techniques to identify patient additives include highlighting or placing an asterisk to identify the additives that are added just prior to administration. See Figure 6-7 for the Home PN Label Template.

Figure 6-3. Standard PN Label Template: Adult Patient

Patient Information

PATIENT NAME	**MEDICAL RECORD #**	**BIRTH DATE/AGE**
PATIENT LOCATION	**HEIGHT (CM)**	**DOSING WEIGHT (KG)**
DIAGNOSIS(ES)/INDICATION(S) FOR PN:	**VAD/CVC TYPE**	
LOCATION	**ADMINISTRATION DATE/TIME**	

Macronutrients — Amount per day

Amino acids[a] _____ g

Dextrose _____ g

ILE[a] _____ g

Electrolytes — Amount per day

Sodium phosphate _____ mmol of phosphate (sodium _____ mEq)

Sodium chloride _____ mEq

Sodium acetate _____ mEq

Potassium phosphate _____ mmol of phosphate (potassium _____ mEq)

Potassium chloride _____ mEq

Potassium acetate _____ mEq

Magnesium sulfate/chloride _____ mEq

Calcium gluconate _____ mEq

Vitamins, trace elements — Amount per day

Multicomponent vitamins[a] _____ mL

Multicomponent trace elements[a] _____ mL

Other additives

(eg, individual vitamins or trace elements, regular insulin): _____

PN Instructions - *For central (peripheral) vein administration only*

Total Volume: _____ mL, Overfill volume: _____ mL

Infusion rate: _____ mL/h, Start and stop times: _____

Cycle information: _____

Do not use after date/time: _____

******Discard any unused volume after 24 h********

Prescriber and contact information:

Institution/pharmacy name: _____

Institution/pharmacy address: _____

Pharmacy telephone number: _____

CVC, central vein catheter; Ht, height; ILE, lipid injectable emulsion. PN, parenteral nutrition; VAD, vascular access device; Wt, weight.
Source: Adapted with permission from Ayers P, Adams S, Boullata J, et al. A.S.P.E.N. parenteral nutrition safety consensus recommendations. *JPEN J Parenter Enteral Nutr.* 2014;38(3):296–333.
[a]Must specify product name.

Figure 6-4. Standard PN Label Template: Pediatric/Neonatal Patient

Patient Information

PATIENT NAME		MEDICAL RECORD #	BIRTH DATE/AGE

PATIENT LOCATION	HEIGHT/LENGTH (CM)	DOSING WEIGHT (KG)

DIAGNOSIS(ES)/INDICATION(S) FOR PN:	VAD/CVC TYPE

LOCATION	ADMINISTRATION DATE/TIME

Macronutrients	Amount/kg/d[b]	
Amino acids[a]	_____	g
Dextrose	_____	g
ILE[a]	_____	g

Electrolytes	Amount/kg/d[b]	
Sodium phosphate	_____	mmol of phosphate (sodium _____ mEq)
Sodium chloride	_____	mEq
Sodium acetate	_____	mEq
Potassium phosphate	_____	mmol of phosphate (potassium _____ mEq)
Potassium chloride	_____	mEq
Potassium acetate	_____	mEq
Magnesium sulfate/chloride	_____	mEq
Calcium gluconate	_____	mEq

Vitamins, trace elements	Amount/kg/d[b]	
Multicomponent vitamins[a]	_____	mL
Multicomponent trace elements[a]	_____	mL

Other additives		
Cysteine	_____	mg/g amino acids
Others (eg, regular insulin)	_____	

PN Instructions - *For central (peripheral) vein administration only*

Total Volume: _____ mL, Overfill volume: _____ mL

Infusion rate: _____ mL/h, Start and stop times: _____

Cycle information: _____

Do not use after date/time: _____

******Discard any unused volume after 24 h********

Prescriber and contact information:

Institution/pharmacy name: _____

Institution/pharmacy address: _____

Pharmacy telephone number: _____

CVC, central vein catheter; Ht, height; ILE, lipid injectable emulsion; PN, parenteral nutrition; VAD, vascular access device; Wt, weight.

Source: Adapted with permission from Ayers P, Adams S, Boullata J, et al. A.S.P.E.N. parenteral nutrition safety consensus recommendations. *JPEN J Parenter Enteral Nutr.* 2014;38(3):296–333.
[a]Must specify product name.
[b]Because the admixture usually contains multiple sources of sodium, potassium, chloride, acetate, and phosphorus, the amount of each electrolyte per kilogram provided by the PN admixture is determined by adding the amount of electrolyte provided by each salt.

Figure 6-5. Standard ILE Label Template: Adult

Patient Information

PATIENT NAME		MEDICAL RECORD #	BIRTH DATE/AGE

PATIENT LOCATION		HEIGHT (CM)	DOSING WEIGHT (KG)

DIAGNOSIS(ES)/INDICATION(S) FOR PN:	VAD/CVC TYPE

LOCATION	ADMINISTRATION DATE/TIME

	Infusion Volume	Amount per day
ILE[a]	_____ mL	_____ g

Instructions - *For central or peripheral vein administration*

Total Volume: _____ mL,(may contain overfill)

Infusion rate: _____ mL/h

Infuse over: _____ h

Do not use after date/time: _____

******Discard any unused volume after 24 h********

Prescriber and contact information:

Institution/pharmacy name: _____

Institution/pharmacy address: _____

Pharmacy telephone number: _____

CVC, central vein catheter; ILE, lipid injectable emulsion; PN, parenteral nutrition; VAD, vascular access device.
Source: Adapted with permission from Ayers P, Adams S, Boullata J, et al. A.S.P.E.N. parenteral nutrition safety consensus recommendations. *JPEN J Parenter Enteral Nutr.* 2014;38(3):296–333.
[a]Specify product name.

Figure 6-6. Standard ILE Label Template: Neonate or Pediatric Patient

Patient Information

PATIENT NAME   **MEDICAL RECORD #**   **BIRTH DATE/AGE**

PATIENT LOCATION   **HEIGHT (CM)**   **DOSING WEIGHT (KG)**

DIAGNOSIS(ES)/INDICATION(S) FOR PN: **VAD/CVC TYPE**

LOCATION   **ADMINISTRATION DATE/TIME**

	Infusion Volume	Amount per day
ILE[a]	_____ mL	_____ g

Instructions - *For central or peripheral vein administration*

Total Volume: _____ mL,(may contain overfill)   ◯ syringe   ◯ bottle

Infusion rate: _____ mL/h

Infuse over: _____ h

Do not use after date/time: _____

******Discard any unused volume after 24 h********

Prescriber and contact information:

Institution/pharmacy name: _____

Institution/pharmacy address: _____

Pharmacy telephone number: _____

CVC, central vein catheter; Ht, height; ILE, lipid injectable emulsion; PN, parenteral nutrition; VAD, vascular access device; Wt, weight.

Source: Adapted with permission from Ayers P, Adams S, Boullata J, et al. A.S.P.E.N. parenteral nutrition safety consensus recommendations. *JPEN J Parenter Enteral Nutr.* 2014;38(3):296–333.

[a]Specify product name.

Patient Information

PATIENT NAME   BIRTH DATE/AGE

PATIENT HOME ADDRESS   HEIGHT (CM)   WEIGHT (KG)

VAD/CVC TYPE   LOCATION

Administration date/time/indication

Infuse 1 bag/d for nutrition.

Infuse at _____ mL/h over _____ h   Start at _____ (time)   Stop at _____ (time)

Macronutrients	Amount per day
Amino acids[a]	_____ g
Dextrose	_____ g
ILE[a]	_____ g

Electrolytes	Amount per day
Sodium phosphate	_____ mmol of phosphate (sodium _____ mEq)
Sodium chloride	_____ mEq
Sodium acetate	_____ mEq
Potassium phosphate	_____ mmol of phosphate (potassium _____ mEq)
Potassium chloride	_____ mEq
Potassium acetate	_____ mEq
Magnesium sulfate/chloride	_____ mEq
Calcium gluconate	_____ mEq

Vitamins, trace elements	Amount per day
Multicomponent vitamins[a]	_____ mL

Add prior to administration

Multicomponent trace elements[a]   _____ mL *to be added immediately prior to administration*

Other additives

Insulin _____ *units to be added immediately prior to administration*

Medications _____ *medication-specific units (mcg, mg, g).*
                                  Specify if requires adding immediately prior to administration.

Total Volume: _____ mL, Overfill volume: _____ mL

Do not use after date/time: _____

Prescriber and contact information:

Institution/pharmacy name: _____
Institution/pharmacy address: _____
Pharmacy telephone number: _____

CVC, central vein catheter; ILE, lipid injectable emulsion; VAD, vascular access device.

Source: Adapted with permission from Ayers P, Adams S, Boullata J, et al. A.S.P.E.N. parenteral nutrition safety consensus recommendations. *JPEN J Parenter Enteral Nutr.* 2014;38(3):296–333.

ªMust specify product name.

References

1. Ayers P, Adams S, Boullata J, et al.; ASPEN. A.S.P.E.N. parenteral nutrition safety consensus recommendations. *JPEN J Parenter Enteral Nutr.* 2014;38(3):296–333.

2. Boullata JI. Overview of the parenteral nutrition use process. *JPEN J Parenter Enteral Nutr.* 2012;36(2 suppl):10S–13S.

3. Boullata JI, Holcombe B, Sacks G, et al; Parenteral Nutrition Safety Committee, ASPEN. Standardized competencies for parenteral nutrition order review and parenteral nutrition preparation, including compounding: the ASPEN model. *Nutr Clin Pract.* 2016;31(4):548–555.

4. Hermanspann T, Schoberer M, Robel-Tillig E, et al. Incidence and severity of prescribing errors in parenteral nutrition for pediatric inpatients at a neonatal and pediatric intensive care unit. *Front Pediatr.* 2017;5:149. doi:10.3389/fped.2017.00149

5. Boullata JI, Guenter P, Mirtallo JM. A parenteral nutrition use survey with gap analysis. *JPEN J Parent Enteral Nutr.* 2013;37(2):212–222.

6. Chapter <797>. *Pharmaceutical Compounding—Sterile Preparations. United States Pharmacopeia Revision Bulletin.* Rockville, MD: The United States Pharmacopeial Convention; 2007:1–61.

7. American Society of Health-System Pharmacists. ASHP guidelines on outsourcing sterile compounding services. *Am J Health Syst Pharm.* 2015;72(19):1664–1675.

8. Mirtallo J, Canada T, Johnson D, et al. Task Force for the Revision of Safe Practices for Parenteral Nutrition. Safe practices for parenteral nutrition. *JPEN J Parenter Enteral Nutr.* 2004;28(6):S39–S70.

9. Kochevar M, Guenter P, Holcombe B, Malone A, Mirtallo J; ASPEN Board of Directors and Parenteral Nutrition Standardization Task Force. A.S.P.E.N. statement on parenteral nutrition standardization. *JPEN J Parenter Enteral Nutr.* 2007;31(5):441–448.

10. Driscoll DF. Total nutrient admixtures: theory and practice. *Nutr Clin Pract.* 1995;10(3):114–119.

11. Barnett MI. Physical stability of all-in-one admixtures: factors affecting fat droplets. *Nutrition* 1989;5(5):348–349.

12. Boullata JI, Gilbert K, Sacks G, et al; ASPEN. A.S.P.E.N. clinical guidelines: parenteral nutrition ordering, order review, compounding, labeling, and dispensing. *JPEN J Parenter Enteral Nutr.* 2014;38(3):334–377.

13. Driscoll DF, Giampietro K, Wichelhaus DP, et al. Physicochemical stability assessments of lipid emulsions of varying oil composition. *Clin Nutr.* 2001;20(2):151–157.

14. Trissel LA. *Trissel's Calcium and Phosphate Compatibility in Parenteral Nutrition.* Houston, TX: TriPharma Communications; 2001.

15. Eggert LD, Rusho WJ, MacKay MW, Chan GM. Calcium and phosphorus compatibility in parenteral nutrition solutions for neonates. *Am J Hosp Pharm.* 1982;39(1):49–53.

16. Schmidt GL, Baumgartner TG, Fischlschweiger W, Sitren HS, Thakker KM, Cerda JJ. Cost containment using cysteine HCl acidification to increase calcium/phosphate solubility in hyperalimentation solutions. *J Parenter Enteral Nutr.* 1986;10(2):203–207.

17. Driscoll DF, Newton DW, Bistrian BR. Precipitation of calcium phosphate from parenteral nutrition fluids. *Am J Hosp Pharm.* 1994;51(22):2834–2836.

18. Department of Health and Human Services. Food and Drug Administration. Aluminum in large and small volume parenterals used in total parenteral nutrition. *Fed Regist.* 2000;65:4103–4111.

19. Bohrer D, do Nascimento PC, Binotto R, Carlesso R. Influence of the glass packing on the contamination of pharmaceutical products by aluminum. Part II: amino acids for parenteral nutrition. *J Trace Elem Med Biol.* 2001;15(2–3):103–108.

20. Bohrer D, do Nascimento PC, Binotto R, Becker E, Pomblum S. Contribution of raw material to the aluminum contamination in parenterals. *JPEN J Parenter Enteral Nutr.* 2002;26(6):383–388.

21. Klein GL. Aluminum in parenteral solutions revisited—again. *Am J Clin Nutr.* 1995;61(3):449–456.

22. Yokel RA, McNamara PJ. Aluminum toxicokinetics: an updated minireview. *Pharmacol Toxicol.* 2001;88(4):159–167.

23. USP General Chapter <17> Prescription Container Labeling, 2012. Rockville, MD: The United States Pharmacopeial Convention; 2012.

Parenteral Nutrition Administration and Monitoring

Introduction

This chapter describes parenteral nutrition (PN) initiation, administration, and monitoring. Adherence to evidence-based guidelines for PN therapy promotes clinical benefits while minimizing risks associated with the therapy. This process begins with recognizing clinical indications for PN as well as situations in which PN is not likely to be of benefit. After the judicious selection of candidates, appropriate PN use continues with developing a prescription that meets individual requirements, monitoring the response to therapy, adjusting the therapeutic plan as indicated, and ensuring a prompt, seamless transition when PN is no longer required.[1]

Initiating PN

Selecting Appropriate Candidates

PN serves as the feeding method of choice for patients who are malnourished or at risk for malnutrition because of an inability to maintain adequate intake through the oral or enteral route. Specific clinical features of the patient's medical condition, not the primary diagnosis, determine the need for PN.[1] Table 7-1 lists examples of circumstances in which PN is indicated.

Table 7-1. Examples of Conditions Likely to Require PN Across the Life Cycle

Category	Example	Clinical Features
Impaired absorption or loss of nutrients	Short bowel syndrome, complications of bariatric surgery, intestinal atresia, gastroschisis, volvulus, meconium ileus, necrotizing enterocolitis, mesenteric thrombosis, trauma	Bowel length—adults: 60 cm with colon in continuity; 120 cm without colon in continuity Neonate and pediatric patients: inability to meet nutrient, electrolyte, and fluid requirements regardless of intestinal length; weight loss, failure to thrive; fluid and electrolyte disturbances
	High-output intestinal fistula (>500 mL/d)	Bypasses significant absorptive mucosal area, location precludes enteral access or high-volume output with EN
	Neutropenic colitis	Typhlitis or opportunistic infection in an immune-compromised patient
	Small bowel mucosal disease • Radiation or chemotherapy-related enteritis • Congenital diseases (microvillus inclusion disease, tufting enteropathy) • Autoimmune enteropathy • Intractable diarrhea of infancy	Intractable diarrhea; weight loss, failure to thrive, unresponsive to medical management
Mechanical bowel obstruction	Intrinsic or extrinsic blockage of intestinal lumen • Stenosis or strictures • Inflammatory disease • Peritoneal carcinomatosis • Severe adhesive disease • Severe superior mesenteric artery syndrome	Recurrent or intractable vomiting; limited oral intake Unamenable to medical, surgical, or interventional treatment (placement of stent or enteral access device)

Category	Example	Clinical Features
Need to restrict oral or enteral intake: bowel rest	Ischemic bowel	Mesenteric artery stenosis; intestinal angina, abdominal compartment syndrome, or low-flow states
	Severe pancreatitis	Increased pain or serum lipase levels with EN; infected pancreatic phlegmon or pseudocyst, complex pancreatic fistula, abdominal compartment syndrome
	Chylous fistula	Increased output with low-fat diet or elemental formula
	Preoperative status	*Severely* malnourished adults with nonfunctional GI tract for 7–10 d prior to surgery
Motility disorders	Prolonged ileus	Diffuse peritonitis; or related to medical treatment or other disease state. Time to intervention varies, based on nutrition and clinical status
	Pseudo-obstruction, scleroderma, visceral organ myopathy, very-long-segment Hirschsprung's disease	Failure to tolerate adequate oral intake or EN
	Severe adhesive disease	"Frozen abdomen" with chronic obstructive symptoms and malnutrition
Inability to achieve or maintain enteral access	Varies with clinical circumstances	Hemodynamic instability, active GI bleeding, severe neutropenic fever, or low-birth-weight infant

EN, enteral nutrition; GI, gastrointestinal; PN, parenteral nutrition.
Source: Adapted with permission from Worthington P, Balint J, Bechtold M, et al. When is parenteral nutrition appropriate? ASPEN Consensus Recommendations. *JPEN J Parenter Enteral Nutr.* 2017;41(3):324–377.

Baseline nutrition status can guide the decision to begin PN. An early study of PN use found that preoperative PN improved outcomes for patients with severe malnutrition, whereas well-nourished individuals gained no advantage by delaying surgery for nutrition support.[2] Additional factors such as vascular access, the potential for clinical benefit, prognosis, and the patient's views regarding artificial feeding also come into play when deciding whether PN is appropriate.

Timing of Nutrition Intervention

The length of time that an individual can withstand an absence of nutrient intake before detrimental clinical effects occur is unknown. Clinically stable, well-nourished adults can be maintained on conventional intravenous (IV) fluids for 7–14 days without negative consequences.[3] However, because of uncertainty about the onset of starvation-related malnutrition, clinical guidelines generally recommend beginning PN (supplemental or full) in patients who have failed to achieve nutrition goals after 7 days.[4-7] Preexisting nutrition deficits and conditions marked by nutrient losses or catabolic illness demand more immediate attention. Table 7-2 lists ASPEN recommendations for the appropriate timing for starting PN.

Table 7-2. ASPEN Recommendations for Starting PN

Adult	Initiate PN after 7 d for well-nourished, stable adult patients who have been unable to receive significant (50% or more of estimated requirements) oral or enteral nutrients.
	Initiate PN within 3–5 d in those who are nutritionally at risk and unlikely to achieve desired oral intake or EN.
	Initiate PN as soon as is feasible for patients with baseline moderate or severe malnutrition in whom oral intake or EN is not possible or sufficient.
	Delay the initiation of PN in a patient with severe metabolic instability until the patient's condition has improved.
Neonatal	Begin PN promptly after birth in the very low-birth-weight infant (birth weight < 1500 g). Insufficient data exist to suggest a specific time frame in which PN is ideally initiated in more mature preterm infants or term neonates with critical illness.
Pediatric	For the infant, child, or adolescent with a self-limited illness, it is reasonable to delay consideration of starting PN for 1 wk. However, initiate PN within 1–3 d in infants and within 4–5 d in older children and adolescents when it is evident that they will not tolerate full oral intake or EN for an extended period.

ASPEN, American Society for Parenteral and Enteral Nutrition; EN, enteral nutrition; PN, parenteral nutrition.
Source: Adapted with permission from Worthington P, Balint J, Bechtold M, et al. When is parenteral nutrition appropriate? ASPEN Consensus Recommendations. *JPEN J Parenter Enteral Nutr.* 2017;41(3):324–377.

Regardless of the clinical circumstances, the initiation of PN should never take on the urgency of an emergency situation. The risk of adverse events can be greatly reduced by first achieving hemodynamic stability, controlling blood glucose levels, and correcting electrolyte abnormalities before initiating PN. Table 7-3 provides examples of clinical situations that warrant a cautious approach to initiating PN. In cases in which multiple metabolic disturbances occur, a delay in starting PN may be warranted. In others, adjustments to the initial PN volume, macronutrient content, and/ or micronutrient profile may allow PN to begin safely. Goals for initiation and advancement of protein, energy, electrolytes, minerals, vitamins, trace elements, and fluid intake are listed in chapter 5.

Table 7-3. Clinical Conditions Warranting Cautious Initiation of Parenteral Nutrition in Adults

Condition	Suggested Criteria
Hyperglycemia	Glucose greater than 180 mg/dL
Azotemia	BUN greater than 100 mg/dL
Hypertriglyceridemia	Serum triglycerides greater than 200 mg/dL
Hyponatremia	Serum sodium less than 130 mEq/L
Hypernatremia	Serum sodium greater than 150 mEq/L
Hypokalemia	Serum potassium less than 3 mEq/L
Hypomagnesemia	Serum magnesium less than 1.3 mEq/L
Hypocalcemia	Ionized calcium less than 4.5 mg/dL
Hypophosphatemia	Serum phosphorus less than 2 mg/dL

Source: Used with permission from Worthington P, Balint J, Bechtold M, Bingham A, Chan LN, Durfee S, Jevenn AK, Malone A, Mascarenhas M, Robinson DT, Holcombe B. When is PN Appropriate? ASPEN Consensus Recommendations. *JPEN J Parenter Enteral Nutr.* 2017 Mar;41(3):324-377.

Recognizing Risk for Refeeding Syndrome

Severe weight loss or longstanding malnutrition poses a risk for refeeding syndrome in response to nutrition intervention.[8-10] Characterized by electrolyte disturbances and fluid shifts, refeeding syndrome occurs early in the course of therapy, often in association with overzealous caloric replacement. With the start of nutrition, glucose stimulates an insulin response, which in turn promotes uptake of intracellular ions and a subsequent drop in serum concentrations. Profound hypophosphatemia, the hallmark of refeeding syndrome, can be life-threatening if not detected and treated promptly. Low levels of potassium and magnesium are also typical of the condition. Fluid overload due to sodium retention is another common manifestation that can lead to pulmonary edema, heart failure, and dysrhythmias.[8-10]

When the potential for refeeding syndrome exists, correction of existing electrolyte disturbances should take place before PN begins. Then, the initial PN should provide a reduced level of energy. Because thiamin deficiency can occur in conjunction with refeeding syndrome, supplementation with this vitamin in the first 3 days of PN is also recommended.[11] Vigilant monitoring of serum electrolytes and aggressive correction of deficits are especially critical in avoiding the serious consequences associated with this condition. Electrolyte supplementation is often required in relatively high doses, over several days, before metabolic stability is achieved.

Frequency of Errors in Administration Phase of PN

Because PN administration errors occur at the point of patient contact, mistakes in this phase of the medication delivery process are less likely than other types of PN errors to be intercepted and more likely to cause harm.[12] In addition, the broad range of healthcare settings in which PN administration takes place — from critical care to home care — raises the potential for disparities to exist in the technology, equipment, and knowledge and skills of the nursing staff and caregivers responsible for PN administration. Although once uncommon, PN is administered with increasing frequency in long-term care and skilled nursing facilities. Regardless of the setting or the number of patients receiving the therapy in a given facility, the classification of PN as a high-alert medication by the Institute for Safe Medication Practices (ISMP) requires healthcare organizations to take steps to mitigate risks. This includes developing evidence-based policies and procedures to promote safe PN administration and to validate the competence of those responsible for delivering this complex form of IV therapy.[13]

Because of underreporting, data pertaining to the incidence of errors during PN administration give an incomplete account of the problem.[14,15] The ISMP reports that only 58% of organizations have precautions in place to prevent errors and patient harm associated with PN.[16] In fact, one survey revealed that 44% of organizations do not track PN-related medication errors and do not know where in the process errors may be occurring.[14]

The literature does provide some insight into the scope of the problem. One prospective observational study of errors associated with PN found that 35% of PN-related errors occurred during the administration process.[16] In a similar audit of 18,588 PN days in a tertiary pediatric hospital, administration-related errors accounted for 30% of all PN errors.[17] More recently, a review of error reports submitted to ISMP from 2006 to 2016 revealed that PN administration errors were the second-highest category in the PN use process.[15] An analysis of 906 errors involving IV medication by the Pennsylvania Patient Safety Authority found that PN ranked third in the list of the top 10 medications involved in errors.[18]

The frequency with which case reports of PN-related errors involve neonatal and pediatric patients suggests that this population may be the most vulnerable to PN administration errors.[19-22] Data gathered over a 5-year period from a national medication error–reporting program revealed 266 errors associated with infusion of lipid injectable emulsion (ILE) in neonatal intensive care units; 93.2% of the errors occurred in the administration phase.[23,24] Another report of quality improvement data from a single 39-bed unit caring for neonates to young adults indicated that in one 6-month period, PN and ILE errors accounted for 25% of all medication errors.[25] A study of the frequency and severity of PN errors at a large children's hospital demonstrated that the most common administration errors occurred with rate changes of PN (34%), adjustments in ILE after the PN started (23%), or PN incompatibilities when medications were administered through a Y-site (13%).[26] In 2017, the National Health System (NHS) of the United Kingdom issued a patient safety alert after learning of 10 incidents over 3.5 years in which infusion of the aqueous and/or fat component of PN were infused at the incorrect rate, resulting in severe harm to babies.[27] A follow-up review using "low harm" and "no harm" keywords (including near misses) in the same time frame suggested that approximately 700 similar incidents had been reported.[26] Two years later, the NHS issued an updated alert following the death of a premature baby who received a free-flow infusion of PN.[28]

System-Based Strategies for Enhancing PN Safety

Standardized Policies and Procedures

PN administration. Failure to follow established procedures plays a prominent role in PN administration errors.[29] Although human factors frequently contribute to PN errors, organizational efforts to strengthen the safety of PN administration must extend beyond a focus on individual performance and center on identifying system-based approaches to reduce errors.[30,31] Fundamental to this process is the development and articulation of nursing policies and procedures for PN administration that standardize nursing practices based on published clinical guidelines.[23,32] These policies and procedures must be reviewed and revised on a regular

A. Role responsibilities, delegation considerations

B. Required equipment

C. Verification procedures

    1. Confirmation of patient identity according to organizational policy

    2. Use of PN formulas prepared in another institution

    3. Checking PN label against the order including formulation components, route, and rate of delivery, expiration date

    4. Inspection of formulation to detect defects or visual changes

    5. Verification of appropriate vascular access prior to initiating PN infusion

      • Tip location: newly inserted lines and those in place on admission

      • Safeguards to avoid tubing misconnections – trace tubing to the body before making the connection

      • Confirm patency

D. Administration

    1. Policy regarding verification of pump settings

    2. Observation of formulation integrity during infusion

    3. Importance of maintaining PN infusions at the prescribed rate—avoid interruptions for routine care or adjustments for infusions that are off schedule

    4. Guidelines for medication administration for patients receiving PN

      • Policies for co-infusing IVFE or other medications with PN

      • Policies prohibiting additions to PN formulations on clinical units

    5. Recognizing a compromised PN formulation

    6. Significance of clogged filters

E. Infection control measures

    1. VAD dressing care procedures, aseptic management of catheter hub

    2. Frequency of tubing and filter change

    3. Hang time

    4. Minimizing manipulations

      • Dedicated line, lumen

      • Blood-drawing practices

F. Monitoring

    1. Appropriate blood glucose monitoring based on clinical condition and infusion schedule (cycled vs continuous infusion)

    2. Laboratory monitoring

    3. Evaluating response to therapy

    4. Recognition and intervention for extravasation

G. Complications and troubleshooting

H. Termination of therapy

I. Patient education

J. Documentation

IVFE, intravenous fat emulsion; PN, parenteral nutrition; VAD, vascular access device.
Source: Reprinted with permission from Ayers P, Adams S, Boullata J, et al. A.S.P.E.N. parenteral nutrition safety consensus recommendations. *JPEN J Parenter Enteral Nutr.* 2014;38:296–333.

basis. Figure 7-1 provides an outline of essential components of nursing procedures for safe PN administration.

Extravasation. Policies and procedures related to PN administration should address management of extravasation of PN formulations into perivascular or subcutaneous tissues.[33-37] Although most often associated with peripheral vein infusions, PN extravasation can occur with all types of vascular access devices (VADs).[36,38] A number of factors influence the extent of tissue damage, including pH, osmolarity, electrolyte content, and duration of tissue exposure.[36] No controlled trials are available for the management of PN extravasations, but consensus-based recommendations include stopping the infusion, aspiration of residual fluid, elevation of the limb, and application of cold therapy.[36,38] Treatment with hyaluronidase has also been described for extravasations of PN and hypertonic dextrose.[36,39] In addition, programming hard and soft osmolarity limits into the computerized prescriber order entry (CPOE) software has been shown to reduce injury related to extravasation of peripheral PN.[26] Education for nursing staff and nutrition support clinicians should include ongoing assessment of the vascular access site and appropriate interventions in the event of an extravasation.

Use of PN *formulations compounded* for home infusion. Organizations should also develop policies pertaining to the administration of PN formulations brought in from home or from another facility. One survey found that 75% of organizations prohibit the use of preparations brought from home.[14] The inability to verify the stability and sterility of the formulation—as required by The Joint Commission standards—raises serious safety concerns.[40] The lack of medical and pharmacy review can potentially lead to the infusion of compromised PN formulations or prescriptions that are not appropriate for the patient's current clinical status. For these reasons, acute care and long-term care facilities should not use PN formulations prepared for administration in another setting. In cases in which omitting a PN infusion could lead to patient harm, using such a PN formulation may be acceptable. However, healthcare organizations should develop explicit policies governing situations in which PN compounded for home use can be administered in an acute care or long-term care facility.

Competency validation. Healthcare organizations, regardless of setting (acute care to home care), must have policies regarding ongoing education of nurses and patients or caregivers. This process includes mechanisms to validate competence in PN administration.[29] At a minimum, competency validation should occur in the following circumstances: as part of orientation for newly hired nurses, when a change in protocol or procedure takes place, with the introduction of new equipment or technology, and when quality improvement monitoring or other data sources reveal a gap in skills or knowledge related to PN administration.[37] Home infusion care providers must establish processes for periodic reassessment of knowledge and techniques used by patients or caregivers in the delivery PN in the home.[41] Chapter 9 provides greater detail concerning standardized competencies for PN administration.

Use of Technological Aids

Computer-assisted systems. Technological advances, such as automated compounding devices, CPOE, and bar code medication administration (BCMA) hold much promise for improving the safety of PN.[14,42,43] Unfortunately, these technological aids do not consistently reduce errors in the PN administration process. CPOE appears to avert errors in the prescription and transcription phases rather than those associated with PN administration.[44,45] BCMA automates the "5 rights" of medication safety that all nurses learn: right patient, right drug, right dose, right route, and right time.[30,46,47] BCMA can reduce medication administration errors not related to timing.[47] However, errors can occur when clinicians bypass the safety features of the system.[46,47] Complex admixtures such as PN present challenges with BMCA systems because current technology cannot validate that the label on a formulation containing multiple ingredients accurately reflects the contents of the PN container.

Infusions pumps. Electronic infusion pumps have long been required for PN administration.[38] Yet despite their widespread use as a safety measure, pump-related mishaps stand out as a frequent factor in PN administration errors.[15,17,19,23,26] Data reported to the ISMP show that many of the errors involved pump programming errors: incorrect infusion rates, failure to turn the pump on, or incorrect infusion times. Inadvertent rate and line mix-ups were among the most common errors reported, particularly when the ILE was administered as a separate infusion from the dextrose/amino acid admixture.[15,16,20-22,27] Data from the Pennsylvania Patient Safety Authority found that the dextrose/amino acid infusion was switched with the rate for ILE in 77.3% of errors reported.[18] Errors involving incorrect infusion rates pose the greatest risk for patient harm because of the potential for causing life-threatening metabolic disturbances such as hyperglycemia or fat overload syndrome.

At a minimum, infusion pumps should feature accurate volume (rate control), anti–free flow controls, and alarms for sensing air and pressure changes in the administration tubing, as well as dose error-reduction software.[38] To promote patient safety, healthcare organizations should have risk-reduction strategies in place to address potential performance failures related to infusion pumps.[48]

Infusion pumps equipped with software designed to detect potential errors are becoming the standard of care in all clinical areas.[49] These "smart pumps" offer a safeguard against programming errors and capture data that can support quality improvement programs.[50] When used properly, smart pumps reduce the potential for error, but this pump technology is not foolproof. An observational study of medication errors involving IV medications suggests that clinical factors, such as noncompliance with organizational procedures, can still circumvent the technological safeguards these devices bring to clinical care.[51] If a smart pump drug library is bypassed or is used incorrectly, or if the infusion rate and volume are manually entered, a dose error can occur.[52,53] One case study, for example, reported an incident in which a PN infusion was administered at 10 times the prescribed rate for 2 hours when a soft-limit alert was bypassed.[54] MacKay et al demonstrated that PN administration errors declined dramatically after infusion limits and bar-coding were introduced into the PN administration process.[26]

The advantages of smart pumps can be offset by the complexity of programming the pumps and maintaining a current drug library, although wireless technology has streamlined this responsibility.[49] Whenever possible, infusion pumps should be standardized throughout the organization to promote user familiarity with the operation of the device. Protocols for safe operation of infusion pumps must stipulate rules regarding silencing alarms and overriding soft and hard limits.

Quality Improvement

A critical step in efforts to improve the safety of PN is the implementation of quality improvement programs designed to track and analyze errors associated with PN administration.[30] However, only 39.9% of organizations report having an ongoing quality improvement process for PN.[14] Proactive and reactive methodologies, failure mode effects analysis, root cause analysis, and the Plan-Do-Study-Act model should all serve as the framework for identifying high-occurrence or high-impact errors, closing practice gaps, and engendering continuous process improvement.[55,56] Multifaceted interdisciplinary approaches must foster a culture of safety, clarify problem areas, involve key stakeholders, test change strategies, and maintain channels of communication. These key concepts are most effective in bringing about and sustaining behavior change.[55]

Creating a Culture of Safety

PN administration errors often stem from failure to adhere to the verification steps of PN administration, which parallel the 5 rights of medication safety that all nurses learn: right patient, right drug, right dose, right route, and right time.[31,38] However, adherence to the 5 rights is not sufficient in preventing medication errors.[57] Although human factors frequently contribute to errors, healthcare organizations have a responsibility to create an infrastructure that supports safe practice and reduces the potential for error.[30,31] This includes deploying more effective types of error-reduction strategies, such as forcing functions and constraints, using automation and computerization, creating standardized protocols, and developing rules and policies that promote safety.[57] Staff education is a critical component of this process and must cover the proper use and effectiveness of double-checks and procedures for reporting errors, near misses, and barriers to safe practice in a nonpunitive environment.[30,31]

Policies and procedures for PN administration should avoid broad directives to "check the label" but instead provide clear procedural guidance for each step in the verification process. This verification process should be presented in a bundle format, which uses a set of evidence-based interventions for a defined patient population or care setting. As with other bundles used in healthcare, all components of the verification process must be implemented together to achieve improvements in care.[58]

Strategies to Prevent Errors When Initiating a PN Infusion

Verification Procedures

PN formulations often resemble other products used in clinical care, such as bladder irrigation fluids, enteral formulas, human breast milk, and cardioplegia solutions, posing the risk for wrong-product or wrong-route errors. Practices related to the delivery and storage of these items can mitigate the likelihood of such errors, but the importance of the verification process as the final step before the point of patient contact cannot be overstated.

Nursing education for PN administration must provide information regarding management of potentially compromised or unstable PN formulations. This includes inspection of PN formulations prior to initiating the infusion and at regular intervals during the infusion. Any formulation that displays evidence of precipitants, particulate matter, or an unstable formulation must be returned to the pharmacy for further investigation.[59] Similarly, a container that is leaking or otherwise damaged should never be used, but should be returned to the pharmacy.

Other examples of lapses in the verification process include PN administration to the wrong patient by the wrong route — infusing a central formulation via peripheral vein or through an incorrect tubing connection — or at the wrong rate.[15] The nurse or caregiver should be provided with access to the complete original PN order to facilitate verification of all elements of the order (ie, patient identifiers, nutrient dosing, infusion rate, etc).[12,14]

Vascular access. As outlined in chapter 3, reliable vascular access fosters effective delivery of PN therapy. A wide array of VADs are available, but some are better suited to PN delivery than others. Meticulous care and adherence to guidelines for catheter insertion and maintenance is a critical for element of safe PN administration.

For all newly inserted central venous access devices (CVADs), correct position of the device should be confirmed radiographically or fluoroscopically before PN administration. Ultrasound and electrocardiogram techniques have been suggested as potential alternatives to chest x-ray for confirming correct placement of CVADs, but further research is needed to better define clinical feasibility of these methods.[60,61] In addition, the position of the catheter should be reassessed before starting PN in adult patients who are admitted to the hospital with a CVAD in place.[62] For children who have CVADs in place for extended periods, verification of the catheter position should be considered to assess whether the catheter tip has retracted proximally as the child has grown.

Tubing Misconnections

Inadvertent catheter tubing misconnections have been recognized as a serious problem in healthcare. Although the administration of enteral feeding through IV devices has been associated with many serious injuries, accidental connections between IV tubing and other systems that rely on Luer connectors have been reported, including epidural, intracranial, intrathecal, and tracheal tubing systems.[63,64] Because tubing used to administer PN must be changed every 24 hours, the potential for a misconnection occurs at more frequent intervals than with conventional IV fluids. Clear labeling on PN containers, tubing, and pump channels can reduce the risk of inadvertent misconnections.[48,65] But the single most important risk-reduction strategy is to trace all tubing back to its origin before connecting devices or infusions and to recheck connections and trace all patient tubes and catheters to their sources at the start of each shift and on the patient's arrival to a new setting or unit as part of the hand-off process.[66,67] The development of standards for new enteral connectors with physical incompatibility with other connectors is completed and the adoption in the market is in progress.

Independent Double-Checks

Reports of PN-related errors often recommend implementation of independent double-checks at critical phases of PN administration, such as order verification or programming the infusion rate into the pump.[12,29,48,68] An independent double-check involves 2 clinicians separately checking the infusion settings in accordance with the prescriber's order, alone and apart from each other, then comparing results.[68] However, if the concern is infusion pump programming errors and possible line mix-ups, then an independent double-check at the bedside may be the best risk-reduction strategy.[68]

Although double-checks serve as a valuable safety mechanism if performed correctly, the process may disrupt workflow and consume nursing time.[68] Other barriers include a lack of clarity regarding the procedure for double-checking and a culture that does not fully support peer review.[69] Furthermore, excessive use of double-checks can dilute the effectiveness of this safety mechanism.[68] Independent double-checks should not be implemented to address problems that could be corrected through system redesign.[68] Nevertheless, organizations that have identified errors in conjunction with a specific component of the PN verification process, such as order verification, patient identification, or pump programming, should implement double-checks strategically to avert potentially harmful errors. For optimal effectiveness, independent double-checks should be used in conjunction with other error-reduction strategies and system changes aimed at reducing the risk of medication errors.[68]

Checklists, such as that shown in Figure 7-2, can reinforce steps in the verification process and serve as an adjunct to independent double-checks in preventing PN administration errors.[29] The PN Administration Checklist addresses failures stemming from distraction or poor concentration rather than errors due to inexperience or lack of training.

Preventing Errors During PN Administration

Safe Use of Medical Devices and Equipment

Filters. In-line filters are required for PN administration to reduce the potential for patient harm due to particulates, microprecipitates,

Figure 7-2.

PN Administration **CHECKLIST**

The **American Society for Parenteral and Enteral Nutrition** (A.S.P.E.N.) champions the best evidence-based practices that support parenteral nutrition therapy in varying age populations and disease states. The appropriate use of this complex therapy aims to maximize clinical benefit while minimizing the potential risks for adverse events.

The **purpose of this checklist** is to promote safe practices by nurses administering parenteral nutrition.

☐ Perform hand hygiene

☐ Use sterile technique when manipulating vascular access device

☐ Inspect PN container, check for:
  ☐ Integrity of container: no defects or leaks present
  ☐ No visible particles or precipitates
  ☐ No oiling, streaking, clumping, or separation

☐ Confirm correct formulation, check for:
  ☐ Patient's name on label
  ☐ Match all components listed on the label against the PN order
  ☐ Route of administration (central vs peripheral)
  ☐ Documentation of proper VAD tip placement
  ☐ Start time
  ☐ Infusion rate with taper if appropriate
  ☐ Beyond use date and time

☐ Verify patient identification
  ☐ Confirm patient identity using two identifiers
  ☐ Inspect armband (not applicable in home care)

☐ Initiate PN infusion
  ☐ Use appropriate size filter on distal end of tubing
  ☐ Spike container
  ☐ Prime tubing
  ☐ Set infusion pump settings using double check
  ☐ Trace catheter system to point of origin
  ☐ Disinfect needleless adapter on VAD hub
  ☐ Connect PN to patient
  ☐ Initiate PN infusion at prescribed rate

☐ Initiate monitoring protocol which includes:
  ☐ Patient response
  ☐ Glucose monitoring
  ☐ Serial weights
  ☐ Intake and Output
  ☐ Bloodwork
  ☐ Vital signs

PN, parenteral nutrition; VAD, vascular access device.
Source: Reprinted with permission from American Society for Parenteral and Enteral Nutrition. PN administration checklist. ASPEN website. http://www.nutritioncare.org/Guidelines_and_Clinical_Resources/Toolkits/Parenteral_Nutrition_Safety_Toolkit/Parenteral_Nutrition_Safety_Consensus_Recommendations_and_Clinical_Guidelines/. Accessed January 13, 2020.

microorganisms, and air emboli.[70] A 0.22-µm filter is recommended for a dextrose/amino acid formulation; a 1.2-µm filter is used for a total nutrient admixture (TNA). These devices should be placed as close to the patient as possible on the administration system. Filters (and the administration sets) should by changed with each new PN container. If an occluded filter triggers pump alarms, the PN infusion should be stopped. Before resuming PN, a pharmacist should review the PN formulation to determine if the incorrect size filter has been used or if incompatibility issues are the cause of the problem. An occluded filter must be removed and replaced with a new filter. No unfiltered PN formulations should be allowed to infuse.[12] Education of nurses, pharmacists, and lay caregivers must include information regarding appropriate actions and troubleshooting in response to high-pressure or occlusion alarms.

Recently, US manufacturers of ILEs revised their administration instructions to include a statement to filter all ILE infusions using a 1.2-µm in-line filter.[71] To comply with this new recommendation 2 filters are necessary when administering PN as dextrose/amino acid (2-in-1) admixture and the IV fat emulsions as a separate infusion. A 0.22-µm in-line filter is used for the dextrose/amino acid solution. The second filter, a 1.2-µm filter, is for the IV ILE, which is infused by means of a Y-connector placed closer to the patient than the 0.22-µm filter or via a separate VAD.[72]

Filters are manufactured for single-patient use and should be changed according to the manufacturer's guidelines. The typical maximum use interval for PN filters is 24 hours. Because of the potential for contamination and subsequent release of endotoxin, filters should not be primed with PN fluid in advance — in the compounding pharmacy, for example. Instead, the filter should be filled with fluid immediately before initiating the infusion.

Administration tubing and containers. PN formulations should be provided in a single daily bag, with the exception of ILE that is administered as a separate infusion. Multichamber PN bags, which are designed to reduce the risk for instability or precipitation, have separate components of the PN formulation with a bar or seal until just prior to administration. The contents of the chambers should be mixed, and additives should be introduced, by pharmacy staff prior to dispensing the formulation.[73] However, if these products are used in home care, patients and/or caregivers must receive thorough training regarding the procedure for properly mixing the product before use. (More detail about multichamber bags is presented in chapter 12.)

The PN admixture should be kept refrigerated and protected from light exposure between the time it is dispensed until just before infusion. Exposure of PN formulations to ambient light generates peroxides and other degradation products, potentially contributing to oxidant stress. Concern regarding the clinical impact of this phenomenon has led to recommendations that PN be shielded from light, especially for neonates.[74] A meta-analysis evaluating the effects of not protecting PN from light reported an elevated risk of mortality for preterm infants.[75] Currently, adequate light protection may not be feasible, depending on the circumstances of whether PN is compounded on-site or at a central location. Partial light protection offers no clinical benefit. To reduce PN degradation, the container and tubing must be protected from light at all points from compounding through administration.

The administration tubing should be attached to the PN container, using sterile techniques, immediately prior to initiating the infusion. Although there may be workflow advantages to spiking the container and priming tubing in advance, no studies have, to our knowledge, examined the safety of this practice. Infection control guidelines for nonnutritional IV fluids stipulate that the infusion begin within 1 hour of inserting the tubing spike into the container.[76] The issue of whether the risk of contamination could be reduced by spiking the PN container in an ISO class 5 environment or higher remains unknown.

ILE administered separately must be appropriately labeled and administered in keeping with the organization's policies and procedures for minimum/maximum hang times. PN containers and administration sets must be free of the plasticizer di-2-ethylhexyl phthalate (DEHP) to prevent DEHP contamination of TNAs and ILEs that are infused separately.[38]

As noted in chapter 3, administration sets and filters should be changed with each new PN container. For continuous infusions, this interval will typically be every 24 hours; cycled PN will require tubing and filter changes based on the hours of the infusion. Administration sets used for ILE infused separately must also be changed with each new infusion (hang time 12 hours). In cases in which a prolonged ILE infusion is desirable to promote tolerance, the daily fat emulsion dose should be divided into 2 parts, with a new container and tubing used every 12 hours.[77,78]

Infusion Practices

Prescribed rate. PN infusions should be administered according to the prescribed rate via an infusion pump. To avoid switch errors when administering the dextrose/amino acid component of the PN and the ILE as separate infusions, nurses must completely set up the first infusion, including programming the pump for that fluid, before the setup for the second infusion begins. In addition, the correct infusion rate must be verified when the PN infusion is initiated, at regular intervals during the infusion, and at hand-offs.[79] Unscheduled interruptions or disconnections of the infusion should be avoided because they may contribute to metabolic disturbances, suboptimal nutrient delivery, and infection risk. In addition, for the PN infusion, no adjustments of the infusion rate should occur in an effort to "catch up" if the infusion falls behind schedule. In cases in which PN is required during transport, it should be discontinued prior to discharge or transport if this would require changing the administration set already attached to the PN container. An appropriate infusion control device and personnel competent in infusion therapy must be available in the transport vehicle.

Cycled infusion. Scheduled changes in the prescribed administration rate should be based on patient tolerance and metabolic stability. In acute care settings, PN is commonly infused continuously over 24 hours. However, a schedule in which the PN is cycled to infuse over 10–14 hours (based on patient tolerance) can offer physiological and psychological benefits to patients in selected circumstances.[78,80] The conversion from a continuous to a cycled administration period typically takes place by reducing the infusion time by 4–6 hours each day until the infusion time has been compressed to the target duration. One study suggests that cycling PN to 12 hours can be accomplished in one step.[81] Reports of adverse events associated with PN cycling underscore the importance of close patient monitoring during the transition to cycled PN.[82] At each stage, the healthcare team must assess tolerance of the cyclic infusion before advancing to the next step.

Hyperglycemia, edema, or symptoms of fluid intolerance signal the need for a more cautious approach to cyclic infusion. Adult patients generally tolerate discontinuation of PN without experiencing rebound hypoglycemia.[83] However, a 30- to 60-minute taper-down period is customarily used with ambulatory PN infusion pumps that perform this function automatically.[84] On the other hand, pediatric patients younger than 2 or 3 years old are prone to developing hypoglycemia with abrupt discontinuation of PN and therefore require more gradual taper-down procedures in conjunction with cycling.[80,82] During the transition to a cycled PN regimen, on-cycle and off-cycle glucose monitoring should take place daily. Once patient tolerance to cycled PN is established, less frequent glucose monitoring may be acceptable, especially in stable home PN patients.[85]

When transitioning to cyclic PN, dosing regimens for insulin should be tailored to avoid abnormal fluctuations in blood glucose levels. In patients for whom PN is the sole source of nutrition, giving a subcutaneous correctional dose of insulin in the final phase of the cycle could lead to hypoglycemia when the PN infusion is discontinued. On the other hand, when PN formulations contain large doses of insulin, patients may require intermediate- or long-acting insulin to prevent hyperglycemia after the PN stops.

Intraoperative PN. The risks of metabolic complications, particularly those related to glycemic control, have raised questions regarding the safety of continuing PN during operative procedures. However, no studies have adequately examined this issue. One survey of pediatric anesthesiologists revealed a high degree of variability in the clinical management of blood glucose levels in patients receiving PN during anesthesia.[86] As with other areas of PN administration, healthcare organizations should develop clear and consistent policies that address intraoperative PN infusion. When the PN infusion is continued during surgery, the prescribed infusion rate should be maintained, with close monitoring of blood glucose levels and insulin administration as needed to maintain glycemic control. The use of PN infusions for fluid resuscitation shall be avoided.

Medication Administration

Historically, PN formulations were viewed as convenient vehicles for delivery of medications such as heparin, insulin, and histamine receptor antagonists. A better understanding of factors that impact the stability of PN formulations and the potential for drug-nutrient interactions warrants a more conservative approach to medication administration with PN formulations. Nonnutrient medication may be included in PN admixtures only when supported by pharmaceutical data describing physicochemical compatibility and stability of the additive medication and the final preparation under conditions of typical use. In addition, clinical data confirming the expected therapeutic actions of the medication must be available. Extrapolation beyond the parameter limits (eg, products, concentrations) of the given data is discouraged. The mixture of medications in PN preparations is addressed more specifically in ASPEN's PN clinical guidelines.[87]

Incompatibility reactions range from discoloration, degradation of nutrients or medication, and formation of precipitates to loss of emulsion integrity in TNAs. Standardized, commercially available PN products that require further additives prior to patient administration should be prepared in the pharmacy under aseptic conditions. Therefore, in acute care settings, policies should be implemented that prohibit the addition of medication outside the compounding pharmacy. In home care settings, stability considerations often require that medication, such as multivitamin preparations or insulin, be added to PN formulations prior to initiating the infusion. In this case, the addition of medication should take place as close to the beginning of the infusion as possible. Patient and caregiver training in the proper technique for adding medication to PN formulations should be documented. The additions should be made as close to the beginning of the infusion as possible to reduce the potential for harm should touch contamination occur during this process.

As noted in chapter 3, the optimal way to administer PN is through an IV line reserved solely for that purpose (or one lumen of a multilumen CVAD). However, maintaining a dedicated line for PN administration may be impractical or impossible in patients who receive multiple IV medications or have limited vascular access. Pharmacists must conduct a comprehensive review of stability and compatibility data from the literature and manufacturer of IV nutrients before a medication is administered in a PN formulation.[87]

As with all high-alert medications, PN should be administered as a primary infusion.[38] Co-infusion of medication through the same tubing used for PN should be avoided if possible. When co-infusion of medications with PN cannot be avoided, pharmacists must review compatibility information for PN that closely matches the formulation in question, as well as the concentration of the medication and the rate of administration. If a compatible medication is not available, the PN admixture must be interrupted but not disconnected so the incompatible medication can be infused. The IV line must be flushed with a compatible fluid before and after administration of the medication. Medication administration policies should explicitly detail safe practices with regard to medication administration in conjunction with PN.

Monitoring

The PN monitoring process aims to detect complications early, optimize attainment of nutrition goals, and evaluate changes in gastrointestinal (GI) function to determine the continued appropriateness of PN.[1] This process includes physical assessment, laboratory data, body weight (or in children, growth), hydration and electrolyte status, glycemic control, performance status, and psychosocial response.[38,88] The frequency of monitoring depends on the severity of illness, level of metabolic stress, and nutrition status, as well as the patient's clinical condition.[88] Table 7-4 shows a suggested schedule for laboratory monitoring for patients of all ages and in all healthcare settings. In cases in which severe malnutrition exists, and for patients receiving long-term PN, monitoring should include periodic measurement of vitamin and trace element levels.[1] Table 7-5 provides an overview of PN clinical monitoring parameters for adult and pediatric hospitalized patients, and Table 7-6 lists monitoring parameters for patients who receive PN at home or alternative sites.

Table 7-4. Laboratory Monitoring During PN (Adult and Pediatric)

	Acute Care PN			Long-term PN			
Parameter	Baseline	Days 1–7	Ongoing, Stable	Initial, Postdischarge	Weeks 1–4 (or until stable)	At 3 mo	Ongoing, Stable
Glucose, BUN, creatinine, electrolytes, calcium, magnesium, phosphorous	√	Daily × 3 or until stable	1–2 times/ wk or as clinically indicated	√	√		Monthly
CBC with differential	√	Daily × 3 or until stable	1–2 times/wk	√	√		Monthly
Total bilirubin, direct bilirubin, AP, AST, ALT,	√		Weekly	√			Monthly
PTT, PT, INR	√		Weekly				Monthly
Triglyceride level	√	Pediatric: daily until stable then weekly	Weekly	√			Monthly
Serum proteins (to monitor inflammation)	√		Weekly	√			Monthly
Iron indices			As clinically indicated			√	Every 3–6 mo
Zinc, selenium, manganese, copper, chromium			As clinically indicated			√	Every 3–6 mo
Vitamin A, 25 (OH)D, vitamin E			As clinically indicated			√	Every 12 mo
Vitamin B12 and folate			As clinically indicated			√	Every 6–12 mo
TSH				As indicated			Every 12 mo
Carnitine			No guideline for adults			√ Pediatric patients	Every 3–12 mo

AP, alkaline phosphatase; ALT, alanine aminotransferase; AST, aspartate aminotransferase; BUN, blood urea nitrogen; CBC, complete blood cell count; INR, international normalized ratio; 25 (OH)D, 25 hydroxyvitamin D; PN, parenteral nutrition; PTT, partial thromboplastin time; PT, prothrombin time; TSH, thyroid-stimulating hormone.
Source: Worthington P, Balint J, Bechtold M, Bingham A, Chan LN, Durfee S, Jevenn AK, Malone A, Mascarenhas M, Robinson DT, Holcombe B. When is PN Appropriate? ASPEN Consensus Recommendations. *JPEN J Parenter Enteral Nutr.* 2017 Mar;41(3):324-377.

Parameter	Approach	Frequency
Physical examination	Including a nutrition-focused approach: • micronutrient abnormalities • muscle and fat stores • fluid accumulation • functional/developmental status	On initial examination (Physical examination should be done initially, then according to hospital nutrition reassessment policy.)
Adults: evaluate weight and height	Use of stadiometer, knee-height calculations, or arm-span measures Weight scales used in a consistent manner; patients should not wear shoes or heavy garments	On initial examination, then weights daily until stable (2-3 times/wk for stable patient)
Neonates/pediatrics: growth parameters measured and documented on z-score charts	Children < 36 mo: • Weight for age • Head circumference for age • Weight for length • Length for age Children ages 2 to 20 y: • Standing height for age • Weight for age • BMI for age • Length/height for age	Neonates: weight daily, length and head circumference weekly Infants: daily weight, monthly head circumference and length Children: weight daily to twice weekly; height monthly
Determine energy and macronutrient needs	Use of appropriate predictive equations, indirect calorimetry, or nitrogen balance	On initial examination, then when changes in medical condition or activity level occur
Evaluate intake and output records	Oral or enteral intake, IV fluids and medications, blood products, urine, stool/ostomy/fistula output, other relevant wound/drain output	On initial examination, then daily until stable
Review vital signs	Blood pressure, respiratory rate, heart rate, temperature	On initial examination, then daily until stable
Blood glucose monitoring	Capillary glucose levels, in addition to correctional-dose insulin program and ancillary orders for appropriate intervention for hypoglycemia	Every 1-24 h, as warranted by clinical status; discontinue once blood glucose values normalize and PN reaches target dextrose dose
Evaluation of micronutrient status	Serum levels of vitamins, minerals, trace elements	When history, physical, and/or clinical evidence suggests an abnormality

Parameter	Approach	Frequency
Examination of VAD	Inspection and palpation to assess for redness, tenderness, or rash under dressing or along subcutaneous tunnel Observe for upper extremity edema Review position on chest x-ray	Daily assessment, x-ray confirmation at VAD placement, when admitted with a VAD in place, whenever concern for catheter displacement exists
Reassess continued need for PN therapy	Intake and output records, nutrition adequacy assessment, physical examination, radiological evaluation	Daily, or with signs indicating return of or improvement in bowel function, or with change in pertinent clinical condition
General response to therapy	Wound healing, stamina, functional status, progress toward weight or growth goals	Ongoing throughout the course of therapy

BMI, body mass index; IV, intravenous; PN, parenteral nutrition; VAD, vascular access device.
Source: Adapted with permission from Worthington P, Balint J, Bechtold M, et al. When is parenteral nutrition appropriate? ASPEN Consensus Recommendations. *JPEN J Parenter Enteral Nutr.* 2017;41(3):324–377.

Table 7-6. Monitoring PN in the Home and at Alternate Sites

Assessment Parameters	Frequency of Monitoring
Signs and symptoms of intolerance to therapy	Weekly, or at each home visit and patient encounter
Home environment assessment (running water, electricity, telephone, safe and sanitary conditions, etc)	Prior to discharge to that environment, then regularly throughout the course of therapy
Vital signs	At each home visit and patient encounter
Weight changes and/or growth as appropriate; maintain weight/growth charts	Weekly and at each home visit and patient encounter
Children < 36 mo: • Length for age • Weight for age • Head circumference for age • Weight for length Children ages 2–20 y: • Standing height for age • Weight for age • BMI for age • Length/height for age	Monthly and at all patient encounters with healthcare providers; documented on z-score growth charts
Hydration status	Baseline and regularly throughout the course of therapy
Review of systems and/or physical examination	Weekly, or at each home visit and patient encounter with healthcare encounter

Table 7-6 continued on next page

Assessment Parameters	Frequency of Monitoring
Clinical signs of nutrient deficiencies or excesses	Baseline, weekly until stable, then monthly
Other disease states or conditions that may affect the nutrition therapy	Baseline and regularly throughout the course of therapy
Dual energy x-ray absorptiometry scan	Baseline when expected duration of PN exceeds 6 mo, then annually
Liver and biliary tract ultrasonography	As clinically indicated
Assess readiness to begin or advance oral and/or enteral intake; provide dietary guidance as indicated	Baseline and at every patient encounter
Interaction between nutrition therapy and medications	Baseline, when medication changes occur, then monthly
Functional status and performance	Weekly
Psychosocial status; quality of life; sleep disturbances, etc.	Weekly
VAD and insertion/exit site	Baseline and weekly
Evaluate patient compliance with techniques and procedures of nutrition therapy, storage of admixtures, and supply inventory	Weekly, or at each home visit

PN, parenteral nutrition; VAD, vascular access device.
Source: Adapted with permission from Worthington P, Balint J, Bechtold M, et al. When is parenteral nutrition appropriate? ASPEN Consensus Recommendations. JPEN J Parenter Enteral Nutr. 2017;41(3):324–377.

Transitional Feeding and Discontinuing PN

The healthcare team should modify the PN prescription as indicated based on ongoing evaluation of GI function, nutrition status, and, for pediatric patients, growth. Initiation of oral or enteral intake requires GI function, minimal risk for aspiration, and patient motivation. In some circumstances, a swallowing evaluation may be useful in determining readiness for oral feeding and can dictate the type and texture of foods introduced.

To successfully wean or transition from PN therapy, return of or improvement in bowel function must occur (eg, as seen with adaptation in short bowel syndrome).[1] For the hospitalized patient, tolerance of oral intake or enteral nutrition (EN) should be confirmed before reducing the PN formulation. PN may have a negative effect on appetite. If >25% of caloric needs are provided as PN, reduced oral intake can be expected.[89] When oral intake equals 500 kcal/d in an adult patient, the carbohydrate and protein in the PN should be reduced by an amount equal to the amount consumed orally. Subsequent decreases in the PN should continue as oral intake increases. Generally, PN is not fully discontinued until the patient consistently consumes at least 50%–75% of energy and protein needs orally or through EN, with signs of continuing improvement.[1]

At times, this process is quite rapid, and PN can be withdrawn in a very short period without significant modification. However, patients with a complicated hospital course and/or malnutrition may require longer weaning periods and should demonstrate higher oral intakes than those not malnourished. Patients with severe GI disease also typically require an extended weaning period or, in some cases, may never successfully transition off PN. For those receiving EN, the transition from PN should use a weaning protocol to prevent overfeeding and fluid overload.[90]

As shown in Table 7-7, metabolically stable adults can be weaned from long-term PN by reducing the number of infusion days each week. This strategy offers benefits in terms of quality of life while limiting manipulation of the CVAD. However, patients must be closely monitored for fluid and electrolyte abnormalities, weight loss, and other evidence of nutrition decline.[91] In pediatric patients, discontinuation of PN is often a more gradual process than in adults. PN is tapered gradually as enteral or oral feedings are advanced. Ideally, the combination of PN and enteral feedings will meet all estimated nutrition goals during the transitional period. In practice, PN is generally continued until about 75%–80% of energy needs are being met enterally.

Table 7-7. Recommendations for Weaning Long-term PN for Adult and Pediatric Patients

- Routinely assess GI function for readiness to begin or advance oral or enteral intake.
- Verify metabolic and clinical stability on current PN regimen.
- Establish clear goals with patient: to reduce or eliminate dependence on PN.
- Optimize pharmacologic management of GI symptoms such as anorexia, nausea and diarrhea.
- Provide nutrition counseling and dietary guidance as indicated.
- Monitor weight and hydration status closely.
- Consider increasing the frequency of weight and laboratory monitoring during the transition.
- Assess the need to provide oral vitamin and mineral supplementation.
- Eliminate 1 or 2 nonconsecutive infusions per wk; in children, consider weaning by a small percentage every wk.
- Adjust PN during the transition to avoid overfeeding.
- Consider further reductions if nutrition and hydration remain stable.
- Evaluate the need for oral or IV fluid and/or electrolyte supplementation.
- Make a nutrition-monitoring plan after PN is stopped to optimize safe transition to full oral nutrition or EN.

EN, enteral nutrition; GI, gastrointestinal; IV, intravenous; PN, parenteral nutrition.

Patients with short bowel syndrome may have ongoing fluid and electrolyte losses despite improved nutrient absorption.[92] Successful attempts to wean or reduce PN in this setting often require supplementation with fluids and/or micronutrients orally or intravenously. The use of oral rehydration fluids either sipped throughout the day or administered nocturnally through a gastrostomy tube may promote nutrition independence.[93]

Documentation

Organizational policies and procedures should define documentation practices related to PN administration in accordance with legal and regulatory requirements. This includes, but is not limited to, initiation and discontinuing times of the infusion, rate, route of administration, results of capillary glucose monitoring and laboratory tests, condition of the VAD, patient's response to therapy, progress toward therapeutic goals, and patient education provided.

Summary

PN is a complex form of IV therapy that has life-preserving potential but also poses risks for serious complications. A multidisciplinary approach that begins with careful selection of candidates and develops PN prescriptions based on clinical status is essential to achieving positive outcomes. Adherence to standards for optimal care of the VAD can reduce infectious complications related to PN. Close monitoring and prompt response to changes in the patient's status are needed to avoid the adverse effects associated with PN.

References

1. Worthington P, Balint J, Bechtold M, et al. When is parenteral nutrition appropriate? ASPEN Consensus Recommendations. *JPEN J Parenter Enteral Nutr*. 2017 Mar;41(3):324–377.

2. Veterans Affairs Total Parenteral Nutrition Cooperative Group. Perioperative total parenteral nutrition in surgical patients. *N Engl J Med*. 1991;325(8):525–532.

3. Koretz RL, Lipman TO, Klein S; American Gastroenterological Association. AGA technical review on parenteral nutrition. *Gastroenterology*. 2001;121(4):970–1001.

4. McClave SA, Taylor BE, Martindale RG, et al. Guidelines for the provision and assessment of nutrition support therapy in the adult critically ill patient: Society of Critical Care Medicine (SCCM) and American Society for Parenteral and Enteral Nutrition (A.S.P.E.N.). *JPEN J Parenter Enteral Nutr*. 2016;40(2):159–211.

5. Canadian Clinical Practice Guidelines Committee. 2015 Canadian clinical practice guidelines: the use of enteral nutrition vs. parenteral nutrition. https://www.criticalcarenutrition.com/docs/CPGs%202015/1.0%202015.pdf. Accessed January 14, 2020.

6. Braga M, Ljungqvist O, Soeters P, et al. ESPEN guidelines on parenteral nutrition: surgery. *Clin Nutr.* 2009;28(4):378–386.

7. McClave SA, DiBaise JK, Mullin GE, Martindale RG. ACG clinical guideline: nutrition therapy in the adult hospitalized patient. *Am J Gastroenterol.* 2016;111(3):315–334.

8. Boland K, Solanki D, O'Hanlon C; Irish Society for Clinical Nutrition & Metabolism. Prevention and treatment of refeeding syndrome in the acute care setting. https://www.irspen.ie/wp-content/uploads/2014/10/IrSPEN_Guideline_Document_No1.pdf. Published November 2013. Accessed January 14, 2020.

9. Pulcini CD, Zettle S, Srinath A. Refeeding syndrome. *Pediatr Rev.* 2016;37(12):516–523.

10. Friedli N, Stanga Z, Culkin A, et al. Management and prevention of refeeding syndrome in medical inpatients: an evidence-based and consensus-supported algorithm. *Nutrition.* 2018;47:13–20.

11. Centers for Disease Control and Prevention. Lactic acidosis traced to thiamine deficiency related to nationwide shortage of multivitamins for total parenteral nutrition—United States, 1997. *MMWR Morb Mortal Wkly Rep.* 1997;46(23):523–528.

12. Ayers P, Adams S, Boullata J, et al.; American Society for Parenteral and Enteral Nutrition. A.S.P.E.N. Parenteral nutrition safety consensus recommendations. *JPEN J Parenter Enteral Nutr.* 2014;38(3):296–333.

13. Institute for Safe Medication Practices. ISMP list of high-alert medications in acute care settings. https://www.ismp.org/sites/default/files/attachments/2018-08/highAlert2018-Acute-Final.pdf. Accessed November 14, 2019.

14. Boullata J, Guenter P, Mirtallo J. A parenteral nutrition survey with gap-analysis. *JPEN J Parenter Enteral Nutr.* 2013;37(2):212–222.

15. Guenter, P Ayers P, Boullata J, Gura KM, Holcome B, Sacks GS. Parenteral nutrition errors and potential errors reported over the past 10 years. *Nutr Clin Pract.* 2017;32(6):826–830.

16. Institute for Safe Medication Practices. Results of ISMP survey on high-alert medications. *ISMP Med Saf Alert!* 2012;7(3):1–4.

17. Narula P, Hartigan D, Puntis JWL. The frequency and significance of errors related to parenteral nutrition in children. *Proc Nutr Soc.* 2010;69(OCE7):E556. doi:10.1017/S0029665110004258

18. Wollitz A, Grissinger M. Aligning the lines: an analysis of IV line errors. *Pa Patient Saf Advis.* 2014;11(1):1–7. http://patientsafety.pa.gov/ADVISORIES/Pages/201403_01.aspx. Accessed November 17, 2019.

19. Sacks GS, Rough S, Kudsk KA. Frequency and severity of harm of medication errors related to the parenteral nutrition process in a large university teaching hospital. *Pharmacotherapy.* 2009;29(8):966–974.

20. Cole C, Robertson S. Nine cases of unintentional rapid infusion of lipid emulsion in children: root cause analysis and changes to practice. *Arch Dis Child.* 2014;99(8):e3. doi:10.1136/archdischild-2014-306798.4

21. Khriesat W, Barham K, Abu-Ekteish F. A fat overload after fat emulsion high dose infusion in an infant. *Pediat Therapeut.* 2015;5(3):246. doi:10.4172/2161-0665.1000246

22. Khasawneh W, Hani SB. Intravenous lipid emulsion overdose in infancy: a case report and overview of opportunities. *Drug Saf Case Rep.* 2018;5(1):13. doi:10.1007/s40800-018-0079-y

23. Chuo J, Lambert G, Hicks RW. Intralipid medication errors in the neonatal intensive care unit. *Jt Comm J Qual Patient Saf.* 2007;33(2):104–111.

24. Hicks RW, Becker SC, Chuo J. A summary of NICU fat emulsion medication errors and nursing services: data from MEDMARX. *Adv Neonatal Care.* 2007;7(6):299–308; quiz 309–310.

25. Colevas AH, Rempe B. Nurse-sensitive indicators: integral to the Magnet journey. *Am Nurse Today.* 2011;6:39–41.

26. MacKay M, Anderson C, Boehme S, Cash J, Zobell J. Frequency and severity of parenteral nutrition medication errors at a large children's hospital after implementation of electronic ordering and compounding. *Nutr Clin Pract.* 2016;31(2):195–206.

27. National Health System. Patient safety alert: risk of severe harm and death from infusing total parenteral nutrition too rapidly in babies. Alert reference number: NHS/PSA/W/2017/005. https://improvement.nhs.uk/documents/1756/Patient_Safety_Alert_-_TPN_in_babies_FINAL.pdf. Published September 27, 2017. Accessed November 14, 2019.

28. National Health System. Rapid over infusion of parenteral nutrition. https://www.sps.nhs.uk/wp-content/uploads/2019/04/Rapid-over-infusion-of-Parenteral-Nutrition.pdf. Accessed November 15, 2019.

29. Guenter P, Worthington P, Ayers P, et al. Standardized competencies for parenteral nutrition administration: the ASPEN model *Nutr Clin Pract.* 2018;33(2):295–304.

30. Sacks GS. Safety surrounding parenteral nutrition systems. *JPEN J Parenter Enteral Nutr.* 2012;36(2 suppl):20S–22S.

31. Institute for Safe Medication Practices. The five rights cannot stand alone. *ISMP Med Saf Alert! Nurse AdviseERR.* 2004;2(11).

32. Boitano M, Bojak S, McCloskey S, McCaul DS, McDonough, M. Improving the safety and effectiveness of parenteral nutrition: results of a quality improvement collaboration. *Nutr Clin Pract.* 2010;25(6):663–671.

33. Gil ME, Mateu J. Treatment of extravasation from parenteral nutrition solution. *Ann Pharmacother.* 1998;32(1):51–55.

34. Kumar RJ, Pegg SP, Kimble RM. Management of extravasation injuries. *ANZ J Surg.* 2001;71(5):285–289.

35. Wilkens CE, Emmerson AJB. Extravasation injuries on regional neonatal units. *Arch Dis Child Fetal Neonatal Ed.* 2004;89(3):F274–F275.

36. Doellman D, Hadaway L, Bowe-Geddes LA, et al. Infiltration and extravasation. *J Infus Nurs.* 2009;32(4):203–211.

37. Benedetta B, Andres C. Extravasation of peripherally administered parenteral nutrition. *N Engl J Med.* 2011;364(10):e20. doi:10.1056/NEJMicm1006399

38. Infusion Nursing Society. Infusion therapy standards of practice. *J Infus Nurs.* 2016;39(1S):S1–S159.

39. Wiegand R, Brown J. Hyaluronidase for the management of dextrose extravasation. *Am J Emerg Med.* 2010;28(28):257.e1–e2. doi:10.1016/j.ajem.2009.06.010

40. Joint Commission Resources. Standard MM. In: DeMase K, ed. 2020 *Comprehensive Accreditation Manual for Hospitals.* Oakbrook Terrace, IL: The Joint Commission; 2020.

41. Konrad D, Mitchell R, Hendrickson E. Home nutrition support. In: Muller CM, ed. *ASPEN Adult Nutrition Support Core Curriculum.* 3rd ed. Silver Spring, MD: American Society for Parenteral and Enteral Nutrition; 2017:765–784.

42. Vanek VW, Ayers P, Charney P, et al. Follow-up survey on functionality of nutrition documentation and ordering nutrition therapy in currently available electronic health record systems. *Nutr Clin Pract.* 2016;31(3):401–415.

43. Vanek VW, Ayers P, Kraft M, et al; American Society for Parenteral and Enteral Nutrition; Academy of Nutrition and Dietetics; American Society of Health-System Pharmacists. A call to action for optimizing the electronic health record in the parenteral nutrition workflow. *Nutr Clin Practice.* 2018;33(5):e1–e21. doi:10.1002/ncp.10095

44. Pederson CA, Schneider PJ, Scheckelhoff DJ. ASHP national survey of pharmacy practice in hospital settings: monitoring and patient education—2012. *Am J Health Syst Pharm.* 2013;70(9):787–803.

45. Hilmas E, Peoples JD. Parenteral nutrition prescribing process using computerized prescriber order entry: opportunities to improve safety. *JPEN J Parenter Enteral Nutr.* 2012;36(2 suppl):32S–35S.

46. Kelly K, Harrington L, Matos P, Turner B, Johnson C. Creating a culture of safety around bar-code medication administration: an evidence-based evaluation framework. *J Nurs Adm.* 2016;46(1):30–37.

47. Shah K, Lo C, Babich M, Tsao NW, Bansback NJ. Bar code medication administration technology: a systematic review of impact on patient safety when used with computerized prescriber order entry and automated dispensing devices. *Can J Hosp Pharm.* 2016;69(5):394–402.

48. US Food and Drug Administration. Infusion pump risk reduction strategies for clinicians. http://www.fda.gov/MedicalDevices/ProductsandMedicalProcedures/ GeneralHospitalDevicesandSupplies/InfusionPumps/ucm205406.htm. Published April 2010. Accessed November 17, 2019.

49. Institute for Safe Medication Practices. Draft guidelines for optimizing safe implementation and use of smart infusion pumps. https://www.ismp.org/resources/draft-guidelines-optimizing-safe-implementation-and-use-smart-infusion-pumps. Published March 27, 2019. Accessed January 14, 2020.

50. Institute for Safe Medication Practices. Guidelines for safe implementation and use of smart pumps. http://ismp.org/Tools/guidelines/smartpumps/default.asp. Published March 7, 2008. Accessed November 16, 2019.

51. Schnock KO, Dykes PC, Albert J, et al. The frequency of intravenous medication errors related to smart infusion pumps: a multihospital observational study. *BMJ Qual Saf.* 2017;26(2):131–140.

52. Hertzel C, Souza VD. The use of smart pumps for preventing medication errors. *J Infus Nurs.* 2009;32(5):257–267.

53. Ohashi K, Dalleur O, Dykes PC, Bates DW. Benefits and risks of using smart pumps to reduce medication error rates: a systematic review. *Drug Saf.* 2014;37(12):1011–1120.

54. Cummings K, McGowan R. "Smart" infusion pumps are selectively intelligent. *Nursing.* 2011;41(3):58–59.

55. Hughes RG. Tools and strategies for quality improvement and patient safety. In: Hughes RG, ed. Patient Safety and Quality: An Evidence-Based Handbook for Nurses. (Prepared with support from the Robert Wood Johnson Foundation). AHRQ Publication No. 08-0043. Rockville, MD: Agency for Healthcare Research and Quality; 2008. https://archive. ahrq.gov/professionals/clinicians-providers/resources/nursing/resources/nurseshdbk/ FrontMatter_NursesHandbook.pdf. Accessed January 14, 2020.

56. Langley GL, Nolan KM, Nolan TW, Norman CL, Provost LP. *The Improvement Guide: A Practical Approach to Enhancing Organizational Performance.* 2nd ed. San Francisco: Jossey-Bass; 2009.

57. Pennsylvania Patient Safety Authority. The five rights: not the gold standard for safe medication practices. *PA-PSRS Patient Saf Advis.* 2005;2(2):9–10. http://patientsafety. pa.gov/ADVISORIES/Pages/200506_09.aspx. Accessed March 8, 2018

58. Resar R, Griffin FA, Haraden C, Nolan TW. Using care bundles to improve health care quality. IHI Innovation Series white paper. Cambridge, MA: Institute for Healthcare Improvement; 2012.

59. Rollins CJ. Total nutrient admixtures: stability issues and their impact on nursing practice. *J Intraven Nurs.* 1997;20(6):299–304.

60. Mundi MS, Edakkanambeth Varayil J, McMahon MT, et al. Accuracy of intravenous electrocardiography confirmation of peripherally inserted central catheter for parenteral nutrition. *Nutr Clin Pract.* 2016;32(2):207–210.

61. Perin G, Scarpa MG. Defining central venous line position in children: tips for the tip. *J Vasc Access.* 2015;16(2):77–86.

62. DeChicco R, Seidner DL, Brun C, Steiger E, Stafford J, Lopez R. Tip position of long-term central venous access devices used for parenteral nutrition. *JPEN J Parenter Enteral Nutr.* 2007;31(5):382–387.

63. The Joint Commission on Accreditation of Healthcare Organizations. Tubing misconnections—a persistent and deadly occurrence. *Sentinel Event Alert.* 2006;(36):1–3.

64. Pennsylvania Patient Safety Advisory. Tubing misconnections: making the connection to patient safety. *Pa Patient Saf Advis.* 2010;7(2):41–45.

65. AAMI Foundation/HTSI. Safety innovations: nine recommendations to prevent multiple line infusion medication errors. https://www.aamifoundation.org/wp-content/ uploads/2018/11/2012_SI_9_Recommendations_Multiple_Line_Infusion.pdf. Accessed November 17, 2019.

66. Guenter P, Hicks RW, Simmons D, et al. Enteral feeding misconnections: a consortium position statement. *Jt Comm J Qual Patient Saf.* 2008;34(5):285–292.

67. Simmons D, Symes L, Guenter P, Graves K. Tubing misconnections: normalization of deviance. *Nutr Clin Pract.* 2011;26(3):286–293.

68. Institute for Safe Medication Practices. Independent double checks: worth the effort used judiciously and properly. I*SMP Med Saf Alert!* 2019;24(11). https://www.ismp.org/resources/independent-double-checks-worth-effort-if-used-judiciously-and-properly. Accessed November 17, 2019.

69. Dickinson, A, McCall E, Twomey B, James N. Paediatric nurses' understanding of the process and procedure of double-checking medications. *J Clin Nurs.* 2010;19(5–6):728–735.

70. Lumpkin MM. Safety alert: hazards of precipitation with parenteral nutrition. *Am J Hosp Pharm.* 1994;51(11):1427–1428.

71. Cohen MR, Smeltzer JL. Selected medication safety risks to manage in 2016–Part I: intravenous fat emulsion needs a filter. *Hosp Pharm.* 2016;51(5):353–357.

72. American Society for Parenteral and Enteral Nutrition. Parenteral nutrition – new recommendations for in-line filters. ASPEN website. http://www.nutritioncare.org/News/General_News/Parenteral_Nutrition_%E2%80%93_New_Recommendations_for_In-line_Filters/. Accessed November 17, 2019.

73. Institute for Safe Medication Practices. Pharmacist supervision is critical for proper preparation of Clinimix multichamber bags. *ISMP Med Saf Alert! Nurse AdviseERR.* 2011;9(4):1–4.

74. Hoff DS, Michaelson AS. Effects of light exposure on total parenteral nutrition and its implications in the neonatal population. *J Pediatr Pharmacol Ther.* 2009;14(3):132–143.

75. Chessex P, Laborie S, Nasef N, Masse B, Lavoie JC. Shielding parenteral nutrition from light improves survival rate in premature infants: a meta-analysis. *JPEN J Parenter Enteral Nutr.* 2017;41(3):378–383.

76. Dolan SA, Felizardo G, Barnes S, et al. APIC position paper: safe injection, infusion and medication vial practices in health care. *Am J Infect Control.* 2010;38(3):167–172.

77. Committee on Nutrition, American Academy of Pediatrics; Kleinman RE, ed. *Pediatric Nutrition Handbook.* 6th ed. Elk Grove Village, IL: American Academy of Pediatrics; 2004.

78. Koletzko B, Goulet O, Hunt J, Krohn K, Shamir R; Parenteral Nutrition Guidelines Working Group; European Society for Clinical Nutrition and Metabolism; European Society of Paediatric Gastroenterology, Hepatology and Nutrition (ESPGHAN); European Society of Paediatric Research (ESPR). Guidelines on paediatric parenteral nutrition of the European Society of Paediatric Gastroenterology, Hepatology and Nutrition (ESPGHAN) and the European Society for Clinical Nutrition and Metabolism (ESPEN), supported by the European Society of Pediatric Research (ESPR). *J Pediatr Gastroenterol Nutr.* 2005;41(suppl 2):S1–S87.

79. Institute for Safe Medication Practices. Lack of standard dosing methods contribute to IV errors. ISMP Med Saf Alert! Nurse AdviseERR. 2007;12(17):1–3.

80. Suryadevara S, Celestin J, DeChicco R, et al. Type and prevalence of adverse events during the parenteral nutrition cycling process in patients being prepared for discharge. Nutr Clin Pract. 2012;27(2):268–273.

81. Austhof SI, DeChicco R, Corrigan ML, et al. Cycling parenteral nutrition from 24 hours to 12 hours in 1 step is safe in patients requiring long-term therapy [published online January 2013]. *JPEN J Parenter Enteral Nutr.* Abstract Data Supplement.

82. Stout SM, Cober MP. Metabolic effects of cyclic parenteral nutrition infusion in adults and children. *Nutr Clin Pract.* 2010;25(3):277–281.

83. Krzywda EA, Andris DA, Whipple JR, et al. Glucose response to abrupt discontinuation of total parenteral nutrition. *JPEN J Parenter Enteral Nutr.* 1993;17(1):64–67.

84. Norman JL, Crill CM. Optimizing the transition to home parenteral nutrition in pediatric patients. *Nutr Clin Pract.* 2011;26(3):273–285.

85. Newton AF, DeLegge MH. Home initiation of parenteral nutrition. *Nutr Clin Pract.* 2007;22(1):57–64.

86. Ayers J, Graves SA. Perioperative management of total parenteral nutrition, glucose containing solutions, and intraoperative glucose monitoring in paediatric patients: a survey of clinical practice. *Paediatr Anesth.* 2001;11(1):41–44.

87. Boullata JI, Gilbert K, Sacks GS, et al; American Society for Parenteral and Enteral Nutrition. A.S.P.E.N. clinical guidelines: parenteral nutrition ordering, order review, compounding, labeling, and dispensing. *JPEN J Parenter Enteral Nutr.*2014;38(3)334–377.

88. Ukleja A, Gilbert K, Mogensen KM, et al; Task Force on Standards for Nutrition Support: Adult Hospitalized Patients, American Society for Parenteral and Enteral Nutrition. Standards for nutrition support: hospitalized adult patients. *Nutr Clin Pract.* 2018;33(6):906–920.

89. Gil KM, Skeie B, Kvetan V, Askanazi J, Freidman MI. Parenteral nutrition and oral intake: effect of glucose and fat infusions. *JPEN J Parenter Enteral Nutr.* 1991;15(4):426–432.

90. Dervan N, Dowsett J, Gleeson E, Carr S, Corish C. Evaluation of over-and underfeeding following the introduction of a protocol for weaning from parenteral to enteral nutrition in the intensive care unit. *Nutr Clin Pract.* 2012;27(6):781–787.

91. DiBaise JK, Matarese LE, Messing B, Steiger E. Strategies for parenteral weaning in adult patients with short bowel syndrome. *J Clin Gastroenterol.* 2006;40(suppl 2):S94–S98.

92. Jeejeebhoy KN. Short bowel syndrome: a nutritional and medical approach. *CMAJ.* 2002;166(10):1297–1302.

93. Nauth J, Chang CW, Mobarhan S, Sparks S, Borton M, Svoboda S. A therapeutic approach to wean total parenteral nutrition in the management of short bowel syndrome: three cases using nocturnal enteral rehydration. *Nutr Rev.* 2004;62(5):221–231.

Complications of Parenteral Nutrition

Introduction

Complications associated with parenteral nutrition (PN) can be categorized as mechanical, metabolic, or infectious. Metabolic complications are more commonly associated with PN than enteral nutrition (EN). Therefore, patients receiving PN require close monitoring for prevention and early detection of complications. Mechanical complications related to the venous access device and infectious complications are presented elsewhere (see chapter 3). This chapter will focus on recognizing, preventing, and treating metabolic complications associated with PN in the adult patient.

Macronutrient-Related Complications

Hyperglycemia

Hyperglycemia is the most common complication associated with PN administration and can be caused by various factors. Stress-associated hyperglycemia in patients with acute illness and sepsis often develops as a result of insulin resistance, increased gluconeogenesis and glycogenolysis, and suppressed insulin secretion.[1] Excess carbohydrate administration has been associated with hyperglycemia, hepatic steatosis, and increased carbon dioxide production. American Society for Parenteral and Enteral Nutrition (ASPEN) clinical guidelines recommend a target blood glucose level of 140–180 mg/dL in the adult hospitalized patient receiving nutrition support.[2] PN should be initiated at half of the estimated energy needs or approximately 150–200 g of dextrose for the first 24 hours. Lesser dextrose delivery (approximately 100 g) is warranted in the patient with hyperglycemia requiring insulin therapy or a hypoglycemic agent. Carbohydrate administration should not exceed a rate of 4–5 mg/kg/min or 20–25 kcal/kg/d.[3] Capillary blood glucose concentrations should be monitored every 6 hours and more frequently in patients with hyperglycemia.

Blood glucose concentrations can be controlled with insulin therapy, which may be administered subcutaneously or intravenously via an insulin infusion or added directly to the PN formulation. An initial regimen of 0.05–0.1 units of insulin per gram of dextrose in the PN formulation is common unless a patient already has hyperglycemia, in which case 0.15–0.2 units of insulin per gram of dextrose is used. Supplemental subcutaneous regular insulin may be administered if needed using a sliding scale/correctional regimen. Two-thirds of the total amount of sliding-scale insulin required over 24 hours may then be added to the next day's PN formulation. Increases in dextrose concentrations in PN should not be implemented until serum glucose concentrations are under good control. Insulin should be proportionally increased and decreased with respect to the PN dextrose concentration. Alternatively, an insulin infusion, which provides a more consistent and safe glucose control, may be instituted. A proportional increase of lipid injectable emulsion (ILE) may be necessary to increase energy. Rarely, hyperglycemia may be due to chromium deficiency. Insulin is ineffective in patients with chromium deficiency. Increasing the chromium dose in the PN formulation beyond the standard amount in the commercially prepared, multiple trace element injections may be necessary.[4,5] Uncontrolled hyperglycemia may result in hyperosmolar hyperglycemia nonketotic dehydration, coma, and death secondary to osmotic diuresis.[6]

Hypoglycemia

PN-associated hypoglycemia can occur from excess insulin administration via the PN formulation or by intravenous (IV) infusion or subcutaneous injection. Excessive or erroneous administration of insulin is a severe medication error, and the resulting hypoglycemia may be life threatening. Treatment includes initiation of a dextrose 10% infusion, administration of dextrose 25 g (dextrose 50% in 50 mL), and/or stopping any source of insulin administration. Abrupt discontinuation of PN formulations has been associated with rebound hypoglycemia.[7] Studies have reported no symptomatic hypoglycemia after abruptly stopping PN infusions given over 16–24 hours.[8,9] However, nonsymptomatic hypoglycemia did occur in some patients. Patients requiring large doses of insulin have a greater propensity for rebound hypoglycemia, but predicting which patients will experience rebound hypoglycemia is difficult. Therefore, to reduce the risk of rebound hypoglycemia in susceptible patients, a 1- to 2-hour taper-down of the infusion, or half the infusion rate, may be necessary. If a PN formulation must be discontinued quickly, a dextrose-containing fluid should be infused for 1 or 2 hours following PN discontinuation to avoid possible rebound hypoglycemia. Obtaining a capillary blood glucose concentration 30 minutes to 1 hour after the PN formulation is discontinued will help identify rebound hypoglycemia.

Essential Fatty Acid Deficiency

ILE is generally provided as a source of essential fatty acids and as a nonprotein energy source. Although the incidence is low, several potential complications are associated with ILE use, such as infusion-related adverse reactions and allergy to the ILE components. Depending on the length of the PN therapy and the nutrition status of the patient, ILE-free PN may result in essential fatty acid deficiency (EFAD). Two polyunsaturated fatty acids, linoleic and α-linolenic acid, cannot be synthesized by the body and are considered essential. Clinical manifestations of EFAD include scaly dermatitis, alopecia, hepatomegaly, thrombocytopenia, fatty liver, and anemia.[10] Biochemical evidence of EFAD is determined by a triene-to-tetraene ratio of >0.2 and can occur within 1–3 weeks in adults receiving ILE-free PN.[11] The adult requirements for linoleic acid are met through exogenous sources or endogenously through the lipolysis of adipose tissue. However, when hypertonic dextrose is infused, insulin is secreted and lipolysis is reduced. Thus, an exogenous source of fat must be provided. To prevent EFAD, 1%–2% of daily energy requirements should be derived from linoleic acid, and about 0.5% of energy should be derived from linolenic acid.[12] This translates into approximately 250 mL of soy oil 20%–based ILE or 500 mL of soy oil 10%–based ILE administered over 8–10 hours, 2 times a week. Alternately, 500 mL of a soy oil 20% ILE can be given once a week. In patients who are intolerant to ILE, a trial of topical skin application or oral ingestion of safflower or sunflower seed oils to alleviate biochemical deficiency of EFAD may be given.[13,14]

The recently approved ILE products have less soy oil, and so proportionately higher volumes will need to be administered to provide the required dose. In general, when ILE is used as an energy source in doses sufficient to provide 15%–30% of total energy, enough essential fatty acids are administered to prevent EFAD.

Hypertriglyceridemia

Hypertriglyceridemia can occur with dextrose overfeeding or with rapid administration rates of ILE (>110 mg/kg/h). Hyperlipidemia may impair immune response, alter pulmonary hemodynamics, and increase the risk of pancreatitis.[15,16] Reducing the dose and/or lengthening the infusion time of soy oil ILE will help minimize these effects. Soy oil ILE intake should be restricted to <30% of total energy or 1 g/kg/d and be provided slowly during 8–10 hours at minimum if administered separately.[15] An alternate action would be to change soy oil ILE to a newer ILE product that has less soil oil and/or fewer medium-chain triglycerides. Serum triglyceride concentrations should be checked in any patient with a known history of hyperlipidemia prior to ILE administration. Acceptable serum triglyceride concentrations are <400 mg/dL.[12,17] Occasionally, serum triglyceride concentrations will rise in a patient who is fat intolerant. In such patients, ILE infusions should be reduced or discontinued. Pancreatitis due to ILE-induced hyperlipidemia is rare unless serum triglyceride concentrations exceed 1000 mg/dL. ILE is considered safe for use in patients with pancreatitis without hypertriglyceridemia.[18] However, ILE should be withheld from the PN regimen if serum triglyceride concentrations exceed 400 mg/dL.

Although rare, allergic reactions to ILE can occur, especially in patients with a history of egg allergy. This is most likely a result of the egg phospholipid that is used as an emulsifier. Soy allergic reactions are also possible with soy oil ILE. Other acute infusion-related adverse reactions include hyperlipidemia, dyspnea, cyanosis, flushing, sweating, dizziness, headache, back or chest pain, nausea, and vomiting.[19]

Azotemia

Excessive protein administration results in an increased metabolic demand on the body for disposing of the byproducts of protein metabolism. Prerenal azotemia can result from dehydration, excess protein, and/or inadequate nonprotein energy intake. Intolerance to the protein load will be exhibited by an increase in blood urea nitrogen. Patients with hepatic or renal disease are prone to developing azotemia because of the impaired ability to metabolize and eliminate urea. When urea clearance is impaired, dialysis may be required to assist with the elimination of urea and allow for the adequate intake of protein.

The incidence of hyperammonemia has been a rare occurrence since the advent of crystalline amino acid solutions. The early protein hydrolysates contained excessive amounts of ammonia and insufficient arginine for urea-cycle metabolism. However, hyperammonemia has been observed with the new crystalline amino acid solutions in patients with urea-cycle defects, such as ornithine transcarbamylase deficiency.[20,21]

Patients who develop an amino acid intolerance such as prerenal azotemia, hepatic encephalopathy, or hyperammonemia may benefit from a reduction in the amount of amino acids provided. In patients with hepatic failure and hepatic encephalopathy, the use of high branched-chain, low aromatic amino acid formulations has provided inconsistent results.

Micronutrient-Related Complications

Fluid and Electrolytes

Once macronutrient tolerance has been established, the routine management of the patient receiving PN centers on fluid and electrolytes. The requirements vary depending on the patient's renal, fluid, and electrolyte and nutrition (refer to refeeding section) status when starting PN as well as his or her underlying disease process and any losses that may incur.[22,23] Daily fluid and electrolyte shifts between the intracellular and extracellular space or changes in total body water or electrolyte content will require changes in the PN formulation composition and volume.

Evaluation of concurrent IV fluids and medications provided during PN therapy is necessary when determining the fluid and electrolyte status. PN formulations should be prescribed with consideration of all fluids being infused. Fluid and electrolyte replacement with separate IV fluids outside of the PN formulation may be necessary when the patient has excessive losses. Treatment involves replacing the lost fluids with IV fluids of similar electrolyte composition. Accurate intake and output records are necessary to show the amount of loss from various body fluids.

Vitamins

Vitamins are essential for effective nutrient utilization. A sustained exogenous intake of vitamins is essential to avoid deficiency. However, excessive intake of lipid-soluble vitamins A, D, E, and K has the potential for accumulation and therefore the capacity for toxicity. Provision of adequate vitamin intake in the patient receiving PN may be complicated by conditions that increase requirements, such as sepsis, trauma, or following surgery. Identifying vitamin deficiency or toxicity states can be difficult because of limitations in correlating serum vitamin concentrations with body stores and often because of vague clinical symptoms. Therefore, adult patients receiving PN should receive a standard daily dose of parenteral multivitamins.[17] Delaying IV multivitamin therapy until development of clinical signs of vitamin deficiency is inappropriate.

Certain clinical situations warrant special attention. Patients receiving both PN and warfarin therapy require close monitoring of the desired anticoagulation level because of the inclusion of vitamin K in some of the multivitamin preparations. PN supplementation with additional thiamin (25–100 mg/d) is reasonable in patients with a history of alcohol abuse, especially if the patient did not receive thiamin on hospital admission. Thiamin supplementation is also recommended on initiation of nutrition support therapy in patients with a prolonged history of poor dietary intake or severe weight loss. During parenteral multivitamin shortages in the United States in the late 1980s and 1990s, several cases of lactic acidosis due to thiamin deficiency were reported, including 3 deaths.[24] ASPEN recommends that the following practices be implemented during periods of short supply: (1) use oral or enterally administered multivitamins whenever possible, especially liquid multivitamins of defined content; (2) when all options to obtain IV multivitamins have been exhausted, ration use by reducing the dose by 50% or giving one dose 3 times a week; and (3) if IV multivitamins are no longer available, administer thiamin, ascorbic acid, pyridoxine, and folic acid daily as individual entities and vitamin B_{12} at least once per month.[25]

Vitamin toxicity, particularly of the fat-soluble vitamins, is also a potential complication of PN. Vitamin A toxicity has been reported in patients with chronic renal failure receiving PN. Therefore, some clinicians have recommended reducing the frequency of fat-soluble vitamin administration to twice per week in patients with renal failure. However, because no injectable multivitamin preparations are available without fat-soluble vitamins, the potential for developing water-soluble vitamin deficiency exists with restricted dosing. In addition, because some water-soluble vitamins may be lost with hemodialysis, provision of water-soluble vitamins to patients receiving dialysis has been recommended.[12] This requires use of an oral vitamin B-complex supplement or individual parenteral vitamin B supplementation, as available.

Several vitamins are known to undergo substantial degradation after addition to the PN admixture. This is not considered a significant problem in the acute care setting because of the relatively short time period between compounding and administration. However, when PN preparations are compounded in a batch fashion for patients in the home setting, this degradation must be considered. The degradation was clearly demonstrated in a home PN patient who developed night blindness within 6 months of receiving PN that was prepared on a weekly basis with the vitamins added to the PN preparation by the pharmacy before delivery.[26]

Although night blindness resolved after a therapeutic dose of vitamin A, symptoms returned 6 months later before the source of the problem was identified. Substantial amounts of vitamin A were likely lost to degradation and adsorption to the plastic matrix of the bag because the vitamins were added to the PN preparation up to a week before administration. Therefore, daily addition of vitamins to the PN preparation immediately before the infusion is recommended.[17]

Trace Elements

Trace element deficiency states are relatively uncommon in patients receiving PN but can occur with insufficient intake or increased utilization or excretion over a prolonged period. For example, zinc deficiency may occur in the patient with high intestinal losses. Cardiomyopathy caused by selenium deficiency has been reported in patients receiving long-term PN without selenium supplementation. The development of trace element excess is also a potential complication in the long-term PN patient and in the patient with hepatobiliary disease. Available parenteral multi-trace preparations may exceed actual requirements in many patients receiving PN.[27] In addition, many of the components of the PN admixture have been shown to be contaminated with trace elements such as zinc, copper, manganese, chromium, selenium, and aluminum.[28] Tissue elevations of copper, manganese, and chromium have been noted on autopsy in patients receiving long-term PN.[29] Although serum trace element monitoring at baseline and routine follow-up is recommended in patients receiving long-term PN, it is an unreliable measure of total body balance.[30] Empiric adjustments in trace element intake may be warranted. Reductions in manganese and copper dosing should be considered in patients with hepatobiliary disease due to impaired excretion. Removal of supplemental manganese from the PN formulation and reduction in the copper dose may be necessary in long-term PN patients.

Refeeding Syndrome

The delivery of energy, particularly in the form of carbohydrate, may induce refeeding syndrome in a patient with malnutrition. Refeeding syndrome refers to the metabolic and physiologic shifts of fluid, electrolytes, and minerals (eg, phosphorus, magnesium, and potassium) that occur as a result of aggressive nutrition support or nutrition repletion of a patient with malnutrition.[31] Carbohydrate delivery stimulates insulin secretion, which causes an intracellular shift of these electrolytes and minerals with the potential for severe hypophosphatemia, hypomagnesemia, and hypokalemia. Refeeding syndrome is characterized by symptoms of generalized fatigue, lethargy, muscle weakness, edema, cardiac arrhythmia, and hemolysis. Thus, for patients who are at risk for refeeding such as those with severe weight loss, prolonged decreased intake, or severe burns, calories should be initiated slowly by providing half of the energy requirements, or approximately 15 kcal/kg/d, on the first day of PN.[31] Recommendations differ with regard to initial protein dosing. The effect of protein on glycolysis is not as concerning as that of dextrose, so some have recommended starting at the goal dose for amounts ≤1.5 g/kg/d. Nutrition should be slowly advanced to full nutrition goal over the next 3–5 days as electrolytes are stabilized.

Hepatobiliary Complications

Disorders of the hepatic and biliary system are complications commonly reported in patients receiving PN. These complications may be life-threatening and are particularly concerning for patients dependent on long-term support. Mechanisms explaining the influence of PN on the development of liver disease are lacking. Historically, it was thought that some existing component of the PN formulation or nutrient not provided by the PN formulation caused the liver disease. However, that simplistic concept has been replaced with the realization that liver dysfunction can result from a complex set of risk factors present in patients receiving PN. The term PN-induced liver disease has therefore been replaced with the term PN-associated liver disease (PNALD).[32] Intestinal failure is a primary risk factor and therefore the term intestinal failure–associated liver disease (IFALD) has also been used.[33] The terms PNALD and IFALD (more commonly) have been used interchangeably to refer to hepatic dysfunction secondary to intestinal failure that occurs in the setting of PN.

Types of Hepatobiliary Disorders

The types of hepatobiliary disorders associated with PN differ among adult and pediatric patients, although the distinction becomes less evident in the patient on long-term PN. Three types of hepatobiliary disorders are associated with PN therapy: steatosis, cholestasis, and gallbladder sludge/stones; however, these disorders may coexist.[34] Steatosis, or hepatic fat accumulation, is predominant in adults and is generally benign. It typically presents as modest elevations of serum aminotransferase concentrations that occur within 2 weeks of PN therapy and may return to normal, even when PN is continued. Most patients are asymptomatic. Steatosis appears to be a complication of overfeeding and has probably decreased in prevalence over the years with the decrease in estimates of PN energy requirements. Although steatosis is generally thought to be a nonprogressive lesion, progression to fibrosis or cirrhosis may become an issue in patients receiving long-term PN.[35]

PN-associated cholestasis (PNAC) is a condition of impaired secretion of bile or frank biliary obstruction that occurs predominantly in children but may also occur in adult patients receiving long-term PN. PNAC typically presents as an elevation of alkaline phosphatase, γ-glutamyl transpeptidase (GGT), and conjugated (direct) bilirubin concentrations with or without jaundice. Although both GGT and alkaline phosphatase are sensitive markers for hepatobiliary disease, they lack specificity because serum levels may be elevated in other diseases as well. An elevated serum level of conjugated bilirubin is considered the prime indicator for cholestasis, typically defined as a concentration >2 mg/dL. PNAC is a serious complication because it may progress to cirrhosis and liver failure.

Gallbladder stasis during PN therapy may lead to the development of gallstones or gallbladder sludge with subsequent cholecystitis. It is related more to the lack of enteral stimulation than to the PN infusion itself. The lack of oral intake results in decreased cholecystokinin (CCK) release and impaired bile flow and gallbladder contractility. The duration of PN therapy appears to correlate with the development of biliary sludge.[36] Biliary sludge may progress to acute cholecystitis in the absence of gallstones. This condition is also referred to as acalculous cholecystitis.

Prevalence of Hepatobiliary Complications

Reported prevalence rates of IFALD vary greatly. In adult patients receiving PN, the reported incidence of abnormal enzyme elevations has varied from 25% to 100%.[34] However, few studies have correlated enzyme changes to permanent hepatic function or histological damage. Development of liver disease in patients receiving long-term PN is particularly concerning because its occurrence and severity appear to increase with longer duration of PN therapy. The prevalence of chronic cholestasis in a group of 90 patients receiving home PN for permanent intestinal failure was 55% at 2 years, 64% at 4 years, and 72% at 6 years.[35]

Many of the studies evaluating prevalence of IFALD also attempted to identify risk factors unrelated to the PN therapy. Bacterial and fungal infections have been documented to be associated with cholestasis. Sepsis likely causes liver inflammation because of the release of proinflammatory cytokines that are activated by endotoxins. This is especially relevant in the patient on long-term PN who may suffer from recurrent catheter-associated bloodstream infections. Many patients receiving PN have disorders that predispose them to developing small intestine bacterial overgrowth, which is considered another risk factor for liver disease. Bacterial overgrowth occurs when large amounts of bacteria normally confined to the colon and lower small bowel populate the upper small intestine. It has been postulated that these anaerobic bacteria in the small intestine may produce hepatotoxins. Massive intestinal resection has also been identified as a risk factor for IFALD.[35,37,38] A small bowel remnant <50 cm in length has been significantly associated with chronic cholestasis.[35]

PN-Related Risk Factors

Although supporting data are limited, various factors related to the nutrient composition of the PN formulation have been suggested to contribute to the development of hepatic complications. Therefore, it is important to evaluate the merits of these potential risk factors to design a PN formulation that minimizes risk of IFALD.

Energy. Clinical studies suggest that the development of steatosis during PN administration is primarily due to excessive energy intake.[34] Overfeeding of either combined or individual energy substrates (carbohydrate, fat, protein) can contribute to liver complications. The administration of excessive energy is thought to promote hepatic fat deposition by stimulating insulin release, which in turn promotes lipogenesis and inhibits fatty acid oxidation.[34]

Carbohydrate. Dextrose-based PN formulations that contain little or no fat have been implicated in the development of steatosis. Not only do excess carbohydrates deposit in the liver as fat, but a dextrose-based PN formulation may result in EFAD. EFAD may lead to impaired lipoprotein formation and triglyceride secretion, resulting in steatosis. Providing balanced dextrose and fat energy seems to decrease the incidence of steatosis, possibly by decreasing hepatic triglyceride uptake, and promoting fatty acid oxidation. A balanced PN formulation should provide 70%–85% of nonprotein energy as carbohydrate and 15%–30% as fat.[17] In addition, carbohydrate content should not exceed 7 g/kg/d in adults.

Protein. Early sources of amino acids for parenteral use included protein hydrolysates that had significant amounts of aluminum contamination. Animal studies suggest that high levels of aluminum contamination may lead to the development of cholestasis. However, the replacement of protein hydrolysates with crystalline amino acids has significantly reduced the overall aluminum contamination in PN admixtures. Although the role amino acids play in the development of cholestasis in adults is unclear, it does not appear to be as significant as it is in infants.

Lipid injectable emulsion. Various concerns exist regarding the role of ILE in the development of liver complications, including fat source, the phytosterol content, and the dose. In the United States, the soybean oil–based ILE contains high concentrations of ω-6 fatty acids and significant quantities of phytosterols. Phytosterols are inefficiently metabolized to bile acids by the liver, and it has been postulated that they may impair bile flow and cause biliary sludge and stones. Adult patients with short bowel syndrome receiving PN containing soybean-based ILE have been shown to have much higher serum phytosterol levels than other short bowel syndrome patients or healthy controls.[39] Case reports of children with PN-related cholestasis have documented high serum phytosterol levels.[40] In addition, concern exists that the high ω-6 fatty acid content of soybean-based ILE may initiate or worsen inflammatory states, and it has been shown to have immunosuppressive effects.[41] The presence of phytosterols and proinflammatory ω-6 fatty acids may contribute to the hepatotoxic effects seen in patients receiving long-term PN with a soybean oil–based ILE. The use of a fish oil–based ILE, primarily composed of ω-3 fatty acids and containing no phytosterols, has shown promising results in reversing IFALD in pediatric patients when used in place of soybean-based ILE.[41] A fish oil 100%–based ILE was recently approved for prevention of PNAC in pediatric patients.[42]

The soy oil ILE dose is another concern. Although liver complications have been associated with EFAD, they can also occur when the ILE dose is excessive. Steatosis can occur when the soy oil ILE infusion rate exceeds the liver's ability to clear the phospholipids and fatty acids, leading to direct deposition in the liver. Cholestasis may also be associated with high ILE doses, especially with long-term use. Multivariate analysis demonstrated that chronic cholestasis and severe IFALD were strongly associated with ILE intake >1 g/kg/d in patients receiving long-term PN.[35] The results demonstrated no association between dextrose intake or nonprotein energy intake and IFALD. In 2016, a 4-oil ILE containing soy, medium-chain triglyceride, olive oil, and fish oil was introduced in the United States market.[43] In late 2018, a soy and olive oil–based ILE was made available for use in adult patients in the United States.[44] Smaller studies have shown potential benefit for using these alternative ILEs in patients with elevated liver function tests.[45,46]

Carnitine. Carnitine plays an important role in fat metabolism. Primary carnitine deficiency has been associated with the development of steatosis. Because carnitine is not routinely added to PN, plasma carnitine concentrations may fall below the reference range within a few weeks of starting PN therapy. Carnitine supplementation has been shown to help mobilize hepatic fat stores and prevent steatosis in neonates receiving PN.[47] However, low serum carnitine concentrations do not necessarily correlate with hepatic dysfunction in adults. In adult home PN patients with abnormal serum liver enzymes and low serum carnitine concentrations, no improvement was shown in liver enzymes after carnitine was supplemented for 1 month, despite normalization of serum carnitine concentrations.[48] The role of carnitine in the prevention and treatment of PN-associated liver complications in adults remains to be established.

Choline. Choline is a nutrient found in many foods that is essential for normal function of all cells and required for lipid transport and metabolism. It is not a component of PN formulations because it is assumed that endogenous synthesis is possible from methionine contained in the crystalline amino acid solution. However, the conversion of methionine to choline may be less efficient when methionine is given parenterally than when given orally.[49] Low free-choline plasma concentrations have been reported in patients receiving long-term PN and have been associated with elevated serum hepatic aminotransferase concentrations. Steatosis reportedly resolved following choline supplementation.[49] Additional studies are needed to further evaluate the role of choline supplementation in the prevention and treatment of IFALD. At present, there is no commercially available injectable choline preparation.

Strategies to Manage PN-Associated Hepatobiliary Complications

When a patient receiving PN develops hepatic complications, a review of all aspects of care is necessary to identify and eliminate or treat other contributing factors. Table 8-1 outlines strategies to consider when a patient receiving PN develops these complications.

Table 8-1. Strategies to Manage PN-Associated Liver Complications

Strategies	Actions
1. Consider non-PN factors	Rule out: • Hepatotoxic medications • Herbal supplements • Biliary obstruction • Hepatitis • Sepsis
2. Consider PN modifications	Decrease dextrose Decrease soy oil ILE (<1 g/kg/d) Provide a balance of dextrose and ILE Cyclic PN infusion Recently available ILE[a]

Strategies	Actions
3. Maximize enteral intake	Encourage oral diet
	Tube feeding, even at slow rate
4. Prevent/treat bacterial overgrowth	Prescribe enteral antibiotics, such as:
	• Metronidazole
	• Neomycin
	• Doxycycline
	• Ciprofloxacin
	• Rifaximin
	In CIPO patients, consider agents to enhance motility:
	• Metoclopramide
	• Erythromycin
	• Tegaserod
	• Octreotide[b]
5. Pharmacotherapy	Prescribe aggressive treatment of infection
	Ursodeoxycholic acid (ursodiol)
	Treatment of pruritis:
	• Cholestyramine
	• Rifampin
	• Phenobarbital
6. Intestinal transplantation	Consider for patients with PN failure

CIPO: chronic intestinal pseudo-obstruction; ILE, lipid injectable emulsion; PN: parenteral nutrition.
[a]Recently available ILEs are SMOF43(Fresenius-Kabi) and Clinolipid44 (Baxter Healthcare).
[b]Octreotide delays gastric emptying but stimulates small intestinal motility.

Oral Nutrition and EN

Oral nutrition and EN should be optimized whenever feasible in the patient on long-term PN because even small amounts of dietary or enteral intake may be beneficial in promoting enterohepatic circulation of bile acids. Oral nutrition is generally preferable to tube feeding for obvious reasons, but tube feeding may offer certain advantages in select patients. For example, a trial of jejunal feeding at a slow infusion rate may be tolerated during a portion of the day or night in the patient with chronic intestinal pseudo-obstruction who is dependent on PN and requires gastric decompression. Medications to enhance motility may be necessary to aid success, and multiple attempts may be required before EN tolerance is achieved. During periods of acute illness, enteral tolerance may be more difficult to achieve, and setbacks can be expected, but attempts should be made to restart EN as soon as possible once the condition has stabilized. Patients with short bowel syndrome should be encouraged to maximize oral intake because at least some of their intake will be absorbed. Depending on the severity of the short bowel syndrome, a reduction in energy provided by PN may be necessary to prevent unwanted weight gain. However, fluid requirements generally remain high because stool output tends to increase when oral intake increases.

Cyclic Infusion

Cyclic PN infusion refers to the infusion of a PN formulation over <24 hours (generally 8–12 hours), allowing a period of time off PN. Continuous PN infusion can result in hyperinsulinemia and fat deposition in the liver and thereby potentially increase risk of liver complications. Cyclic PN infusion has been shown to reduce serum liver enzyme and conjugated bilirubin concentrations in comparison with continuous PN infusion.[50] Allowing a period of time each day off PN may reduce the risk of IFALD, especially in the patient dependent on long-term PN.

Pharmacotherapeutic Options

In addition to enteral intake, medications can also be used to help stimulate bile flow and maintain gallbladder contractility. Ursodiol (ursodeoxycholic acid) is a form of bile acid that has been widely used in the treatment of various chronic cholestatic liver diseases and has been shown to improve biochemical markers of cholestasis. When given orally at therapeutic doses, it becomes the predominant biliary bile acid and is thought to displace potentially hepatotoxic bile salts. Experience using ursodiol to treat PNAC is limited, but it may improve biochemical markers and symptoms of pruritis.[51] However, no evidence exists that the progression of disease is delayed. In addition, ursodiol has limited use in patients who cannot absorb oral medications because no IV form is available. CCK-octapeptide is a synthetic fragment of CCK that produces the biologic activities of CCK and is available in an injectable form. However, there is not enough evidence at this time to support its use in the prevention or treatment of PNAC. Phenobarbital has been used in relieving pruritis in patients with cholestasis and has been used in the treatment of other types of cholestatic liver disease. However, evidence supporting use for treating PNAC remains lacking.

Transplantation

In the patient receiving long-term PN with significant or progressive liver disease, an isolated intestinal or combined liver/intestinal transplant may be the only remaining treatment option.[52,53] Medicare has approved payment for intestinal transplantation in patients who fail PN therapy. One of the criteria used by Medicare to define PN failure is the development of impending or overt liver failure. The choice of isolated small bowel vs combined small bowel and liver transplantation depends on the extent of liver disease. Although many patients are able to discontinue PN after receiving intestinal transplantation, other life-threatening complications and quality-of-life issues must be considered before deciding on this option.

Metabolic Bone Disease

Osteoporosis and osteomalacia have been associated with long-term PN use. Osteoporosis is the most common form of metabolic bone disease and is defined as a loss of bone mass and microarchitectural deterioration of the skeleton leading to increased risk of fractures.[54] According to World Health Organization criteria, the diagnosis of osteoporosis is based on a bone mineral density measurement that is >2.5 standard deviations below the mean score of young adult ethnicity- and sex-matched controls. It is reported as a T-score below −2.5. A T-score that ranges between −1 and −2.5 is considered low bone mass, or osteopenia. Osteomalacia is characterized as softening and bending of the bones that occurs because the bones contain osteoid tissue that has failed to calcify. This generally occurs because of vitamin D deficiency. Bone biopsy for histologic examination of bone tissue is necessary for the diagnosis of osteomalacia and is, therefore, more difficult to identify. A combination of osteoporosis and osteomalacia may also occur.

Prevalence of Metabolic Bone Disease

The prevalence of PN-associated metabolic bone disease is unknown but is a concern in all patients requiring long-term PN. Osteoporosis was reported in 41% of patients after at least 6 months of home PN in one group[55] and in 67% of patients receiving long-term PN because of intestinal failure in another group.[56] Many diseases, conditions, and medications have been associated with bone loss (Table 8-2). Essentially all patients receiving long-term PN manifest at least one of these risk factors, and thus it is unclear whether or not PN actually contributes to accelerated bone loss. A follow-up study in a relatively large patient group receiving long-term PN showed moderate bone loss that was not statistically larger than in age- and sex-matched healthy patients.[57]

Table 8-2. Diseases or Conditions Associated with Bone Loss

General Diseases, Conditions, or Therapy	Specific Examples
Postmenopausal osteoporosis	NA
Long-term PN	NA
Endocrine disease	Cushing's syndrome Hypogonadism Amenorrhea Hyperthyroidism Hyperparathyroidism
GI disease	Crohn's disease Short bowel syndrome Malabsorption
Malignancy	Multiple myeloma Leukemia
Medications	Corticosteroids Heparin Warfarin Levothyroxine overreplacement Phenytoin Phenobarbital Leuprolide Methotrexate
Genetic disease	Osteogenesis imperfecta
Immobilization	Spinal cord injury Prolonged bed rest
Other	Alcohol abuse Anorexia nervosa

GI, gastrointestinal; NA, not applicable; PN, parenteral nutrition.

PN-Related Factors

Various factors related to the nutrient composition of the PN admixture have been suggested to interfere with bone metabolism.[58,59] Therefore, designing a PN formulation that minimizes the risk is important.

Calcium. Calcium plays a vital role in maintaining bone integrity by decreasing bone turnover and slowing bone loss. Patients receiving PN are particularly vulnerable to negative calcium balance because of limited intake and increased urinary calcium loss. Not only is calcium supplementation in the PN formulation limited by physical compatibility with phosphorus, but there also seems to be a threshold for calcium uptake when given parenterally. Higher calcium doses provided in the PN formulation are offset by higher urinary calcium losses. Therefore, the recommended daily intake of calcium gluconate added to the PN formulation is 10–15 mEq.[17] An inadequate phosphorus dose may also increase urinary calcium excretion. Phosphorus seems to enhance calcium reabsorption by the renal tubules and thereby promote a positive calcium balance. The recommended daily intake of phosphorus added to the PN formulation is 20–40 mmol.[17] Higher protein doses (2 g/kg/d as compared with 1 g/kg/d) in PN formulations have been associated with increased urinary calcium excretion, so reducing protein intake to maintenance doses whenever possible has been recommended. Chronic metabolic acidosis has also been associated with hypercalciuria and metabolic bone disease. Correction of the acidosis with acetate salts in the PN formulation has been shown to reduce urinary calcium excretion, so adequate amounts of acetate salts should be added to the PN formulation to avoid metabolic acidosis. Finally, cycling the PN infusion has been shown to result in higher urinary calcium losses in comparison with continuous infusion. However, this potential disadvantage associated with cyclic infusion should be weighed against its potential benefits to the liver and quality of life in patients receiving long-term PN in comparison with continuous infusion.

Vitamin D. Data regarding vitamin D requirements in patients receiving PN are controversial. Both vitamin D deficiency and vitamin D toxicity can result in bone disease. The adult multivitamin preparation used for PN formulations contains 200 international units of vitamin D (ergocalciferol or cholecalciferol). Vitamin D can be detrimental to the bone when excessive doses are given because it can suppress parathyroid hormone (PTH) secretion and directly promote bone resorption. Short-term removal of vitamin D from the PN formulation has been reported to result in decreased hypercalciuria and an improvement in osteomalacia, although the results may have been influenced by the presence of significant aluminum contamination. Removal of vitamin D for an average of 4.5 years in 9 long-term PN patients with low serum PTH and low

1,25-hydroxyvitamin D resulted in normal PTH and 1,25-hydroxyvitamin D concentrations and improvement in bone mineral density of the spine.[59] Although vitamin D removal may be beneficial in certain patients, such as those with a low serum PTH concentration, it is impractical because there are no commercially available injectable multivitamin preparations without vitamin D. Because vitamin D deficiency can also result in bone disease, it seems reasonable to provide PN patients with the maintenance vitamin D dose contained in the injectable multivitamin preparation. Excessive supplementation should be avoided.

Aluminum toxicity. Osteomalacia had been associated with PN formulations that once contained significant aluminum contamination because of protein hydrolysates. A low turnover bone disease and decreased bone formation was described in patients with elevated plasma, urine, and bone aluminum concentrations. Aluminum contamination of PN formulations is significantly lower now that crystalline amino acids have replaced protein hydrolysates. However, aluminum contamination is still a concern and has prompted the US Food and Drug Administration to establish labeling requirements. Manufacturers of large-volume parenterals, small-volume parenterals (SVPs), and pharmacy bulk packages (PBPs) used in PN compounding are required to measure the aluminum content of their product and disclose the concentration on the label.[55] LVPs, including amino acid and concentrated dextrose solutions, ILE, and sterile water for injection, are required to contain no more than 25 mcg/L of aluminum. There is no limit for the aluminum content in SVPs (ie, electrolyte salts) and PBPs (ie, parenteral multivitamins and trace element solutions), but manufacturers are required to provide the maximum aluminum level at expiry in the products' labeling.

Magnesium deficiency. Hypocalcemia is a prominent manifestation of magnesium deficiency. Magnesium deficiency results in decreased mobilization of calcium from bone through several mechanisms. Hypomagnesemia causes an increased release of magnesium ions at the bone surface in exchange for increased bone uptake of calcium ions from the serum. In addition, chronic severe hypomagnesemia inhibits PTH release, resulting in inappropriately low PTH levels for the degree of hypocalcemia. The response of bone to PTH can also be diminished, resulting in functional hypoparathyroidism. Hypomagnesemic hypocalcemia should be treated with magnesium supplementation because it is often refractory to calcium therapy alone. Magnesium deficiency can also lead to hypophosphatemia because of increased phosphorus excretion.

Copper deficiency. Copper deficiency impairs bone formation and can cause osteoporosis. Bone disease has been reported in infants receiving a copper-free PN formulation.[60]

Prevention and Management

Because most patients with osteoporosis are asymptomatic, a screening process is important to identify patients at risk. A thorough history, physical examination, and laboratory assessment should be performed to identify risk factors. Decreased height may occur as a result of compression fractures of the vertebral bodies in patients receiving long-term PN. A baseline dual energy x-ray absorptiometry scan is recommended for all patients who require long-term PN therapy. If results are normal, then follow-up bone mineral density measurements may be considered in 2–3 years.[61] If osteopenia or osteoporosis is present, repeat measurement should be considered in 1–2 years.

In addition to routine laboratory monitoring, patients with low bone mineral density may require further diagnostic testing, including measurement of thyroid-stimulating hormone, intact PTH, 25-hydroxyvitamin D, 24-hour urine calcium and magnesium, urine markers of bone turnover (such as N-teliopeptide collagen), and serum markers of bone turnover (such as osteocalcin and C-teliopeptide collagen).

Strategies to prevent and treat osteoporosis should be considered in all patients who require long-term PN therapy, as outlined in Table 8-3. The PN formulation should be designed to minimize hypercalciuria; provide adequate magnesium, calcium, and phosphorus; avoid metabolic acidosis; provide vitamins and trace elements; and minimize aluminum contamination.[62] Selection of individual products with the lowest reported maximal aluminum content should be used in PN compounding whenever possible, such as the use of sodium phosphate instead of potassium phosphate.[57]

Patients with osteoporosis should be educated on lifestyle modifications, low-intensity exercises, and fall prevention measures to minimize risk. Medications are available that have shown safety and efficacy in improving bone mineral density and decreasing fracture risk in patients with osteoporosis. Medications used for the prevention or treatment of osteoporosis that decrease bone resorption include bisphosphonates, raloxifene (a selective estrogen-receptor modulator), calcitonin, estrogen, and the newly approved monoclonal antibody denosumab. Teriparatide is the only approved medication that stimulates bone formation.

Table 8-3. Strategies to Prevent and Treat Osteoporosis in Long-term PN Patients

Strategy	Considerations
PN modifications	Avoid high doses of protein.
	Avoid excessive doses of sodium.
	Provide calcium 10–15 mEq/d.
	Provide phosphorus 20–40 mmol/d.
	Treat metabolic acidosis.
	Maintain adequate magnesium intake.
	Maintain adequate copper intake.
	Minimize aluminum contamination.
	Avoid adding heparin.
Lifestyle modification	Do weight-bearing exercise
	Stop smoking.
	Reduce caffeine.
	Reduce alcohol.
Fall prevention measures	Ensure home safety.
	Discontinue medications that may increase risk of falls, if possible.
Calcium	Consider oral supplementation.
Antiresorptive agents	Avoid oral route because of malabsorption and tolerance issues.
	Consider IV bisphosphonate (ie, zoledronic acid 5 mg IV once yearly).
Estrogen	Estrogen is approved for prevention of postmenopausal osteoporosis but may not be safest option.
	Raloxifene, a selective estrogen-receptor modulator, is approved for prevention and treatment of postmenopausal osteoporosis.
Nasal calcitonin	Shown to reduce risk of vertebral fractures, but not hip fractures.
Teriparatide	Recombinant human PTH.
	Stimulates bone formation.
	Dose approved for osteoporosis is 20 mcg subcutaneously daily for up to 2 y.

IV, intravenous; PN, parenteral nutrition; PTH, parathyroid hormone.

Special considerations are required in the pharmacologic approach to the treatment of osteoporosis in PN-dependent patients because of impaired gastrointestinal (GI) absorption of oral medications. Oral bisphosphonate therapy, including alendronate and risedronate, are considered first-line treatment options in the general population but are problematic in PN patients. Oral bioavailability of these agents is <1% in the fasting state of normal patients and requires special measures to ensure adequate absorption even when GI anatomy and function are normal. The ability to achieve adequate absorption in patients with impaired absorptive capacity is questionable. In addition, oral bisphosphonates can cause mucosal inflammation and ulceration, which may lead to GI intolerance. IV bisphosphonate therapy provides a therapeutic option for PN patients. Zoledronic acid is approved for the treatment of postmenopausal osteoporosis, and pamidronate has been effectively used off-label for the treatment of postmenopausal osteoporosis.[62-66] Teriparatide, recombinant human PTH, is approved for treatment of glucocorticoid-induced osteoporosis, postmenopausal osteoporosis, and osteoporosis in men. Its subcutaneous route of administration offers a therapeutic option for patients unable to take oral medications. Although IV bisphosphonate agents and teriparatide may provide a safe and effective therapeutic option for the treatment of PN-associated metabolic bone disease, further study is warranted. To date, only a single randomized controlled study has evaluated the use of bisphosphonate therapy in patients on home PN.[67]

Summary

Patients receiving PN therapy are at risk of developing metabolic complications and therefore require close monitoring. Refeeding syndrome and hyperglycemia are particular concerns in patients receiving PN in the acute care setting. In patients receiving long-term PN, the development of micronutrient abnormalities, hepatobiliary complications, and metabolic bone disease are concerns. Although the PN itself may not be the sole cause of these complications, efforts to minimize contributing risk factors from the PN formulation should be taken. A thorough monitoring plan is required to identify and prevent the development of both short and long-term metabolic complications in all patients receiving PN.

References

1. Lewis KS, Kane-Gill SL, Bobek MB, Dasta JF. Intensive insulin therapy for critically ill patients. *Ann Pharmacother.* 2004;38(7–8):1243–1251.

2. McMahon MM, Nystrom E, Braunschweig C, Miles J, Compher C; American Society for Parenteral and Enteral Nutrition (A.S.P.E.N.) Board of Directors; American Society for Parenteral and Enteral Nutrition. A.S.P.E.N. clinical guidelines: nutrition support of adults with hyperglycemia. *JPEN J Parenter Enteral Nutr.* 2013;37(1):23–36.

3. McMahon MM. Management of parenteral nutrition in acutely ill patients with hyperglycemia. *Nutr Clin Pract.* 2004;19(2):120–128.

4. Hopkins LL Jr, Ransome-Kuti O, Majaj AS. Improvement of impaired carbohydrate metabolism by chromium (III) in malnourished infants. *Am J Clin Nutr.* 1968;21(3):203–211.

5. Jeejeebhoy KN, Chu RC, Marliss EB, Greenberg GR, Bruce-Robertson A. Chromium deficiency, glucose intolerance, and neuropathy reversed by chromium supplementation, in a patient receiving long-term total parenteral nutrition. *Am J Clin Nutr.* 1977;30(4):531–538.

6. McCurdy DK. Hyperosmolar hyperglycemia nonketotic diabetic coma. *Med Clin North Am.* 1970;54(3):683–699.

7. Stout SM, Cober MP. Metabolic effects of cyclic parenteral nutrition infusion in adults and children. *Nutr Clin Pract.* 2010;25(3):277–281.

8. Krzywda EA, Andris DA, Whipple JK, et al. Glucose response to abrupt initiation and discontinuation of total parenteral nutrition. *JPEN J Parenter Enteral Nutr.* 1993;17(1):64–67.

9. Eisenberg PG, Gianino S, Clutter WE, Fleshman JW. Abrupt discontinuation of cycled parenteral nutrition is safe. *Dis Colon Rectum.* 1995;38(9):933–939.

10. Hamilton C, Austin T, Seidner DL. Essential fatty acid deficiency in human adults during parenteral nutrition. *Nutr Clin Pract.* 2006;21(4):387–394.

11. Holman RT, Smythe L, Johnson S. Effect of sex and age on fatty acid composition of human serum lipids. *Am J Clin Nutr.* 1979;32(12):2390–2399.

12. A.S.P.E.N. Board of Directors and The Clinical Guidelines Task Force. Guidelines for the use of parenteral and enteral nutrition in adult and pediatric patients [erratum in *JPEN J Parenter Enteral Nutr.* 2002;26(2):144]. *JPEN J Parenter Enteral Nutr.* 2002;26(1 suppl):1SA–138SA.

13. Miller DG, Williams SK, Palombo JD, Griffin RE, Bistrian BR, Blackburn GL. Cutaneous application of safflower oil in preventing essential fatty acid deficiency in patients on home parenteral nutrition. *Am J Clin Nutr.* 1987;46(3):419–423.

14. Friedman Z, Shochat SJ, Maisels MJ, Marks KH, Lamberth EL Jr. Correction of essential fatty acid deficiency in newborn infants by cutaneous application of sunflower-seed oil. *Pediatrics* 1976;58(5):650–654.

15. Seidner DL, Mascioli EA, Istfan NW, et al. Effects of long-chain triglyceride emulsions on reticuloendothelial system function in humans. *JPEN J Parenter Enteral Nutr.* 1989;13(6):614–619.

16. Carpentier YA, Kinney JM, Sidedrova VS, et al. Hypertriglyceridemia clamp: a new model for studying lipid metabolism. *Clin Nutr.* 1990:9(suppl 1):1–9.

17. Mirtallo J, Canada T, Johnson D, et al.; Task Force for the Revision of Safe Practices for Parenteral Nutrition. Safe practices for parenteral nutrition [erratum in JPEN J Parenter Enteral Nutr. 2006;30(2):177]. *JPEN J Parenter Enteral Nutr.* 2004;28(6):S39–S70.

18. Adamkin DH, Gelke KN, Andrews BF. Fat emulsions and hypertriglyceridemia. *JPEN J Parenter Enteral Nutr.* 1984;8(5):563–567.

19. Warshawsky KY. Intravenous fat emulsions in clinical practice. *Nutr Clin Pract.* 1992;7(4):187–196.

20. Kapila S, Saba M, Lin CH, Bawle EV. Arginine deficiency-induced hyperammonemia in a home total parenteral nutrition-dependent patient: a case report. *JPEN J Parenter Enteral Nutr.* 2001;25(5):286–288.

21. Felig DM, Brusilow SW, Boyer JL. Hyperammonemic coma due to parenteral nutrition in a woman with heterozygous ornithine transcarbamylase deficiency. *Gastroenterology.* 1995;109(1):282–284.

22. Sacks GS, Mayhew S, Johnson D. Parenteral nutrition implementation and management. In: Merritt RM, ed. *The A.S.P.E.N. Nutrition Support Practice Manual.* 2nd ed. Silver Spring, MD: American Society for Parenteral and Enteral Nutrition; 2005:108–117.

23. Kraft MD, Btaiche IF, Sacks GS, Kudsk KA. Treatment of electrolyte disorders in adult patients in the intensive care unit. *Am J Health Syst Pharm.* 2005;62(16):1663–1682.

24. Centers for Disease Control and Prevention. Lactic acidosis traced to thiamine deficiency related to nationwide shortage of multivitamins for total parenteral nutrition—United States, 1997 [erratum in *JAMA.* 1997;278(5):380]. JAMA. 1997;278(2):109, 111.

25. American Society for Parenteral and Enteral Nutrition. A.S.P.E.N. Information to use in the event of an intravenous multivitamin shortage—May 2012. ASPEN website. http://www.nutritioncare.org/guidelines_and_clinical_resources/clinical_practice_library/information_to_use_in_the_event_of_an_iv_multivitamin_shortage/. Accessed January 14, 2020.

26. Howard L, Chu R, Feman S, Mintz H, Oversen L, Wolf B. Vitamin A deficiency from long-term parenteral nutrition. *Ann Intern Med.* 1980;93(4):576–577.

27. Vanek VW, Borum P, Buchman A, et al; Novel Nutrient Task Force, Parenteral Multi-Vitamin and Multi–Trace Element Working Group; American Society for Parenteral and Enteral Nutrition (A.S.P.E.N.) Board of Directors. A.S.P.E.N. position paper: recommendations for changes in commercially available parenteral multivitamin and multi-trace element products. *Nutr Clin Pract.* 2012;27(4):440–491.

28. Pluhator-Murton MM, Fedorak RN, Audette RJ, Marriage BJ, Yatscoff RW, Gramlich LM. Trace element contamination of total parenteral nutrition.1. Contribution of component solutions. *JPEN J Parenter Enteral Nutr.* 1999;23(4):222–227.

29. Howard L, Ashley C, Lyon D, Shenkin A. Autopsy tissue trace elements in 8 long-term parenteral nutrition patients who received the current U.S. Food and Drug Administration formulation. *JPEN J Parenter Enteral Nutr.* 2007;31(5):388–396.

30. Buchman AL, Howard LJ, Guenter P, Nishikawa RA, Compher CW, Tappenden KA. Micronutrients in parenteral nutrition: too little or too much? The past, present, and recommendations for the future. *Gastroenterology.* 2009;137(5 suppl):S1–S6.

31. Solomon SM, Kirby DF. The refeeding syndrome: a review. *JPEN J Parenter Enteral Nutr.* 1990;14(1):90–97.

32. Kumpf VJ. Parenteral nutrition-associated liver disease in adult and pediatric patients. *Nutr Clin Pract.* 2006;21(3):279–290.

33. Kelly DA. Intestinal failure-associated liver disease: what do we know today? *Gastroenterology.* 2006;130(2 suppl 1):S70–S77.

34. Quigley EM, Marsh MN, Shaffer JL, Markin RS. Hepatobiliary complications of total parenteral nutrition. *Gastroenterology.* 1993;104(1):286–301.

35. Cavicchi M, Beau P, Crenn P, Degott C, Messing B. Prevalence of liver disease and contributing factors in patients receiving home parenteral nutrition for permanent intestinal failure. *Ann Intern Med.* 2000;132(7):525–532.

36. Messing B, Bories C, Kunstlinger F, Bernier JJ. Does total parenteral nutrition induce gallbladder sludge formation and lithiasis? *Gastroenterology.* 1983;84(5 pt. 1):1012–1019.

37. Luman W, Shaffer JL. Prevalence, outcome and associated factors of deranged liver function tests in patients on home parenteral nutrition. *Clin Nutr.* 2002;21(4):337–343.

38. Buchman A. Total parenteral nutrition-associated liver disease. *JPEN J Parenter Enteral Nutr.* 2002;26(5 suppl):S43–S48.

39. Ellegård L, Sunesson A, Bosaeus I. High serum phytosterol levels in short bowel patients on parenteral nutrition support. *Clin Nutr.* 2005;24(3):415–420.

40. Btaiche IF, Khalidi N. Parenteral nutrition-associated liver complications in children. *Pharmacotherapy.* 2002;22(2):188–211.

41. de Meijer VE, Gura KM, Meisel JA, Le HD, Puder M. Parenteral fish oil monotherapy in the management of patients with parenteral nutrition-associated liver disease. *Arch Surg.* 2010;145(6):547–551.

CHAPTER 8

42. Onegevan [package insert]. Graz, Austria: Fresenius Kabi; 2018. FDA website. https://www.accessdata.fda.gov/drugsatfda_docs/label/2018/0210589s000lbledt.pdf. Accessed December 10, 2019.

43. Smoflipid [package insert]. Smoflipid website. Uppsala, Sweden: Fresenius Kabi; 2016. https://smoflipid.com/wp-content/themes/smoflipid/Smoflipid-PI.pdf. Accessed December 10, 2019.

44. Clinolipid [package insert]. Deerfield, IL: Baxter Healthcare; 2016.http://www.baxterpi.com/pi-pdf/Clinolipid+PI.pdf. Accessed December 10, 2019.

45. Klek S, Szczepanek K, Scislo, et.al. Intravenous lipid emulsions and liver function in adult chronic intestinal failure patients: results from a randomized clinical trial. *Nutrition.* 2018;55–56:45–50.

46. Cai W, Calder PC, Cury-Boaventurs MF, et.al. Biological and clinical aspects of an olive oil-based lipid emulsion-a review. *Nutrients* 2018;10(6):E776. doi:10.3390/nu10060776

47. Bowyer BA, Miles JM, Haymond MW, Fleming CR. L-carnitine therapy in home parenteral nutrition patients with abnormal liver tests and low plasma carnitine concentrations. *Gastroenterology.* 1988;94(2):434–438.

48. Chawla RK, Berry CJ, Kutner MH, Rudman D. Plasma concentrations of transsulfuration pathway products during nasoenteral and intravenous hyperalimentation of malnourished patients. *Am J Clin Nutr.* 1985;42(4):577–584.

49. Buchman AL. The addition of choline to parenteral nutrition. *Gastroenterology.* 2009;137(5 suppl):S119–S128.

50. Hwang TL, Lue MC, Chen LL. Early use of cyclic TPN prevents further deterioration of liver functions for the TPN patients with impaired liver function. *Hepatogastroenterology.* 2000;47(35):1347–1350.

51. San Luis VA, Btaiche IF. Ursodiol in patients with parenteral nutrition-associated cholestasis. *Ann Pharmacother.* 2007;41(11):1867–1872.

52. Buchman AL, Scolapio J, Fryer J. AGA technical review on short bowel syndrome and intestinal transplantation. *Gastroenterology.* 2003;124(4):1111–1134.

53. Staun M, Pironi L, Bozzetti F, et al; ESPEN. ESPEN guidelines on parenteral nutrition: home parenteral nutrition (HPN) in adult patients. Clin Nutr. 2009;28(4):467–479.

54. Consensus development conference: diagnosis, prophylaxis and treatment of osteoporosis. *Am J Med.* 1993;94(6):646–650.

55. Pironi L, Labate AM, Pertkiewicz M, et al; ESPEN-Home Artificial Nutrition Working Group. Prevalence of bone disease in patients on home parenteral nutrition. *Clin Nutr.* 2002;21(4):289–296.

56. Cohen-Solal M, Baudoin C, Joly F, et al. Osteoporosis in patients on long-term home parenteral nutrition: a longitudinal study. *J Bone Miner Res.* 2003;18(11):1989–1994.

57. Haderslev KV, Tjellesen L, Haderslev PH, Staun M. Assessment of the longitudinal changes in bone mineral density in patients receiving home parenteral nutrition. *JPEN J Parenter Enteral Nutr.* 2004;28(5):289–294.

58. Seidner DL. Parenteral nutrition-associated metabolic bone disease. *JPEN J Parenter Enteral Nutr.* 2002;26(5 suppl):S37–S42.

59. Buchman AL, Moukarzel A. Metabolic bone disease associated with total parenteral nutrition. *Clin Nutr.* 2000;19(4):217–231.

60. Hurwitz M, Garcia MG, Poole RL, Kerner JA. Copper deficiency during parenteral nutrition: a report of four pediatric cases. *Nutr Clin Pract.* 2004;19(3):305–308.

61. Verhage AH, Cheong WK, Allard JP, Jeejeebhoy KN. Harry M. Vars Research Award. Increase in lumbar spine bone mineral content in patients on long-term parenteral nutrition without vitamin D supplementation. *JPEN J Parenter Enteral Nutr.* 1995;19(6):431–436.

62. Reid IR, Brown JP, Burckhardt P, et al. Intravenous zoledronic acid in postmenopausal women with low bone mineral density. *N Engl J Med.* 2002;346(9):653–661.

63. Department of Health and Human Services; US Food and Drug Administration. Amendment of regulations on aluminum in large and small volume parenterals used in total parenteral nutrition; delay of effective date. *Fed Regist.* 2003;68(106):32979–32981.

64. Smith BS, Kothari H, Hayes BD, et al. Effect of additive selection on calculated aluminum content of parenteral nutrient solutions. *Am J Health Syst Pharm.* 2007;64(7):730–739.

65. Miller RG, Chreitien KC, Meoni LA, Liu YP, Klag MJ, Levine MA. Comparison of intravenous pamidronate to standard therapy for osteoporosis. Use in patients unable to take oral bisphosphonates. *J Clin Rheumatol.* 2005;11(1):2–7.

66. Vis M, Bultink IEM, Dijkmans BA, Lems WF. The effect of intravenous pamidronate versus oral alendronate on bone mineral density in patients with osteoporosis. *Osteoporos Int.* 2005;16(11):1432–1435.

67. Haderslev KV, Tjellesen L, Sorensen HA, Staun M. Effect of cyclical intravenous clodronate therapy on bone mineral density and markers of bone turnover in patients receiving home parenteral nutrition. *Am J Clin Nutr.* 2002;76(2):482–488.

CHAPTER 8

Competency in Parental Nutrition: Prescribing, Order Writing, and Administration

Introduction

Parenteral nutrition (PN) provision requires careful interpretation of clinical and laboratory data, multidisciplinary communication, and vigilant surveillance for unintended complications. The process is prone to a variety of potential errors during each step, from PN prescription to order writing to delivery. The practices and safeguards surrounding this process are critical to maintaining patient safety.

Competencies in PN Prescribing[i]

In 2012, patients received PN during approximately 320,000 hospital stays, whereas many others received it in the home or in long-term care settings.[1] Compared with most other medications, ordering PN varies considerably among organizations, as reported in a survey of current PN practices performed in 2011, in which a number of trends were reported.[2] In this survey, members of the primary medical or surgical

---

i   **Source:** Adapted with permission from Guenter P, Boullata JI, Ayers P, et al; Parenteral Nutrition Safety Task Force, ASPEN. Standardized competencies for parenteral nutrition prescribing: The American Society for Parenteral and Enteral Nutrition Model. *Nutr Clin Pract.* 2015;30(4):570–576.

service prescribed PN most often (71.6%), with nutrition support team members (30.5%), pharmacists (28.3%), dietitians (20.9%), advanced practice nurses (14.7%), or physician assistants (PAs; 12.8%) also involved in ordering PN. In organizations with a smaller daily census (<200), PN was also most commonly ordered by the primary clinical service members (75.3%), followed by pharmacists (29.8%), nutrition support team members (21.8%), and dietitians (21.5%). This trend was similar in organizations with ≤5 PN orders daily (76%, 27.8%, 23.5%, and 21.1%, respectively). The PN order was most often communicated in handwriting using a standard order form (62.1%), with an additional 5.1% communicating with handwriting using a nonstandardized order. Electronic order entry was only available in 32.7% of organizations, and just over half of those used a standardized process. When standardized order entry occurred, it was available to adult patients (96.7%) much more often than for pediatric patients (36.5%) or neonates (46%).[2]

American Society for Parenteral and Enteral Nutrition (ASPEN) PN clinical guidelines addressed the education of prescribers as a way to improve PN ordering.[3] The prescriber should be well versed in the appropriate indications for PN, formulation design (volume, macronutrient and micronutrient composition) for patients of differing weights, medical and surgical conditions, and metabolic management. Prescribers should also be knowledgeable about vascular access devices (VADs; peripheral and central) and their associated complications. There is scant literature evaluating the direct impact of safe prescribing education programs on the outcomes of patients receiving PN. However, interdisciplinary teams applying education as part of an overall quality intervention have been successful in reducing unnecessary PN use and decreasing errors.[4]

Judicious PN order review and appropriate modification of daily orders is also critical to optimize patient safety. On the basis of pharmacists' survey responses, the pharmacy receiving the PN order may have been onsite or at a remote location and commonly dedicated a pharmacist to verify, review, and clarify PN orders. Most facilities (60.2%) dedicate 0.6 full-time equivalents or more to this effort, although 23.1% of respondents did not have any dedicated pharmacist time for these processes. According to this survey, when a pharmacist was involved, both a clinical review (eg, allergy, indication for PN, dosing; 88.2%) and a pharmaceutical review (eg, stability and compatibility of the formulation; 92.8%) of the PN order took place. According to 68.5% of survey respondents, clarification is required for ≤10% of PN orders, another 20.6% reported that clarifications are required for 11%–25% of PN orders, and the remaining 10.9% of respondents reported that clarifications are needed for 26%–100% of orders.

There are many reasons for requiring clarification of the PN order, although no specific component of the PN admixture stands out more than another. When a prescribed PN order is expected to be unstable on order review, the responsibility to rewrite the order is relegated to the pharmacist twice as often as to the original prescriber. In 69.7% of organizations, a pharmacist can adjust electrolyte additives most commonly as per guideline or protocol (64.2%) or with individual prescriber approval (35.8%).[2] Therefore, competent PN prescribers would reduce the need for order clarification and revision. Permanent and easily retrievable documentation is required to further determine appropriate prescribing processes.

Adding to the complexity of PN prescribing are 3 inconsistencies in PN practices. First, nutrient dosing in PN orders may follow a number of different formats from amount per day, amount per volume, or amount per liter to percent final concentration. Second, the error-prone step of PN order transcription is still required in the majority of organizations. Third, for transitions in patient care, PN orders are communicated by a number of individuals, including the case manager, dietitian, nurse, pharmacist, or physician.

Recently, changes have occurred in PN prescribing patterns with the increase in midlevel prescribers such as nurse practitioners (NPs) and PAs. The 2014 Centers for Medicare and Medicaid Services (CMS) final rule permitting clinically qualified nutrition professionals, including registered dietitians (RDs), to be privileged to prescribe patient diets under the hospital conditions of participation states that patient diets, "including therapeutic diets, must be ordered by a practitioner responsible for the care of the patient, or by a qualified dietitian or qualified nutrition professional as authorized by the medical staff and in accordance with state law governing dietitians and nutrition professionals."[5]

With these prescribing trends, changes in the CMS rules, and the recent publication of prescribing recommendations from the ASPEN PN clinical guidelines and safety consensus recommendations, the next logical step was to develop a model for standardized competencies around PN prescribing that all institutions may use.[3,6] A model for PN standardized competencies would allow for consistency among institutions and offer a template for a variety of nutrition professionals to identify a minimum standard level of knowledge and skills for prescribing this complex drug therapy. Regardless of whether PN is compounded onsite, outsourced to a compounding vendor, or makes use of multichamber fixed-dose products, a standardized model for PN prescribing could be applied in a multidisciplinary fashion and be used to educate and assist institutional privileged physicians in training (residents and fellows); medical students;

nutrition support RDs, NPs, and PAs; clinical nurse specialists; and nutrition support pharmacists, as appropriate. A secondary gain from this competency model might be more standardized prescribing patterns, which also could help educate providers, improve patient care and safety, and decrease prescribing-related errors.

The competency recommendations within this chapter are intended for discussion and adoption over time by organizations involved in the prescribing for patients requiring PN. The competency recommendations are not intended to supersede the judgment of the employing institution, in light of the individual circumstances of each case.

General Nutrition Competencies

A competency is a quality or characteristic of a person that is related to effective performance. Competencies can be described as a combination of knowledge, skills, motives, and personal traits. Competencies help individuals and their organizations look at how they do their jobs.[7] Competencies define expectations for knowledge, skills, and traits for effective role implementation. Without documented competencies, an assessment of an individual at regular intervals cannot be performed, and, therefore, the ability to effectively and safely perform a role within their job is compromised.

In 1999, ASPEN published interdisciplinary core competencies to help nutrition support clinicians meet performance expectations in job descriptions and demonstrate the knowledge and skills necessary to adapt care to the physical, psychosocial, cultural, and age-related needs of patients. These core competencies are examples of critical aspects of job performance that supervisors, managers, or directors may use and/or adapt for performance appraisal of nutrition support practitioners.[8] There are many ways to gather data to evaluate practitioner performance, which include but are not limited to one or more of the following[8]:

1. Direct observation of a practitioner demonstrating skills or tasks.

2. Observation of participation in interdisciplinary clinical rounds.

3. Evaluation of an approach to practice in clinical simulations.

4. Evaluation of care plans for specific case examples.

5. Review of results of written examinations.

6. Verification of nutrition support certification.

7. Analysis of performance on nutrition support-related self-assessment programs.

8. Evaluation of educational presentations on nutrition support-related topics.

9. Confirmation of participation in local or national professional organization activities.

10. Documentation of continuing education in activities related to nutrition support practice.

11. Confirmation of participation in mentoring or peer review programs.

12. Confirmation of participation in quality improvement programs.

Building programs and tools for patient safety and professional accountability has long been a goal for ASPEN. In his presidential address, Philip Schneider stated, "the tools that can be used to improve patient safety include self-assessment of practitioners who routinely use nutrition support in their practice, curricular-based continuing education programs, board certification in nutrition support practice, and the use of clinical guidelines to assist in making clinical decisions. By developing and promoting these tools, ASPEN is committed to building a safe nutrition system so every patient receives optimal nutrition care."[9] Competencies are a strong evaluation tool to build that safe PN system.

Prescribing Competencies Framework

A competency framework is a collection of competencies thought to be central to effective performance and includes guiding principles to optimize patient safety. Development of competencies should help individuals to continually improve their performance and work more effectively.[10] If acquired and maintained, the prescribing competencies in this framework should help healthcare professionals to be safe and effective prescribers. This competency framework underpins the clinician's personal responsibility for prescribing.[7] Selected tenets of the British National Health Service framework[7] on prescribing effectively that are particularly pertinent to PN prescribing can be found in Table 9-1.[7]

Examples of PN Prescribing Practices

A full assessment of the patient and PN prescribing system is important in order for the competent clinician or interdisciplinary nutrition support team to prescribe appropriate PN.[11] A British report specifically found that patients with prescription-related complications were often inadequately assessed before beginning PN.[12] A patient's current and past medical conditions, physical examination findings, nutrition status and requirements, fluid and electrolyte requirements, venous access, and current medication therapy must be evaluated.[11] Several studies indicated a need for prescribing education, as well as revision of PN

Table 9-1. Selected Competencies Pertinent to PN Prescribing

Competency	Tenets
A: Safe	Knows the limits of her/his own knowledge and skill and works within them.
	Knows when to refer to or seek guidance from another member of the team or a specialist.
	Only prescribes a medicine if he or she has adequate up to date awareness of its actions, indications, dose, contraindications, interactions, cautions, and side effects.
	Accurately calculates doses and routinely checks calculations when relevant, such as for children.
	Keeps up to date with advances in practice and emerging safety concerns related to prescribing.
	Knows about common types of medication errors and how to prevent them.
	Ensures confidence and competence to prescribe are maintained.
	Makes accurate, legible, and contemporaneous records and clinical notes of prescribing decisions.
	Effectively uses the systems necessary to prescribe medicines (eg, medicine charts, electronic prescribing, decision support).
	Writes legible, unambiguous, and complete prescriptions that meet legal requirements.
B: Professional	Accepts personal responsibility for prescribing and understands the legal and ethical implications of doing so.
	Makes prescribing decisions based on the needs of patients and not the prescriber's personal considerations.
	Knows and applies legal and ethical frameworks affecting prescribing practice (eg, misuse of drugs, regulations, prescribing of unlicensed/off label medicines).
	Takes responsibility for her/his own learning and continuing professional development.
	Maintains patient confidentiality in line with best practices, regulatory standards, and contractual requirements.
C: Always improving	Learns and changes from reflecting on practice.
	Shares and debates her/his own and others' prescribing practice and acts on feedback and discussion.
	Acts on colleagues' inappropriate prescribing practice using appropriate mechanisms.
	Understands and uses tools to improve prescribing (eg, review of prescribing data, audit, and feedback).
	Reports prescribing errors and near misses, reviews practice to prevent recurrence.

PN, parenteral nutrition.

ordering processes, including standardized order forms.[13] Although the appropriateness of the PN order is ultimately up to the competent practitioner who examines the patient and determines whether PN is indicated, the content and presentation of the order form (or template) can positively influence the prescription.[14]

Physicians. Several studies report the need for additional nutrition education and training in nutrition assessment and intervention for physicians.[15] Vanek and colleagues[16] specifically assessed the physicians' ability to prescribe PN in the community teaching hospital setting. The authors found that medical and surgical residents need more education in the area of nutrition support, particularly in determining nutrient requirements.

Pharmacists. The concept of pharmacists taking on new patient care roles such as disease management and prescribing is contingent on the determination of the pharmacist's competency. Competency can be addressed in part by obtaining continuing education credits, maintaining licensure, and becoming certified in a clinical specialty,[17] such as through the Board of Pharmacy Specialties (BPS), which has a nutrition support specialty certification program, or through certification by the National Board of Nutrition Support Certification (NBNSC). Traditionally, pharmacists have been heavily involved in the PN order-writing process, and these interactions have led to more appropriate PN therapy, earlier transition to enteral nutrition (EN) therapy, and recognition of pharmacists as resources for physicians.[18-20] There have also been reports of pharmacists as prescribers of PN.[18,21,22] In 1996, 12.1% of pharmacist survey respondents in Canada were prescribing PN,[23] and a more recent study in the United States showed that 28.3% of respondents reported pharmacists prescribing PN.[2]

Dietitians. In the mid-1990s, 1 institution developed clinical privileges for RDs as prescribers of clinical nutrition therapy. These privileges included ordering PN along with the monitoring studies needed with this therapy. The competencies for PN included evaluation of appropriateness of the therapy, recommendation of the PN admixture, advancement of the PN, evaluation of specialty formulas, cycling regimens, and transitioning to oral or enteral feedings.[24] In 2002, this practice was extended to the long-term acute care hospital setting, where competencies included maintenance of certification such as an RD, documentation of certification by NBNSC, demonstration of competence to write PN and EN orders as verified by nutrition experts in the organization, and continued professional education with an emphasis in nutrition support.[25] In 2013, Roberts[26] described the RD order-writing program using a nutrition management protocol and the positive patient outcomes associated with such a program. In this program, a minimum of 10 PN orders were written and evaluated prior to sign-off on privileges. Positive patient outcomes using an electronic order entry program with clinical decision support and monitoring were also demonstrated.[27]

PAs/NPs. Like physicians, PAs and NPs have varied and limited amounts of nutrition education in their basic curriculums. Attempts have been made to improve nutrition instruction,[28-30] yet there are no articles in the literature on PN prescribed by PAs and NPs and the competencies needed for this care management knowledge and skill. Many of these clinicians are in the primary care setting, but greater numbers are practicing in the acute care environment and need PN prescribing competencies.

PN Prescribing Model

This model is intended for use by organizations to train and assist in privileging the following healthcare professionals: physicians in training (residents and fellows); medical students; nutrition support RDs, NPs, and PAs; clinical nurse specialists; and nutrition support pharmacists. An experienced prescriber of PN can serve as preceptor for this training and privileging process. The model should be implemented as a 7-day process.

Communication between PN prescribers and the primary provider team (if they are not the same) is essential to maintain congruent goals in management of the individual patient. Because the PN prescriber and primary provider each may be providing volume and metabolic management (eg, insulin, electrolyte replacement), the PN prescriber must know the goals of the primary provider. Documentation of PN changes are important.

Based on the recommendations from ASPEN's consensus recommendations and clinical guidelines (Table 9-2),[3,6] the following competencies should be met for institutions to privilege the prescriber:

1. The prescriber may be certified as a nutrition support clinician or other related nutrition board certification (eg, NBNSC, BPS, National Board of Physician Nutrition Specialists).

2. If not certified in nutrition support, the prescriber should complete a didactic/interactive course such as the ASPEN PN Order-Writing Workshop or a facility-developed or organization-developed program for initial competency. Such a program should include the following:
   a. PN indications.
   b. PN venous access.
   c. Volume, macronutrient requirements, and micronutrient requirements.

d. Fluid, electrolyte, and acid-base balance basic concepts and principles.

e. Drug-nutrient interactions.

f. PN ordering.

g. Monitoring and complication prevention and management. The didactic course should also include a pretest and post-test to evaluate learning.

3. The prescriber will complete at least 10 PN orders for the initial competency evaluation (via patient case scenarios and/or actual patients) under the supervision of an experienced preceptor. These cases should reflect the spectrum of medical and nutrition conditions, body weights, and age ranges.

4. The prescriber should follow these patients and modify daily PN orders over a period of several days. This allows demonstration of the ability to modify PN orders as needed for changing clinical conditions.

5. During evaluation of competency, the preceptor should use the PN Order-Writing Competency Tool (Figure 9-1).

6. For annual or every-other-year competency reevaluation, completion of ongoing continuing education requirements on nutrition support combined with PN order assessment of at least 5 cases or patients should be reviewed using the PN Order-Writing Competency Tool (Figure 9-1). Communication with the primary provider is essential throughout the process.

Table 9-2. ASPEN Recommendations for Safe PN Prescribing

Question	Recommendations
Does a standardized process for PN prescribing increase clarity and reduce PN-related errors? What are the essential elements of a PN order that minimize errors?	1. Healthcare organizations shall use a standardized process for PN management, and this process shall include clinicians with expertise in the area of nutrition support, preferably from multiple disciplines.
	2. The primary healthcare team, in collaboration with nutrition support professionals, shall evaluate, clearly define, and accurately document the patient's medical problem(s) and indication(s) for PN.
	3. The primary healthcare team, in collaboration with nutrition support professionals, shall specify and document the therapeutic goal(s) of PN therapy.
	4. PN shall be prescribed using a standardized PN order format and review process applicable to patients of every age and disease state within a healthcare organization.
	5. Institutions shall create an HPN order template/format that provides a safe plan for multiple days of therapy. The prescription for HPN therapy should be written in a format that specifically reflects trends in laboratory values and previous days of PN therapy. An institutional daily PN order format should not be used as an HPN prescription.
	6. The most appropriate nutrition modality, in collaboration with nutrition support professionals, should be prescribed for the patient. Healthcare organizations should determine the most appropriate types of PN formulation(s) for their patient population(s) (eg, standardized compounded, standardized commercially available PN products, or customized compounded PN admixtures) or methods of delivery (eg, dextrose/amino acid admixtures vs TNAs), and should develop criteria for each formulation that will be used in their patients.
How can education be provided to nonnutrition support specialist clinicians to improve PN prescribing and safety?	1. Prescribers from all disciplines, including physicians, pharmacists, NPs, PAs, and dietitians, should be educated on basic PN prescribing and monitoring.
	2. Introductory didactic and experiential education/training about PN should be included in the core curriculum. Knowledge and skills should be evaluated for all clinicians in each discipline involved with PN as determined by the individual institution. Education and assessment materials and processes shall be developed and led by clinicians with expertise in the area of nutrition support, preferably from multiple disciplines.
	3. In-depth education on PN should be included as a standard component of acute care and home care pharmacy and physician residency training. This is also applicable to all pharmacists, nurses, dietitians, physicians, physician extenders, and other clinicians involved in caring for patients who receive PN.

ASPEN, American Society for Parenteral and Enteral Nutrition; HPN, home parenteral nutrition; NP, nurse practitioner; PA, physician assistant; PN, parenteral nutrition; TNA, total nutrient admixture.

Figure 9-1. ASPEN Parenteral Nutrition (PN) Order-Writing Competency Tool

Adult / Pediatric / Neonatal
(Circle applicable patient population)

Case #_____

Pharmacist_____

Verified by_____

Date	Competency	Competency Met	Review Needed	Evaluator's Initials
	Verify PN order elements for:			
	Patient name and other identifiers			
	Birth date and or age			
	Allergies and associated manifestations			
	Height and dosing weight (metric units)			
	Diagnoses			
	Indication(s) for PN			
	Administration route and vascular access device			
	Prescriber contact information			
	Date and time the PN order was submitted			
	Administration date and time			
	Volume and infusion rate			
	Infusion schedule (continuous vs cyclic)			
	Rate of infusion tapered up/down if appropriate			
	Type of formulation (dextrose/amino acids or total nutrient admixture)			
	Verify PN ingredients for:			
	Amounts per day (adults); Amounts per kg per day (pediatrics, neonates)			
	Electrolyte ion doses as a salt form			
	A dose for each macronutrient			
	A dose for each electrolyte salt			
	A dose for fixed-dose multi-trace element product			
	A dose for individual trace element salt			
	A dose for fixed-dose multivitamin product			
	A dose for individual vitamins			
	A dose for insulin (if ordered)			
	A dose for other non-nutrient medications (if ordered)			
	Performs clinical review of the PN order for:			
	Indication consistent with published guidelines or scientific literature			
	Appropriate dose of each macronutrient for the patient given indication, body weight, organ function, and concurrent medications			
	Appropriate dose of each micronutrient for the patient given indication, body weight, organ function, and concurrent medications			
	Appropriate osmolarity for route of administration			
	Changes from previous PN order			
	Any prescriber over-ride to alerts generated by clinical decision support within a CPOE system are addressed			
	Performs pharmaceutical review of the PN order for:			
	Compatibility of all ingredients at ordered doses and volume			
	Stability of the final PN admixture at ordered doses and volume			
	Performs independent double-check for:			
	Transcription from PN order to pharmacy system			
	Transcription from PN order or pharmacy system to the ACD			
	Transcription of PN order to/from a pharmacy vendor			
	Any calculations or conversion of units-of-measure			
	Documents all steps as required for record keeping			

A.S.P.E.N./ASPEN, American Society for Parenteral and Enteral Nutrition; PN, parenteral nutrition.

The model of standards for competency in PN prescribing described here will require time and resources at the organizational level. Interventions to achieve this level of competence may require customized solutions at individual institutions on the basis of their existing PN prescribing structure. Each institution needs to incorporate this model in a way that is practical within its resources and capacity.

The competency program may not be the same for each type of prescriber, even within a single institution. Individual medical institutions may have developed an oversight system for PN order prescribing, in which case this privileging approach for physician trainees may not be necessary. For instance, some medical institutions provide specific nutrition rotations and training to residents and fellows or may have systems in which individuals who are not physicians prescribe PN through a collaborative agreement.

The ultimate goal is to achieve a culture of safe PN prescribing that is based on evaluation of individual patients and achieved by multidisciplinary collaboration among physicians, dietitians, nurses, and pharmacists. The role of electronic health records (EHRs) in providing a layer of safety with built-in checks cannot be overstated (see chapter 13).

Competencies for PN Order Review and Preparation[ii]

Compared with most other medications, the order review and the preparation steps for PN are time and effort intensive. Competence needs to be shown by pharmacists and pharmacy technicians involved in reviewing and preparing PN. Organizations vary in how they verify and the degree to which they review PN orders. A national survey indicated that 60% of organizations dedicate at least 0.6 full-time equivalents to verify, review, and clarify PN orders.[2] Unfortunately, 23% do not dedicate any pharmacist time to this critical activity. For those who do review PN orders, 90% of respondents report that clarifications are required for up to 25% of all PN orders. These range from illegible orders and missing information to dosing, compatibility, and stability concerns.[2]

Judicious PN order review and modification are critical to optimizing patient safety. Therefore, competent pharmacists should identify and clarify inappropriate PN orders prior to preparation. Interventions pursuant to this significant workload are often considered inherent to the workflow and are therefore rarely documented (eg, "near-miss" errors). Permanent and easily retrievable documentation is valuable to further determine appropriate practices. The review step is often not described or is otherwise subsumed within the compounding step. This is clearly an independent step that may occur at a distant site from compounding. This task requires competence, especially given that 19%–21% of organizations outsource PN preparation to a vendor.[2,31]

---

ii   **Source:** Adapted with permission from Boullata JI, Holcombe B, Sacks G, et al; ASPEN. Standardized competencies for parenteral nutrition order review and parenteral nutrition preparation, including compounding: the ASPEN model. *Nutr Clin Pract.* 2016;31(4):548–555.

The preparation step can also vary among organizations. PN preparation includes compounding — whether customized to a patient's specific needs or meeting an organization-specific standard formulation with fixed proportions of macronutrients. Preparation also includes the activation of a standardized commercially available PN product (often referred to as a multichamber bag) with admixture of additional additives as required. Automated compounding devices (ACDs) are used to prepare PN in up to 64% of organizations, especially in larger institutions.[2,31] Standardized commercially available PN products are used by 21%–43% according to recent surveys.[2,31] These products are used more often in smaller institutions, although it is not clear whether the use of the commercially available PN product, let alone PN, is always indicated.[2,31] At least 10% of organizations still use a gravity method to prepare PN.[31] The "gravity" method refers to combining of the major ingredients from their original source container into the final PN container through tubing by the force of gravity without automated means. ACDs infrequently (18%) interface electronically with the order entry system, requiring manual transcription by a pharmacist or pharmacy technician. If any transcription steps remain in place (diverging from recommended best practices), an independent double-check and documentation of the same needs to take place. Regardless of method, PN preparation also requires appropriate labeling, dispensing, and storage. The beyond-use date assigned to PN preparations seems to vary considerably among organizations.[2]

Recently published ASPEN PN clinical guidelines and safety consensus recommendations addressed the current limitations in education and training of pharmacists. Until this is remedied, it is incumbent on organizations to provide in-depth training programs for staff involved in PN order review and compounding. Regulatory oversight of PN compounding is extensive,[32–35] and best PN practices described in ASPEN guidance documents include order review and compounding.[3,6] Regardless of where the order is being reviewed or where the admixture is being prepared, the individuals directly involved are expected to meet basic initial competencies and undergo competency assessments at regularly set intervals.

Although there has been growth of pharmacy specialists through postdoctoral training programs and board certification, this growth has not been seen in the nutrition support specialty in recent years. Given the limited number of board-certified pharmacists in positions overseeing PN, the lack of widespread regulatory requirements for pharmacy technician certification, and the recent publication of the ASPEN PN clinical guidelines and safety consensus recommendations, the next logical step is to develop a model for standardized competencies around PN order review and PN preparation available for organizations to use.[3,6] A model for PN standardized competencies would allow for consistency among institutions and offer a template for those involved in PN order review and PN preparation.

Pharmacy Competencies

Pharmacists reviewing PN orders need to be knowledgeable in all aspects of PN, including VADs, clinical indications, interpretation of physical examination and laboratory findings, appropriate dosing, clinical and metabolic complications, physicochemical principles, interpreting stability, and compatibility data.[36] The pharmacists and pharmacy technicians involved in preparing the PN have a significant role to play in ensuring safe and appropriate use. They make sure that each dispensed PN is appropriate for the patient and prepared using the best compounding practices. Unfortunately, there are a multitude of case reports detailing adverse outcomes, including sentinel events from inappropriate preparation.[3,6,37–50] Attention has been given to prescribing errors that are reflected in the compounded PN without shedding significant light on the critical review step that in some cases did not exist.

The use of checklists in healthcare has expanded in recent years to complement reliance on memory and experience in the complex care of patients. The airline industry has long used checklists as a safety tool—not just for the infrequent emergency condition, but as an important step in routine, everyday situations. Free-to-access checklists are available from ASPEN to help standardize and streamline the process of PN order review and PN preparation.[51,52]

Regardless of whether PN is prepared onsite, is outsourced to a compounding vendor, or makes use of multichamber fixed-dose products, a standardized process for PN order review and preparation is an important safety process that can then be used to train and assist in privileging pharmacists, pharmacy residents, pharmacy students, pharmacy technicians, and technician students as appropriate. A secondary gain from this competency model might be more standardized patterns of order review and preparation that could help improve patient safety by decreasing related errors.

The competency recommendations within this chapter are intended for discussion and adoption over time by organizations involved in the reviewing and/or preparing of PN. These recommendations are not intended to supersede the judgment of the healthcare professional or employing institution based on the circumstances of the individual patient.

Pharmacists. The pharmacist involved in PN therapy is an integral part of the multidisciplinary nutrition care team, whether a formal nutrition support service is in place or not.[36] This critical team member serves as an important resource, and every attempt should be made to have the pharmacist involved in full-team clinical patient care rounds. The concept of pharmacists expanding patient care roles such as disease management and prescribing is contingent on the determination of the pharmacist's competency. Competency can be addressed in part by obtaining continuing education credits, maintaining licensure, and becoming certified in a clinical specialty.[21,53]

The BPS has a nutrition support pharmacy specialty certification program, and the NBNSC identifies the certified as a qualified nutrition support provider.[54,55] Each certifying board has specific processes in place for maintaining certification and for recertification. A BPS task force is also considering whether sterile compounding may qualify for its own specialty certification.[55] Pharmacists have been heavily involved in the PN compounding process, and these collaborations have led to more appropriate PN therapy, earlier transition to EN therapy, and recognition of pharmacists as a resource for providers.[56]

Pharmacy Technicians. Pharmacy technicians involved in preparing PN should complete a standardized training program, whose curriculum should include compounding sterile preparations, validation of sterile compounding techniques, pharmacy calculations related to PN, training with ACDs if used, and education pertinent to PN. The degree of practical experience may vary, but certification of pharmacy technicians should be a minimum requirement for involvement in PN preparation. The Pharmacy Technician Certification Board (PTCB) oversees certification of these healthcare professionals.[57] Although all states accept PTCB certification, pharmacy technicians are currently regulated in 45 states. A PTCB task force is now considering advanced certification for sterile compounding.

Based on the recommendations from the ASPEN Consensus Recommendations and Clinical Guidelines that addressed specific questions,[3,6] the following competencies should be met for the institutions to privilege the pharmacist and/or pharmacy technician involved with PN:

1. Pharmacist shall have the appropriate licensure or credential for his or her profession.

2. The pharmacist should be board-certified, preferably as a nutrition support pharmacy specialist. An alternative is to have a board-certified nutrition support pharmacy specialist on staff who develops and oversees competencies for colleagues in the organization who review and/or prepare PN.

3. If not board-certified in nutrition support, the pharmacist shall complete a didactic/interactive course such as the ASPEN professional development material (eg, Interdisciplinary Review Course, Nutrition Support Fundamentals & Review Course, the module-based Self-Assessment program, or any of a number of on-demand webinars) in addition to the American Society of Health-System Pharmacists resources for sterile compounding.[58-60] An alternative course would be a facility or organizationally developed program for initial competency. The course should also include a pretest and posttest to assess learning. Such a program must include the following:

- PN indications.

- PN venous access.

- Macronutrient and micronutrient requirements in health but also based on age, disease states, clinical conditions, organ dysfunction, and concurrent interventions, including pharmacotherapy.

- Fluid, electrolyte, and acid-base balance basic concepts and principles.

- PN ordering.

- Monitoring and complication prevention and management.

- United States Pharmacopeia (USP) Chapter <797>.

- ACD setup and verification.

- Managing PN component shortages and outages.

- Evaluating and selecting an outsource compounding facility.

- Pharmaceutical considerations for nutrition support formulations.

- Nutrition support interventions for various disease states and clinical conditions/settings, including therapeutic goals.

- Documenting and tracking adverse drug reactions and medication (including nutrient products) errors.

4. The pharmacy technician should be certified and receive in-depth training in PN preparation to include the following:

- Proper personal hygiene and protective equipment.

- Cleaning of the ACD and compounding environment.

- Setup and verification of the ACD and individual components.

- Review formulation, review label, and select appropriate bag.

- Scan and check barcodes, check pump admixture, or activate multichamber bag.

- Be familiar with dosing differences between PN components intended for neonatal, pediatric, and adult patients, as institutionally appropriate.
- Verify ingredients, including those that require manual admixture.
- Safely combine components of PN, including the manual addition of ingredients.
- Affix patient-specific label and auxiliary labels.
- Store properly.
- Inventory management for individual PN components.

5. Pharmacist shall review at least 10 PN orders for the initial competency evaluation (via patient case scenarios and/or actual patients) under the supervision of an experienced pharmacy preceptor.

6. Pharmacist and pharmacy technician shall prepare at least 10 PN orders for each patient population managed by the organization (eg, adult, pediatric, or neonate).

7. During evaluation of competency, the preceptor should use the PN Order-Writing Competency Tool (Figure 9-1) or the PN Compounding Competency Tool (Figure 9-2) as appropriate.

8. For annual competency, completion of ongoing continuing education requirements on nutrition support should be combined with the following:
   - PN order assessment of at least 2 cases or patients reviewed using the PN Order-Writing Competency Tool (Figure 9-1) or
   - PN preparation of at least 2 population-specific PN orders using the PN Compounding Competency Tool (Figure 9-2).

The questions addressed by the ASPEN recommendations for PN order review include the following[3,6]:

1. What are the essential components or attributes for safely transmitting PN orders to pharmacists for review and verification?

2. What is the maximum safe osmolarity of PN admixtures intended for peripheral vein administration?

3. What macronutrient dosing limits are expected to provide for the most stable total nutrient admixtures (TNAs; 3-in-1 admixtures)?

4. What are the most appropriate recommendations for optimizing calcium (gluconate) and (sodium [Na–] or potassium [K–]) phosphate compatibility in PN admixtures?

5. Is it safe to use the PN admixture as a vehicle for nonnutrient medication delivery?

6. What improvements in the PN review and verification processes will enhance the safety of PN therapy?

7. What processes can healthcare organizations implement to improve the safety of PN therapy during shortages of PN components?

Figure 9-2. Parenteral Nutrition (PN) Compounding Competency Tool

Adult / Pediatric / Neonatal

(Circle applicable patient population)

Case #_____

Pharmacist / Pharmacy Technician_____

Verified by_____

Date	Competency	Competency Met	Review Needed	Evaluator's Initials
	Automated Compounding Device			
	Uses vendor-validated setup			
	Includes a second staff member for initial setup • Uses independent double-check • Uses printed check • Verbally affirms all components including name, concentration, container size			
	Uses barcode technology to verify products during initial setup			
	Uses barcode technology to verify products during replacement of each ingredient			
	Traces tubing from the source container to the port attached to the ACD during initial setup			
	Traces tubing from the source container to the port attached to the ACD during replacement of each source container			
	Requests independent pharmacist or supervisor verification when multiple source containers of a single additive are used			
	Completely affixes patient-specific and auxiliary labels			
	Places completed PN in refrigeration prior to delivery			
	Multi-chamber PN Product			
	Identifies the correct product and volume to meet the PN order			
	Inspects the product for any damage or deterioration prior to removing the overwrap			
	Completely activates and agitates the product to mix all components together			
	Able to identify inappropriate additives			
	Makes manual additives as ordered			
	Completely affixes patient-specific and auxiliary labels			
	Places completed PN in refrigeration prior to delivery			
	Manual Compounding			
	Uses manual compounding technique when • Ingredient volume is too small for ACD to measure accurately • Interaction potential between ingredient and ACD component • Chemical reaction potential cannot be mitigated by altering sequence of addition, or • There is a shortage/outage of a PN component and conservation measures are in place			
	Requests independent pharmacist or supervisor verification for manually additives prior to adding to the PN			
	All PN Preparations			
	Environment for PN preparation complies with USP <797>			
	Verifies PN order • After initial order entry • Prior to injecting manual additive • After compounding			
	Visually inspects PN prior to dispensing			
	Reviews and compares PN order, patient-specific PN label, and compounding formulation prior to dispensing			
	Documents all steps as required for record keeping			

ACD, automated compounding device; PN, parenteral nutrition; USP, United States Pharmacopeia.

The questions addressed by the ASPEN recommendations for PN compounding include the following[3,6]:

1. What compounding errors have been caused by deficits in knowledge, lack of training, competency, and proficiency?

2. What compounding errors have been caused by a lack of standardized educational curriculum in schools of pharmacy or pharmacy technician programs?

3. How can organizations avoid PN errors by implementing soft and hard limits on an ACD?

4. What role does USP Chapter <797> play in preventing PN errors?

5. What are the steps healthcare organizations can take to improve the PN label and labeling system?

PN is a complex therapeutic modality reflected in complex prescriptions with dozens of ingredients, each with clinical rationales, dosing implications, and interaction potential. As such, the pharmacist reviewing the PN order should demonstrate competency to optimize the delivery of safe and effective therapy. Additionally, the pharmacist and/or the pharmacy technician preparing or directly supervising the preparation of the PN should demonstrate competency to prepare an appropriate and safe admixture for each patient. Institutions should implement policies and procedures addressing determination of competent PN order review and PN preparation. This should be assessed initially and on an annual basis at a minimum. Any identified medication errors related to PN order review or PN preparation will necessitate more frequent competency assessment — in addition to a systematic review of the PN use process.

Competencies for PN Administration[iii]

PN is a high-alert medication and prone to a variety of potential errors. In 2014, patients received PN during approximately 300,000 hospital stays, about 25,000 patients received home PN (HPN), and many others received it in a long-term care setting.[61,62] Because many PN administration errors occur at the point of patient contact, mistakes in this phase of the medication delivery process are less likely to be intercepted and more likely to cause harm than other types of PN errors. In addition, the broad

---

iii **Source:** Adapted with permission from Guenter P, Worthington P, Ayers P, et al; Parenteral Nutrition Safety Committee, ASPEN. Standardized Competencies for parenteral nutrition administration: the ASPEN model. *Nutr Clin Pract.* 2018;33(2):295–304.

range of healthcare settings in which PN administration takes place — from critical care to home care — creates the potential for disparities to exist in technology and equipment, as well as in the knowledge and skills of the nursing staff and other caregivers responsible for administering PN.

Regardless of the setting or the number of patients receiving this therapy in a facility, the classification of PN as a high-alert medication requires healthcare organizations to develop evidence-based policies and procedures designed to promote safe PN administration and to validate the competence of those responsible for delivering this complex form of intravenous (IV) therapy.[6]

Safe provision of PN therapy requires standardized protocols, interprofessional communication, and vigilant surveillance for complications. The PN use process is associated with a variety of potential errors, from ordering the PN prescription to administering the therapy to a patient. Appropriate practices and safeguards are critical to assuring patient safety. ASPEN recognizes that all healthcare institutions may not currently meet the aspirational goals of this chapter. This section will focus on those competencies required for PN administration, which are generally performed by nurses. This chapter will not address the specifics of PN administration by patients and/or caregivers.

PN administration errors have been well documented. A recently published paper by members of the ASPEN PN Safety Committee, based on data from the Institute for Safe Medication Practices (ISMP) Medication Errors Reporting Program reports, noted that the greatest number of errors were associated with compounding and dispensing PN. The second most common errors were those associated with the administration process.[63] Many of the errors reported involved infusion pump programming: incorrect infusion rates, failure to turn the pump on, or incorrect infusion times. Inadvertent rate and line mix-ups were among the most common errors reported, particularly when the lipid injectable emulsion (ILE) was administered as a separate infusion from the dextrose/amino acid admixture.[64,65]

In another series by Sacks et al,[66] 67% of the errors associated with patient harm occurred during PN administration. For example, infusing the PN over 12 hours instead of the prescribed 24 hours resulted in hyperglycemia and fluid overload in patients who cannot tolerate a cycled infusion. Data from MacKay et al[67] demonstrated that the most common administration errors were associated with PN infusion rate changes (34%), adjustments in ILE after the PN infusion started (23%), or PN component incompatibilities (13%). As a result of these findings, McKay's organization implemented smart pump administration of PN with hard and soft limits for infusion, as well as barcoding for PN order administration.

PN admixtures are prepared and sent to the bedside in a variety of delivery systems, which can contribute substantially to staff member confusion. In a study by Boullata and colleagues[2] conducted in 2011, PN was administered as compounded admixtures by 72% of institutions, whereas 21% used standardized commercially available multichamber PN products; the remainder of the respondents used both types. Forty-five percent used 2-in-1 (dextrose/amino acid admixtures with separate ILE infusions), whereas 28% used 3-in-1 admixtures (TNAs), with the remainder using both types.2 Multichamber-bag PN admixture systems have been associated with reported infusion errors caused by lack of activation of the individual chambers.[68] The variety of PN delivery types requires that the nurse be competent with all types of PN products in use by their institution or agency.

General PN Safety

The 2014 ASPEN PN Safety Consensus Recommendations document provides guidance on using in-line filters for PN administration to reduce the potential for patient harm due to particulates, microprecipitates, microorganisms, and air emboli. The recommendations are to use a 0.22-µm filter for dextrose/amino acid admixtures and to use a 1.2-µm filter for TNAs.[6] The filter should be placed as close to the patient as possible on the administration system. The filter and administration set should be changed with each new PN container or every 24 hours for 3-in-1 admixtures or TNAs and 2-in-1 admixtures or dextrose/amino acid admixtures. An occluded filter should be removed and replaced with a new filter. An unfiltered PN admixture should not be infused.[6]

Since the publication of the ASPEN PN Safety Consensus Recommendations document, the manufacturers of ILE products for use in the United States have revised their administration instructions to include a statement to filter all ILE infusions using a 1.2-µm in-line filter.[09] To comply with this new recommendation, practitioners must use 2 filters when administering PN as a dextrose/amino acid (2-in-1) admixture and the ILE as a separate infusion. A 0.22-µm in-line filter is used for the dextrose/amino acid solution. The second filter, a 1.2-µm filter, is for the ILE, which is infused by means of a Y-connector placed closer to the patient than the 0.22-µm filter for the dextrose/amino acid admixtures or via a separate VAD such as a peripheral catheter. The recommendation for filtering TNAs using a single 1.2-µm in-line or add-on filter has not changed.[69] In a recent survey on ILE use, the issue of filters was raised, and the findings demonstrated a gap in knowledge regarding the appropriate use of filters and an opportunity for continued education and further research.[69] Up to 20% of respondents did not filter ILE when administered as a separate infusion despite a recent call by the US Food and Drug Administration to do so.[69]

Point-of-care drug administration systems may also decrease administration errors. For example, interfacing computerized provider order entry systems with ACD technologies can permit checking the dose of PN components, and the PN label barcode can provide information for administration to prevent wrong-patient errors. Beyond root cause analysis, which allows response to isolated errors, a methodical systems review of the full PN use process can enhance contextual learning and allow for system improvements to advance safety.[70] Healthcare institutions must emphasize reporting of PN medication errors to enhance safe use of this important therapeutic intervention. Error reporting is a vital tool that can be used as a mechanism to identify opportunities for improvements in the medication management processes. Medication error reporting provides insight and assists institutions in improving all aspects of medication management. The World Health Organization notes medication error reporting can be summarized and prioritized for action using the following categories listed by ISMP[71]:

- Patient outcome.
- Medication use process.
- Medication problem.
- Therapeutic group or individual medicine.

Many of the individuals involved in administering PN may be unaware of best-practice standards. Using ASPEN best-practice recommendations and professional competencies for all steps in the PN use process should assist with decreasing PN-related errors.[3,6,72,73]

The competency recommendations within this chapter are intended for discussion and adoption over time by organizations involved in the delivery of PN for patients requiring this therapy. The competency recommendations are not intended to supersede the judgment of the employing institution or individual clinicians in light of the circumstances of each case.

Administration Competencies Framework

General competencies for PN administration were outlined in the recently published ASPEN nurse standards of practice.[74] These standards were set at the following levels: nutrition support nurse specialist, NP, and bedside nurse. The competencies listed below are for the bedside nurse who most often performs PN administration:

- Administers PN and EN in a safe, comfortable, and effective manner.
- Cares for the EN and PN access devices according to evidence-based and institutional guidelines.
- Uses evidence-based interventions designed to prevent, detect, and manage complications related to the feeding formulation, infusion rate, equipment and supplies, and/or access devices.
- Uses technology and electronic health systems for nutrition implementation.

A model for PN standardized competencies would allow for consistency between institutions and offer to a variety of nutrition professionals a template to use to identify a minimum standard level of knowledge and skills for administering this complex medication. Regardless of whether PN admixtures are compounded or activated from multichamber fixed-dose products, a standardized model for PN administration could be applied in an interprofessional fashion, used to educate physicians in training (residents and fellows), medical students, dietitians, NPs, clinical nurse specialists, PAs, pharmacists, and others, as appropriate. Although many of these clinicians will not directly administer PN, knowledge of the correct process and the associated care concepts are important. For example, although physicians, NPs, dietitians, and pharmacists may not perform PN tubing and dressing changes, all clinicians should have some knowledge about central venous catheter infection prevention.

The competency recommendations within this chapter are intended for discussion and adoption over time by organizations involved in the administration of PN. The competency recommendations are not intended to supersede the judgment of the employing institution considering the individual circumstances of each case.

ASPEN Model for PN Administration Competencies

Based on the recommendations from the ASPEN PN Safety Consensus Recommendations (Table 9-3) and the Essential Components of Nursing Policies and Procedures for PN Administration (Table 9-4), the following competencies should be met for the institutions to sign off on the administration competency:

1. If not certified in nutrition support, a clinician should complete a facility- or organization-developed program (such as 1 from ASPEN) for initial competency with content including the following:

- PN indications/appropriate use.

- PN VADs and care.

- Volume/fluid, macronutrient and micronutrient components, and usual dosing range.

- Fluid, electrolyte, and acid-based balance basic concepts and principles.

- Drug-nutrient interactions.

- Nutrient-nutrient interactions.

- PN ordering and labeling.

- Types of PN admixtures and correct use/placement of associated medical devices such as filters and infusion pumps.

- Common complications associated with PN and appropriate monitoring, prevention, and management strategies.

2. The program should assess prior knowledge and effective learning using tools such as a pretest and posttest or interactive question and answer session. Some of this content may be included in other programs such as medication and IV management.

3. The nurse will administer a minimum of 6 PN admixtures for the initial competency evaluation (via patient case scenarios and/or actual patients) under the supervision of an experienced preceptor. These cases should reflect the spectrum of medical and nutrition conditions, body weights, and age ranges cared for by the institution or home care company.

4. The nurse should follow these patients over a period of several days when possible. In home care, follow-up visits or telephone contacts are crucial to optimize patient and caregiver understanding and mastery of HPN administration procedures. This follow-up step allows the nurse to demonstrate the ability to monitor the effectiveness and tolerance of the PN in the event of changing clinical conditions.

5. During evaluation of competency, the preceptor should use the PN Administration Competency Tool (Figure 9-3).

6. For annual (preferred) or periodic competency re-evaluation, completion of institutional-set required number of ongoing continuing education hours on PN therapy, and review of 3 patients should be performed using the Competency Tool (Figure 9-3).

Table 9-3. ASPEN Recommendations for Safe PN Administration

Question	Recommendations
What system-based measures can organizations implement to enhance the safety of PN administration?	1. Written policies and procedures shall be developed to standardize nursing practices for the administration of PN throughout the organization.
	2. Education and competency assessment shall be provided to newly hired nurses and patients or caregivers who are responsible for PN administration.
	3. Healthcare organizations should conduct ongoing validation of competency in PN administration based on changes in practice related to PN administration, results of medication error monitoring, and/or the vulnerability of the patient population (eg, high-acuity patients, including neonates and those with critical illness).
	4. Healthcare organizations that provide nursing services related to home infusion shall establish mechanisms for periodic reassessment of knowledge and techniques used by patient or caregivers for HPN.
	5. Interdisciplinary quality improvement programs shall incorporate analysis of medication errors associated with PN administration and knowledge of errors that occur in other institutions.
	6. Safeguards shall be implemented to address specific problem areas as indicated by analysis of PN administration errors.
	7. An interdisciplinary process should be employed for selecting and evaluating equipment and technological aids, such as smart pumps and barcoding to reduce errors in PN administration.
	8. Healthcare organizations shall develop policies and procedures that address extravasation of PN formulations.
	9. Acute care facilities should establish a policy that prohibits the use of a PN formulation prepared for administration at home or in subacute or long-term care facilities.
	10. Protocols for safe operation of infusion pumps shall stipulate rules regarding alarm silencing, modification, and disabling.
	11. Healthcare organizations should purchase infusion pumps with capacity to reduce errors due to incorrect programming. Whenever possible, infusion pumps should be standardized throughout the organization.
What strategies can prevent errors in the verification phase of PN administration?	1. The verification process of PN administration should be presented in a bundle format, which uses a set of evidence-based interventions for a defined patient population or care setting.
	2. Nurses, caregivers, and patients shall visually inspect the integrity of the PN container and formulation before spiking the container.

Table 9-3 continued on next page

Question	Recommendations

	3. The PN label shall be verified against the original prescriber order. No verbal orders shall be accepted.
	
	  a. Check the patient identifiers, product name, route of administration (central vs peripheral), designated initiation time, infusion rate, and beyond-use date and time.
	
	  b. Match all components listed on the label of the admixture to the PN order.

	4. A printed copy of the PN prescription shall be provided to HPN consumers initially and with each formulation change to allow this verification step.
	5. Patient identity shall be confirmed using 2 identifiers according to organizational policy.
What practices maintain patient safety during the infusion of PN?	1. PN shall be administered by or under the supervision of trained, competent personnel.
	2. Organizations shall establish evidence based policies to guide the selection, insertion, care, and maintenance of VADs used to administer PN.
	3. PN protocols shall include measures to reduce contamination through manipulation of the catheter hub.
	4. VADs used for PN administration should not be used to obtain blood samples for laboratory tests unless no peripheral access is available.
	5. PN infusions shall be infused through a filter appropriate for the type of formulation.
	6. An occluded filter shall never be removed in response to occlusion alarms, thus allowing the unfiltered formulation to continue to infuse.
What practices maintain patient safety during the infusion of PN?	7. Administration tubing should be attached to PN containers immediately prior to use.
	8. Administration tubing and filters shall be changed with each new PN container (every 24 hours for TNAs and dextrose/amino acid admixtures; 12 hours for ILE infused separately).
	9. For prolonged infusions of ILE (20–24 h), the daily dose should be divided into 2 parts, with a new container and tubing every 12 h.
	10. Policies regarding PN multichamber bags should be developed using a multidisciplinary approach.

What practices maintain patient safety during the infusion of PN?	11. The PN infusion shall be maintained at the prescribed rate:
	
	  a. Correct pump settings shall be verified at regular intervals and at each hand-off.
	
	  b. The PN infusion rate shall not be adjusted if the infusion is off schedule.
	
	  c. The rate of PN shall not be increased in response to changes in fluid needs; additional hydration should be provided as a separate infusion.
	
	  d. The PN should not be interrupted for routine care or patient transport for diagnostic studies.
	
	  e. Organizations shall develop policies regarding PN infusion and appropriate metabolic monitoring during surgery.

Question	Recommendations
	12. The timing and frequency for blood glucose monitoring shall be based on clinical status and performed in a manner appropriate for the PN infusion schedule (cycled vs continuous).
	13. Caution shall be used when administering subcutaneous insulin coverage prior to a scheduled interruption of the PN infusion.
	14. In acute care acute settings (including long-term acute care), no additions should be made to PN formulations outside the compounding pharmacy; in home settings, additions to PN formulations should be limited in number and be made as close as possible to initiating the infusion.
	15. In long-term care facilities and in home care, education should be provided and caregiver competency regarding proper technique for the addition of prescribed additives to PN formulations should be verified.
	16. Co-infusion of medications through PN lines shall require a review of compatibility and stability data by a pharmacist.
	17. PN should be discontinued prior to transfer to another facility.
	18. The administration of PN and the patient's tolerance shall be documented in the medical record.

HPN, home parenteral nutrition; ILE, lipid injectable emulsion; PN, parenteral nutrition; TNA, total nutrient admixture; VAD, vascular access device.
Source: Adapted with permission from Ayers P, Adams S, Boullata J, et al. A.S.P.E.N. parenteral nutrition safety consensus recommendations. *JPEN J Parenter Enteral Nutr.* 2014 38(3):296–333.

Table 9-4. Essential Components of Nursing Policies and Procedures for PN Administration

A. Role responsibilities, delegation considerations

B. Required equipment

C. Verification procedures

    1. Confirmation of patient identity according to organizational policy

    2. Use of PN formulas prepared in another institution

    3. Checking PN label against the order including formulation components, route, and rate of delivery, expiration date

    4. Inspection of formulation to detect defects or visual changes

    5. Verification of appropriate vascular access prior to initiating PN infusion

      • Tip location: newly inserted VADs and those in place on admission

      • Safeguards to avoid tubing misconnections—trace tubing to the body before making the connection

      • Confirm patency

D. Administration

    1. Policy regarding verification of pump settings

    2. Observation of integrity during infusion

    3. Importance of maintaining PN infusions at the prescribed rate—avoid interruptions for routine care or adjustments for infusions that are off schedule

    4. Guidelines for medication administration for patients receiving PN

      • Policies for co-infusing ILE or other medications with PN

      • Policies prohibiting additions to PN formulations on clinical units

    5. Recognizing a compromised PN formulation

    6. Significance of clogged filters

E. Infection control measures

    1. VAD dressing care procedures, aseptic management of catheter hub

    2. Frequency of tubing and filter change

    3. Hang time

    4. Minimizing manipulations

      • Dedicated line, lumen

      • Blood-drawing practices

F. Monitoring

    1. Appropriate blood glucose monitoring based on clinical condition and infusion schedule (cycled vs continuous infusion)

    2. Laboratory monitoring

    3. Evaluating response to therapy

    4. Recognition and intervention for extravasation

G. Complications and troubleshooting

H. Termination of therapy

I. Patient education

J. Documentation.

ILE, lipid injectable emulsion; PN, parenteral nutrition; VAD, vascular access device.
Source: Adapted with permission from Ayers P, Adams S, Boullata J, et al. A.S.P.E.N. parenteral nutrition safety consensus recommendations. *JPEN J Parenter Enteral Nutr.* 2014 38(3):296–333.

Fig 9-3. ASPEN Parenteral Nutrition (PN) Administration Competency Tool

Adult/Pediatric/Neonatal (Circle applicable patient population)

Case #_____

Nurse _____

Verified by (enter preceptor)_____

Date	Competency/Critical Behaviors	Competency met	Review needed	Evaluator's Initials
	Confirm patient identity according to policy			
	Identify appropriate administration route for type of PN, confirm catheter tip placement and patency			
	Identify pertinent allergies such as egg allergies for patients receiving ILE and acknowledge review by prescriber			
	Check PN label against the original PN order via standardized form/EHR PN template			
	Inspect PN admixture to detect defects or visual changes initially and then during the infusion for recognition of compromised admixture			
	Accurately program PN infusion pump including correct rate and infusion time			
	Express knowledge of policy on verifying pump settings during the infusion and at handoffs			
	Demonstrate accurate use of IV filters on PN administration tubing, express knowledge of occluded filter policy			
	Trace PN tubing to the catheter/body prior to attaching PN, label PN tubing to pump(s) to verify infusion source			
	Express knowledge of need to flush VAD with normal saline prior to connecting PN			
	Express knowledge of maintaining PN infusion at prescribed rate (avoid interruptions)			
	Demonstrate knowledge of medication			

ASPEN, American Society for Parenteral and Enteral Nutrition; EHR, electronic health record; IV, intravenous; PN, parenteral nutrition; VAD, vascular access device.

The model of standards for competency described in this paper will require time and resources for implementation at the organizational level. Processes and interventions to achieve this level of competence may require customized solutions at individual institutions, based on their existing PN administration structure. Each institution needs to incorporate this model in a way that is practical within its resources and capacity.

The competency program may be slightly different for each nurse, even within a single institution. At a minimum, competency validation should occur in the following circumstances: as part of orientation for newly hired nurses, when a change in protocol or procedure takes place, with the introduction of new equipment or technology, and when quality improvement monitoring or other data sources reveal a gap in skills or knowledge related to PN administration.[6]

The ultimate goal is to achieve safe PN administration, based on evaluation of individual patients, which is achieved by an interprofessional collaboration among physicians, dietitians, nurses, and pharmacists. The role of EHRs in providing a layer of safety with built-in checks cannot be overstated. See Figure 9-4 for the PN administration checklist. This checklist can serve as an adjunct to the competency tool.[6]

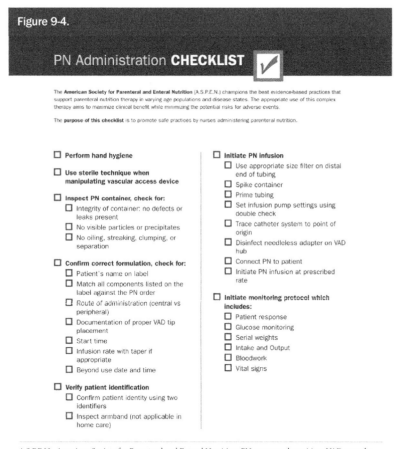

Figure 9-4.

PN Administration **CHECKLIST**

The **American Society for Parenteral and Enteral Nutrition** (A.S.P.E.N.) champions the best evidence-based practices that support parenteral nutrition therapy in varying age populations and disease states. The appropriate use of this complex therapy aims to maximize clinical benefit while minimizing the potential risks for adverse events.

The **purpose of this checklist** is to promote safe practices by nurses administering parenteral nutrition.

☐ Perform hand hygiene

☐ Use sterile technique when manipulating vascular access device

☐ Inspect PN container, check for:
  ☐ Integrity of container: no defects or leaks present
  ☐ No visible particles or precipitates
  ☐ No oiling, streaking, clumping, or separation

☐ Confirm correct formulation, check for:
  ☐ Patient's name on label
  ☐ Match all components listed on the label against the PN order
  ☐ Route of administration (central vs peripheral)
  ☐ Documentation of proper VAD tip placement
  ☐ Start time
  ☐ Infusion rate with taper if appropriate
  ☐ Beyond use date and time

☐ Verify patient identification
  ☐ Confirm patient identity using two identifiers
  ☐ Inspect armband (not applicable in home care)

☐ Initiate PN infusion
  ☐ Use appropriate size filter on distal end of tubing
  ☐ Spike container
  ☐ Prime tubing
  ☐ Set infusion pump settings using double check
  ☐ Trace catheter system to point of origin
  ☐ Disinfect needleless adapter on VAD hub
  ☐ Connect PN to patient
  ☐ Initiate PN infusion at prescribed rate

☐ Initiate monitoring protocol which includes:
  ☐ Patient response
  ☐ Glucose monitoring
  ☐ Serial weights
  ☐ Intake and Output
  ☐ Bloodwork
  ☐ Vital signs

A.S.P.E.N., American Society for Parenteral and Enteral Nutrition; PN, parenteral nutrition; VAD, vascular access device.

Summary

PN is a complex therapeutic modality and should be administered by those clinicians with demonstrated competency in PN administration, order writing, and prescribing to optimize the delivery of safe and effective therapy. Participation in interdisciplinary rounds to discuss patients requiring PN is an excellent way to develop knowledge about the therapy. To deliver safe and competent care for patients receiving PN, institutions must implement policies and procedures that assure assessment of staff members' ability to perform competent PN administration and prescribing. The ASPEN models presented in this chapter can be used to develop and implement such policies and procedures.

References

1. Agency for Healthcare Research and Quality. All listed ICD-9-CM procedure codes for parenteral nutrition infusion, 2012. In: Healthcare Utilization Project (HCUP) National Inpatient Survey. www.hcupnet.ahrq.gov. Accessed January 10, 2015.

2. Boullata JI, Guenter P, Mirtallo JM. A parenteral nutrition use survey with gap analysis. *JPEN J Parenter Enteral Nutr.* 2013;37(2):212–222.

3. Boullata JI, Gilbert K, Sacks G, et al; ASPEN. A.S.P.E.N. clinical guidelines: parenteral nutrition ordering, order review, compounding, labeling, and dispensing. *JPEN J Parenter Enteral Nutr.* 2014;38(3):334–377.

4. Boitano M, Bojak S, McCloskey S, McCaul DS, McDonough M. Improving the safety and effectiveness of parenteral nutrition: results of a quality improvement collaboration. *Nutr Clin Pract.* 2010;25(6):663–671.

5. Centers for Medicare & Medicaid Services, Department of Health and Human Services. Medicare and Medicaid Programs; regulatory provisions to promote program efficiency, transparency, and burden reduction; part II. *Fed Regist.* 2014;79(91):27105–27157.

6. Ayers P, Adams S, Boullata J, et al; ASPEN. A.S.P.E.N. parenteral nutrition safety consensus recommendations. *JPEN J Parenter Enteral Nutr.* 2014;38(3):296–333.

7. National Prescribing Centre; National Institute for Health and Clinical Excellence. *A Single Competency Framework for All Prescribers.* https://v3.pebblepad.co.uk/v3portfolio/cumbria/File/OpenFile/94jgbwqMpZdkm83yzzxsRgdZwh. Published May 2012. Reviewed May 2014. Accessed March 23, 2015.

8. Board of Directors, ASPEN. Interdisciplinary nutrition support core competencies. *Nutr Clin Pract.* 1999;14(6):331–333.

9. Schneider PJ. Crossing the quality chasm: building a safe nutrition system. *JPEN J Parenter Enteral Nutr.* 2002;26(4):219–225.

10. Whidden S, Hollyforde S. *The Competencies Handbook.* London, UK. Chartered Institute of Personnel and Development; 1999.

11. White R. Parenteral nutrition for adults—an overview of the basic principles. *Clin Pharm.* 2011;3:183–184.

12. Stewart JAD, Mason DG, Smith N, Protopapa K, Mason M; National Confidential Enquiry into Patient Outcome and Death. A mixed bag: an enquiry into the care of hospital patients receiving parenteral nutrition. http://www.ncepod.org.uk/2010report1/downloads/PN_report.pdf. Published June 2010. Accessed March 23, 2015.

13. Quercia RA, Keating KP. A CQI program for prescribing and dispensing total parenteral nutrition. *Nutr Clin Pract.* 1998;13(5):219–224.

14. Storm HM, Young SL, Sandler RH. Development of pediatric and neonatal parenteral nutrition order forms. *Nutr Clin Pract.*1995;10(2):54–59.

CHAPTER 9

15. Adams KM, Kohlmeier M, Powell M, Zeisel SH. Nutrition in medicine: nutrition education for medical students and residents. *Nutr Clin Pract.* 2010;25(5):471–480.

16. Vanek VW, Sharnek LK, Snyder DM, Kupensky DT, Rutushin AL. Assessment of physicians' ability to prescribe parenteral nutrition support in a community teaching hospital. *J Am Diet Assoc.* 1997;97(8):856–859.

17. Gourley DR, Fitzgerald WL, Davis RL. Competency, board certification, credentialing, and specialization: who benefits? *Am J Manag Care.*1997;3(5):795–801.

18. Mulholland P. Pharmacist prescribing in neonatal intensive care units in the UK. *Arch Dis Child.* 2013;98(6):e1. doi:10.1136/archdischild-2013-303935b.6

19. Seres D, Sacks GS, Pederson CA, et al. Parenteral nutrition safe practices: results of the 2003 ASPEN Survey. *JPEN J Parenter Enteral Nutr.* 2006;30(3):259–265.

20. Ragab MH, Al-Hindi MY, Alrayees MM. Neonatal parenteral nutrition: review of the pharmacist role as a prescriber. *Saudi Pharm J.* 2016;24(4):429–440.

21. Faber EM. Program for training staff pharmacists in total parenteral nutrition. *Am J Hosp Pharm.* 1991;48(5):980–986.

22. Ahmed M, Irwin S, Tuthill DP. Education and evidence are needed to improve neonatal parenteral nutrition practice. *JPEN J Parenter Enteral Nutr.* 2004;28(3):176–179.

23. Pearson G, Yuksel N, Card D, et al; Task Force on Pharmacist Prescribing. An information paper on pharmacist prescribing within a healthcare facility. *Can J Hosp Pharm.* 2002;55(1):56–62.

24. Davis AM, Baker SS, Leary RA. Advancing clinical privileges for nutrition support practitioners: the dietitian as a model. *Nutr Clin Pract.* 1995;10(3):98–103.

25. Moreland K, Gotfried M, Vaughan L. Development and implementation of the clinical privileges for dietitian nutrition order writing program at a long-term acute-care hospital. *J Am Diet Assoc.* 2002;102(1):72–81.

26. Roberts SR. Improving patient outcomes through registered dietitian order writing. *Nutr Clin Pract.* 2013;28(5):556–565.

27. Holaska JC. Parenteral nutrition web-based order writing: educating prescribers utilizing a network-wide computerized e-learning tool. *J Am Diet Assoc.* 2012;112:139.

28. DiMaria-Ghalili RA, Mirtallo JM, Tobin BW, Hark L, Van Horn L, Palmer CA. Challenges and opportunities for nutrition education and training in the health care professions: intraprofessional and interprofessional call to action. *Am J Clin Nutr.* 2014;99(5 suppl):1184S–1193S.

29. Sullivan SY. Nutrition education in physician assistant programs: a national survey. *J Physician Assist Educ.* 2000;11(1):18–24.

30. Maillet JOS, Fixelle R, Thornton J. What physician assistants should know about nutrition. *Top Clin Nutr.* 1997;12(3):49–57.

31. Pedersen CA, Schneider PJ, Scheckelhoff DJ. ASHP national survey of pharmacy practice in hospital settings: dispensing and administration-2014. *Am J Health Syst Pharm.* 2015;72(13):1119–1137.

32. American Society of Health-System Pharmacists. ASHP guidelines on the safe use of automated compounding devices for the preparation of parenteral nutrition admixtures. *Am J Health Syst Pharm.* 2000;57(14):1343–1348.

33. American Society of Health-System Pharmacists. ASHP guidelines on compounding sterile preparations. *Am J Health Syst Pharm.* 2014;71(2):145–166.

34. Rich DS, Fricker MP Jr, Cohen MR, Levine SR. Guidelines for the safe preparation of sterile compounds: results of the ISMP sterile preparation compounding safety summit of October 2011. *Hosp Pharm.* 2013;48(4):282–294, 301.

35. United States Pharmacopeia. *USP Chapter <797>; Pharmaceutical Compounding — Sterile Preparations.* Rockville, MD: United States Pharmacopeial Conv37ention; 2015.

36. Tucker A, Ybarra J, Bingham A, et al; Standards of Practice for Nutrition Support Pharmacists Task Force; ASPEN. American Society for Parenteral and Enteral Nutrition standards of practice for nutrition support pharmacists. *Nutr Clin Pract.* 2015;30(1):139–146.

37. Food and Drug Administration. Safety alert: hazards of precipitation associated with parenteral nutrition. *Am J Hosp Pharm.* 1994;51(11):1427–1428.

38. Frean JA, Arntzen L, Rosekilly I, Isaäcson M. Investigation of contaminated parenteral nutrition fluids associated with an outbreak of Serratia odorifera septicaemia. *J Hosp Infect.* 1994;27(4):263–273.

39. Carey LC, Haffey M. Incident: home TPN formula order misinterpreted after hospital admission. *Home Care Highlights.* 1995;2(2):7.

40. Hill SE, Heldman LS, Goo EDH, Whippo PE, Perkinson JC. Fatal microvascular pulmonary emboli from precipitation of a total nutrient admixture solution. *JPEN J Parenter Enteral Nutr.* 1996;20(1):81–87.

41. Shay DK, Fann LM, Jarvis WR; Hospital Infections Program, Centers for Disease Control and Prevention. Respiratory distress and sudden death associated with receipt of a peripheral parenteral nutrition admixture. *Infect Control Hosp Epidemiol.* 1997;18(12):814–817.

42. Tresoldi AT, Padoveze MC, Trabasso P, et al. Enterobacter cloacae sepsis outbreak in a newborn unit caused by contaminated total parenteral nutrition solution. *Am J Infect Control.* 2000;28(3):258–261.

43. Mirtallo J, CanadaT, Johnson D, et al. Safe practices for parenteral nutrition [erratum in *JPEN J Parenter Enteral Nutr.* 2006;30(2):177]. *JPEN J Parenter Enteral Nutr.* 2004;28(6):S39–S70.

44. Habsah H, Zeehaida M, Van Rostenberghe H, et al. An outbreak of Pantoea spp. in a neonatal intensive care unit secondary to contaminated parenteral nutrition. *J Hosp Infect.* 2005;61(3):213–218.

45. Institute for Safe Medication Practices. Fatal 1,000-fold overdoses can occur, particularly in neonates, by transposing mcg and mg. *ISMP Med Safety Alert.* 2007;12(18):1–4.

46. Bergman KA, Arends JP, Schölvinck EH. Pantoea agglomerans septicemia in three newborn infants. *Pediatr Infect Dis J.* 2007;26(5)453–454.

47. Institute for Safe Medication Practices. Another tragic parenteral nutrition compounding error. *ISMP Med Safety Alert.* 2011;16(8):1–3.

48. Institute for Safe Medication Practices. Parenteral nutrition deaths tied to drug shortage. *ISMP Med Safety Alert!* 2011;16(8):4.

49. Institute for Safe Medication Practices. Mismatched prescribing and pharmacy templates for parenteral nutrition (PN) leads to data entry errors. *ISMP Med Saf Alert!* 2012;17(13):1–3.

50. Gupta N, Hocevar SN, Moulton-Meissner HA, et al. Outbreak of Serratia marcescens bloodstream infections in patient receiving parenteral nutrition prepared by a compounding pharmacy. *Clin Infect Dis.* 2014;59(1):1–8.

51. Ayers P, Adams S, Boullata J, et al. A.S.P.E.N. safety consensus recommendations: translation into practice. *Nutr Clin Pract.* 2014;29(3):277–282.

52. ASPEN. Safety checklists, 2016. http://www.nutritioncare.org/Guidelines_and_Clinical_ Resources/Toolkits/Parenteral_Nutrition_Safety_Toolkit/Parenteral_Nutrition_Safety_ Consensus_Recommendations_and_Clinical_Guidelines/. Accessed February 4, 2020.

53. Gourley DR, Fitzgerald WL Jr, Davis RL. Competency, board certification, credentialing, and specialization: who benefits? *Am J Manag Care.* 1997;3(5).795–801; quiz 805–807.

54. Board of Pharmacy Specialties. BPS press release, September 10, 2015. http://www.bpsweb.org/news/pr_091015.pdf. Accessed January 10, 2016.

55. The National Board of Nutrition Support Certification. Home: National Board of Nutrition Support Certification. http://www.nutritioncare.org/nbnsc/. Accessed April 10, 2016.

56. Seres D, Sacks GS, Pederson CA, et al. Parenteral nutrition safe practices: results of the 2003 American Society for Parenteral and Enteral Nutrition Survey. *JPEN J Parenter Enteral Nutr.* 2006;30:259–265.

57. Pharmacy Technician Certification Board. Home: Pharmacy Technician Certification Board. www.ptcb.org. Accessed January 10, 2016.

58. ASPEN. Professional development, 2016. http://www.nutritioncare.org/Continuing_
Education/Professional_Development/. Accessed January 10, 2016.

59. American Society of Health-System Pharmacists. Tools for sterile compounding, 2016.
http://www.ashp.org/menu/PracticePolicy/ResourceCenters/Compounding/Tools-for-
Sterile-Compounding.aspx. Accessed January 10, 2016.

60. American Society of Health-System Pharmacists. Sterile compounding resource center,
2016. http://www.ashp.org/menu/PracticePolicy/ResourceCenters/Compounding.
Accessed January 10, 2016.

61. Agency for Healthcare Research and Quality. All listed ICD-9-CM procedure code for
parenteral nutrition infusion, 2014. In: *Healthcare Utilization Project (HCUP) National
Inpatient Survey.* http://www.hcupnet.ahrq.gov. Accessed August 9, 2017.

62. Mundi MS, Pattinson A, McMahon MT, Davidson J, Hurt RT. Prevalence of home
parenteral and enteral nutrition in the United States. *Nutr Clin Pract.* 2017;32(6):799–805.

63. Guenter P, Ayers P, Boullata JI, Gura KM, Holcombe B, Sacks GS. Parenteral
nutrition errors and potential errors reported over the past 10 years. *Nutr Clin Pract.*
2017;32(6):826–830.

64. Wollitz A, Grissinger M. Aligning the lines: an analysis of IV line errors. *Pa Patient Saf
Advis.* 2014;11(1):1-7.

65. Hicks RW, Becker SC, Chuo J. A summary of NICU fat emulsion medication errors and
nursing services: data from MEDMARX. *Adv Neonatal Care.* 2007;7(6):299–308.

66. Sacks GS, Rough S, Kudsk KA. Frequency and severity of harm of medication errors
related to the parenteral nutrition process in a large university teaching hospital.
Pharmacotherapy. 2009;29(8):966–974.

67. MacKay M, Anderson C, Boehme S, Cash J, Zobell J. Frequency and severity of parenteral
nutrition medication errors at a large children's hospital after implementation of
electronic ordering and compounding. *Nutr Clin Pract.* 2016;31(2):195–206.

68. Institute for Safe Medication Practices. Pharmacist supervision is critical for proper
preparation of Clinimix multichamber bags. *ISMP Med Saf Alert!* Nurse AdviseERR.
2011;9(4):1–2.

69. Christensen ML, Ayers P, Boullata JI, et al; ASPEN PN Safety Committee. Lipid injectable
emulsion survey with gap analysis. *Nutr Clin Pract.* 2017;32(5):694–702.

70. Boullata JI. Safe practices for enteral and parenteral nutrition. In: Seres DS, Way CW, eds.
Nutrition Support for the Critically Ill. New York, NY: Springer; 2016:229–241.

71. World Health Organization. Reporting and learning systems for medication errors: the
role of pharmacovigilance centres. http://www.who.int/medicines/areas/quality_safety/
safety_efficacy/emp_mes/en/. Published 2014. Accessed September 15, 2016.

72. Guenter P, Boullata JI, Ayers P, et al. Standardized competencies for parenteral nutrition
prescribing: the American Society for Parenteral and Enteral Nutrition model. *Nutr Clin
Pract.* 2015;30(4):570–576.

73. Boullata JI, Holcombe B, Sacks G, et al; Parenteral Nutrition Safety Committee, ASPEN.
Standardized competencies for parenteral nutrition order review and parenteral
nutrition preparation, including compounding: the ASPEN model. *Nutr Clin Pract.*
2016;31(4):548–555.

74. DiMaria-Ghalili RA, Gilbert K, Lord L, et al; ASPEN Nurses Standards Revision Task
Force, ASPEN. Standards of nutrition care practice and professional performance for
nutrition support and generalist nurses. *Nutr Clin Pract.* 2016;31(4):527–547.

Medication-Related Interactions

Introduction

Interactions between parenteral nutrition (PN) and other medications are likely to occur and should be evaluated as part of the PN order review process. Patient outcomes may be influenced by some of these interactions (eg, because of loss of infusion access or an inappropriate response to a drug). Numerous factors must be considered to prevent or mitigate drug and nutrition interactions (DNIs).

DNIs generally result from physical, chemical, physiologic, or pathophysiologic relationships not only between a drug and a nutrient but also between a drug and multiple nutrients, food in general, specific foods or components, or nutrition status, which is clinically significant if the drug response is altered or nutrition status is compromised.[1,2] Although one group is the object of the interaction, another is the precipitating factor; for example, food may reduce absorption of bisphosphonates (ie, a food-drug interaction). or some antiepileptic drugs may reduce vitamin D status (ie, a DNI). Regardless of the precipitant or object, a DNI is clinically significant if it modifies drug response and/or compromises nutrition status. Interactions can be classified mechanistically as pharmaceutical (ie, physicochemical reactions), pharmacokinetic, or pharmacodynamic.[1]

DNIs with PN present a unique situation; PN and its many components can be considered drugs as well as nutrients.[3] In some cases, PN contains nonnutrient drugs (eg, insulin). Interactions may occur within the PN bag, the administration set, and the intravascular access device, as well as within the patient. These can involve not only the typical components of PN but also other medications administered to the patient. Administering other medications by Y-site infusion sets up the potential for pharmaceutical interactions, whereas systemic exposure to other drugs has the potential for pharmacokinetic or pharmacodynamics interaction. The route and method of drug administration, the dosage form, and pharmacokinetic properties, as well as the stability and compatibility characteristics of a drug, must be evaluated. Factors related to nutrition support that may influence DNIs include the type and site of access, method of administration, and components in the PN.

Unfortunately, few DNIs are well studied in patients receiving PN therapy, and studies that do exist often focus on in vitro physical compatibility interactions or use small numbers of healthy volunteers. Studies in patients are typically unblinded, not placebo controlled, and retrospective in nature; observational studies and case reports from very small numbers of patients are often the only data available. Thus, an understanding of the mechanism of interaction is often poor, and the strength of evidence supporting methods to prevent or mitigate interactions in patients receiving PN therapy is seldom strong. Even the limited data available in the literature are sometimes conflicting, leading to multiple approaches to manage an interaction. Despite these limited and conflicting data, it is often possible to identify general principles that apply to the management of DNIs. This chapter will present general principles to consider with DNIs and discuss specific issues related to the concurrent administration of nonnutrient drugs with PN therapy. This chapter is not intended to be inclusive of all potential DNIs that the clinician may encounter but to illustrate certain common clinical dilemmas.

Table 10-1 illustrates one system for classifying DNIs; other systems using somewhat different categories and terminology are also in use. The focus of this chapter is primarily on the pharmaceutical, pharmacokinetic, and pharmacodynamic interactions because these types are the most likely to present problems specific to PN therapy. Other types of interactions, such as electrolyte alterations related to specific medications, also occur in patients receiving nutrition support, but they tend to be independent of the route of nutrition and will occur whether the patient receives PN, enteral nutrition (EN), or an oral diet.

Table 10-1. Classification of DNIs With PN

Type of Interaction	Effect of Interaction	Associated Factors
Pharmaceutical	Precipitation in PN preparations; disruption of emulsion for ILE preparation; altered viscosity; loss of drug activity; toxicity	Drug and preparation pH; reactive chemical moieties; protein complexity; time; temperature; duration of exposure
Pharmacokinetic	Loss of drug activity; toxicity	Occurs at the sites where drug and nutrient are transported, metabolized, and eliminated
Pharmacodynamic	Loss of drug activity; toxicity	Occurs at the site of action; binding sites or receptors usually involved

DNI, drug and nutrition interaction; ILE, lipid injectable emulsion; PN, parenteral nutrition.

Pharmaceutical Interactions

Pharmaceutical interactions are physical or chemical interactions that alter the characteristics of the nutrition formulation or the medication and typically take place before the drug and nutrient involved have entered the body.[4] These can involve physical or chemical incompatibility, as well as stability concerns for individual components or the PN system.

Interactions that result in altered physical characteristics of the nutrition formulation or the drug occur with PN therapy. Occlusion of the feeding access device is frequently the outcome from physical interactions. Physical interactions typically occur in the preparation or infusion before the drug or nutrients reach the patient.[4] Variables that are important to consider in assessing the risk of physical interactions include the pH at which the drug and the PN formulation are most stable, the presence of cations and anions known to react chemically, the concentration and chemical complexity of nutrients, the container matrix, time, temperature, and the duration of exposure to one another. This latter factor is one reason admixture of drugs with a PN formulation is very different than Y-site administration or coadministration.

Additives to PN Formulation

Many drug studies with PN focus on physical interactions and are generally referred to as compatibility studies. Incompatibility with PN formulations most commonly results in precipitate formations that are occasionally visible to the unaided eyes. Drugs that show no evidence of physical interaction with PN are generally classified as compatible. However, they may not be stable with PN. Although the terms are frequently interchanged in the medical literature, stability is distinct from compatibility. Instability typically results in loss of drug or nutrient activity. For example, injectable multivitamin preparations are compatible with PN preparations, although some vitamins, such as thiamin and ascorbic acid, have limited stability and begin to decompose and lose their activity very quickly once added to the PN formulation because of hydrolysis, photodegradation, or other forms of chemical degradation.

Safety guidelines that address the stability and compatibility of PN formulations have been developed.[5-7] Administration of drugs with PN, either by admixture or co-infusion, should provide a safe product that is stable and free from incompatibility. General principles for evaluating compatibility of drugs with a PN formulation include obtaining data for both physical compatibility and chemical stability of the drug and PN components whenever possible. Unfortunately, studies often evaluate only physical compatibility (eg, precipitate formation, haze, cloudiness) and provide no data on chemical compatibility or the stability of either the drug or PN components. Details related to the specific drug formulation (eg, with or without preservative, salt form) and drug concentrations evaluated, as well as specific components in the PN formulation, should also be considered. Dextrose and amino acid concentration; the specific amino acid product used for compounding; the inclusion of a lipid injectable emulsion (ILE) and the type of ILE product (eg, soybean oil–based); electrolyte concentrations and specific electrolytes added; and the addition of trace elements, unfractionated heparin, regular insulin, and other components can all influence compatibility and stability of PN formulations. Information regarding ILEs new to the US market and compatibility are being studied. Efficacy and toxicity profiles must be acceptable for administration by continuous infusion rather than intermittent infusion.

Reviewing the package insert for the pH and pKa of a medication may provide information for predicting compatibility with a PN preparation. Medications that are weak acids or bases are formulated at a pH that optimizes their solubility. Intravenous (IV) medications that produce extreme changes in the final pH of the reconstituted product, such as phenytoin, tend to be most reactive and therefore capable of significant incompatibilities. Injectable medications that contain cosolvents, such as propylene glycol or ethanol, have the greatest potential for interaction if coadministered with a PN formulation or other large-volume parenteral infusion. Examples include furosemide, diazepam, digoxin, phenytoin, and etoposide.

Physicochemical interactions are best avoided by not allowing drugs to mix with PN formulations. Ideally, drugs should be administered via a route other than the lumen of the vascular access device (VAD) used for PN administration, although this is not always possible. There are a few exceptions in which products are added directly to the PN preparation, including drugs such as regular insulin or histamine 2 (H_2)-receptor antagonists. When a drug that has been determined to be incompatible with PN must be administered through the same IV catheter as the PN, the PN admixture should be stopped, and the access device should be flushed with fluid that is compatible with the PN preparation, as well as the drug. The lumen of the VAD should be flushed before and after drug administration and between drugs if >1 is administered. The "flush" volume must be adequate to eliminate all of the PN formulation or the drug from the lumen of the VAD. Sodium chloride 0.9% is the usual fluid of choice for flushing IV catheters, but a dextrose 5% in water solution is sometimes required. The minimum flush volume for VADs is typically specified by the manufacturer based on catheter size and type. For incompatible drugs that have prolonged administration times (ie, > 30 minutes) and depending on the patient (eg, infant or adult) and the dextrose infusion rate of the PN formulation, the PN formulation may need to be tapered off prior to administering the drug to offset any potential for rebound hypoglycemia.

Other potential methods of preventing physical interactions with PN formulations include altering the formulation or the drug. For PN, an interacting component of the formulation that is not essential, such as heparin, could be omitted. Alternative dosage forms or drugs that are therapeutic equivalents (different drug with the same therapeutic effect) but have a different potential to interact may be viable options in some cases.

ASPEN's clinical safety guidelines recommend that nonnutrient medication can only be included in PN admixtures when supported by (1) pharmaceutical data describing physicochemical compatibility and stability of the additive medication and of the final preparation under conditions of typical use and (2) clinical data confirming the expected therapeutic actions of the medication.[7] The extrapolation beyond the published parameter limits (eg, products and concentrations) of the given data is discouraged.

Medications Co-infused Into PN Tubing

Usually, secondary or IV piggyback medications are co-infused at a Y-site simultaneously with a primary infusion. In most cases, the primary IV infusion contains relatively low concentrations of electrolytes and poses few compatibility problems. Also, the time for contact with the secondary IV infusion is relatively short. Most significant interactions are dependent on time and concentration. The situation becomes more complicated if a PN formulation is used as the primary IV infusion. This should be avoided unless physical and chemical compatibility of the medication with the PN formulation is ensured prior to its administration in this manner.

Studies of medication compatibility with PN found that the compatibility differed for amino acid/dextrose/ILE (3-in-1) vs amino acid/dextrose (2-in-1) formulations, emphasizing that compatibility in 1 formulation does not predict compatibility in the other.[8-10] As such, compatibility information should be derived for PN that closely matches the formulation prescribed for the patient in question. If the medication is not compatible with PN, the PN infusion should not be interrupted for medication administration. The medication should be administered via another IV route (ie, other lumen of a VAD or peripheral IV, if available). An example is the interaction between ceftriaxone and calcium-containing IV fluids when they are coadministered via a Y-site. The result is the formation of a ceftriaxone/calcium precipitant that has been associated with neonatal fatalities. Ceftriaxone should be avoided in neonates who are receiving calcium-containing fluids, including PN. Finally, the compatibility of some medications with a 3-in-1 preparation may be dependent on the drug concentration. For example, morphine sulfate is compatible with 3-in-1 preparation at a concentration of 1 mg/mL, but not 15 mg/mL. See Tables 10-2 through 10-5 for compatibility of selected medications with PN.[8-10] Keep in mind that the number of formulations tested and the study conditions are usually limited, with most results based on physical compatibility only. In one study, only 5 of 131 drugs studied were found to be compatible with PN by Y-site.[11]

Table 10-2. Commonly Used Drugs That Are Compatible With Specific PN (Dextrose/Amino Acid Formulations)

Amikacin	Erythromycin	Nafcillin
Aminophylline	Famotidine	Nitroglycerin
Ampicillin	Fentanyl	Nitroprusside
Ampicillin/sulbactam	Fluconazole	Norepinephrine
Aztreonam	Gentamicin	Octreotide
Calcium gluconate	Heparin	*10 mcg/mL diluted*
0.19 mEq/mL diluted	*100 units/mL undiluted*	Ondansetron
Cefotetan	Haloperidol	Pentobarbital
Cefotaxime	Hydrocortisone	Piperacillin
Cefoxitin	Hydromorphone	Piperacillin/tazobactam
Ceftazidime	Imipenem/cilastatin	Propofol
Cefuroxime	Insulin, regular	Ranitidine
Cimetidine	Iron dextran	Tacrolimus
Clindamycin	Leucovorin	Ticarcillin/clavulanate
Dexamethasone	Lorazepam	Tobramycin
Digoxin	Magnesium sulfate	Trimethoprim/
Diphenhydramine	*0.81 mEq/mL diluted*	sulfamethoxazole
Dobutamine	Meperidine	Vancomycin
Dopamine	Metronidazole	Zidovudine
Enalaprilat	Morphine	

PN, parenteral nutrition.

Table 10-3. Commonly Used Drugs That Are Compatible With Specific PN (3-in-1 Containing Soybean Oil–Based Fat Emulsion)

Amikacin	Dobutamine	Nitroglycerin
Aminophylline	Enalaprilat	Nitroprusside
Ampicillin	Famotidine	Norepinephrine
Ampicillin/Sulbactam	Fentanyl	Octreotide *10 mcg/mL diluted*
Aztreonam	Fluconazole	Piperacillin
Calcium gluconate *0.19 mEq/mL diluted*	Gentamicin	Piperacillin/tazobactam
	Hydrocortisone	
Cefotetan	Imipenem/cilastatin	Potassium chloride *0.1 mEq/mL diluted*
Cefotaxime	Insulin, regular	Ranitidine
Cefoxitin	Leucovorin	Tacrolimus
Ceftazidime	Magnesium sulfate *0.81 mEq/mL diluted*	Ticarcillin/clavulanate
Cefuroxime		Tobramycin
Cimetidine	Meperidine	Trimethoprim/ sulfamethoxazole
Clindamycin	Meropenem	
Dexamethasone	Metronidazole	Vancomycin
Digoxin	Morphine[a]	Zidovudine
Diphenhydramine	Nafcillin	

PN, parenteral nutrition.

[a]Morphine sulfate incompatible at a concentration of 15 mg/mL but compatible at a concentration of 1 mg/mL.

Table 10-4. Commonly Used Drugs That Are Incompatible With Specific PN (Dextrose/Amino Acid Preparations)

Acyclovir	Fluorouracil	Mitoxantrone
Amphotericin B	Furosemide	Phenytoin
Cefazolin	Ganciclovir	Potassium phosphate *3 mmol/mL undiluted*
Ciprofloxacin	Immune globulin	
Cisplatin	Methotrexate	Promethazine
Cyclosporin	Metoclopramide	Sodium bicarbonate
Cytarabine	Midazolam	Sodium phosphate *3 mmol/mL undiluted*
Doxorubicin	Minocycline	

PN, parenteral nutrition.

Table 10-5. Commonly Used Drugs That Are Incompatible With Specific PN (3-in-1 Containing Soybean Oil–Based Fat Emulsion)

Acyclovir	Haloperidol	Ondansetron
Albumin	Heparin	Pentobarbital
Amphotericin B	*100 units/mL undiluted*	Phenobarbital
Cyclosporin	Hydromorphone	Phenytoin
Dopamine	Iron dextran	Potassium phosphate
Doxorubicin	Levorphanol	*3 mmol/mL undiluted*
Doxycycline	Lorazepam	Sodium phosphate
Droperidol	Midazolam	*3 mmol/mL undiluted*
Erythromycin	Minocycline	
Fluorouracil	Morphinea	
Ganciclovir	Nalbuphine	

PN, parenteral nutrition.
aMorphine sulfate incompatible at a concentration of 15 mg/mL, but compatible at a concentration of 1 mg/mL.

Pharmacokinetic Interactions

The term *pharmacokinetics* refers to studies of the time course for drug absorption, distribution, metabolism, and excretion.[12] However, the term can also be applied to nutrients because these same processes occur. Pharmacokinetic DNIs are characterized by alterations in ≥1 pharmacokinetic parameter of a drug or nutrient because of an interaction between them. Changes in drug absorption and metabolism are most often reported. The effects of drugs on nutrient pharmacokinetics are rarely evaluated.

Pharmacokinetic DNIs occur as the result of multiple factors, including those related to administration of PN and the drug. The disease process underlying the requirement for PN therapy can also contribute to pharmacokinetic DNIs, especially as it affects protein status, organ perfusion, and gastrointestinal (GI) motility.

Pharmacodynamic Interactions

Pharmacodynamics refers to the relationship between drug concentration at the site of action and the resulting effect, including the time course and intensity of therapeutic and adverse effects. The effect of a drug present at the site of action is determined by that drug's binding with a receptor.[12] Few examples of the pharmacodynamics of DNIs exist, with the most common being the interaction between the anticoagulant warfarin and vitamin K.

Administration-Related Factors

Tubing and Bag Characteristics

Adsorption of a drug or nutrient to a container or administration tubing results in product loss without changes in the physical appearance of the products and is difficult to separate from chemical instability without sophisticated analysis. Products with high fat solubility are more likely to undergo adsorption with plastics, but other drugs (eg, insulin) can also be adsorbed. The classic example of nutrient loss to the container is vitamin A loss into diethylhexyl phthalate (DEHP)-containing plastics.[13] Desorption can also occur. For example, ILE actually leaches DEHP from the bags into the emulsion, as does the Cremophor (castor oil emulsion) used in formulating certain fat-soluble drugs, such as cyclosporine A. Although not DNIs in the usual sense, these interactions are concerning because the solubilized DEHP and other plasticizers may pose a significant health risk.

Site of Delivery

The site of drug delivery has minimal effect on PN-associated DNIs but can be a major administration-related factor for EN therapy. For PN therapy, the delivery sites are the peripheral vein or central venous circulation, with the primary difference in PN formulations being a lower osmolarity of peripheral PN.

Formula-Related Factors

Macronutrients

Protein may also influence drug metabolism through effects on enzymes of the mixed-function oxidase system (MFOS) in the liver.[14,15] Activity of the MFOS appears to be stimulated with high protein intake and with riboflavin, niacin, and large ascorbic acid doses, thereby increasing clearance of drugs metabolized by these enzymes. Protein intake may also influence blood flow, with low intake reducing flow to the kidney and lowering renal elimination of some drugs. However, most data on protein effects are specific to oral protein intake in animal studies, and more research is required before any definitive statement or recommendations can be made regarding the effect of parenteral amino acids on DNIs in the clinical setting.

Micronutrients

Micronutrients in EN formulations have the potential to cause DNIs. For example, divalent and trivalent minerals (calcium, magnesium, zinc, and iron) are known to form complexes with certain drugs, such as tetracycline and ciprofloxacin, which results in poor absorption of the drugs. Degradation products from micronutrients have also been reported to cause physical interactions. For instance, oxalate from ascorbic acid degradation has been reported to interact with calcium in PN formulations, forming an insoluble precipitate.[16]

Disease-Related Factors

Malnutrition is a disease associated with alterations in body composition that may affect the risk of pharmacokinetic DNIs. Pharmacokinetic parameters can be affected by decreased serum concentrations of visceral proteins, especially albumin, which can bind many drugs (eg, phenytoin, valproic acid, and warfarin). Edema, increased body water, and decreased lean muscle mass may also affect pharmacokinetic parameters. Other disease-related factors include alterations in organ function and perfusion, as well as effects on GI motility.

Medication Additives with PN

In general, the PN formulation should not be used as a medication delivery vehicle because of potential DNIs and limited compatibility and stability data.[7] However, in some situations, the concurrent administration of medications with PN may be appropriate. If the medication will come into direct contact with the PN formulation, either through administration in a single container or co-infusion through the same IV tubing, the compatibility and stability of the various components should be validated. If an incompatible or unstable condition exists or information is not available, the medication should be administered separately from the PN preparation.[4,7]

Medications Added Directly to the PN Formulation

H2-receptor antagonists. Cimetidine, ranitidine, and famotidine have been added to PN formulations to reduce gastric acid secretion. Clinical evidence supports the efficacy of administering H_2-receptor antagonists via a continuous infusion. Compatibility and stability of cimetidine, ranitidine, and famotidine when added to PN formulations have been studied in both amino acids/dextrose and 3-in-1 formulations. In the home setting, the addition of H_2-receptor antagonists to PN formulations should be done by the patient or caregiver immediately prior to administration, but only when the PN formulation being used closely matches those studied for compatibility, stability, and clinical effect.

Insulin. Insulin is commonly administered with PN. Only regular human insulin is compatible with PN formulations. Other insulin products, such as neutral protamine Hagedorn, lispro, aspart, detemir, glulisine, degludec, and glargine are incompatible with PN. Insulin requirements are generally higher and most variable during the first 24 hours of intensive care for patients with critical illness. Because of the potential for serious adverse events, the addition of insulin in PN should be done in a consistent manner that adheres to a defined protocol, of which healthcare personnel have adequate knowledge. Hyperglycemia and insulin resistance occur frequently in patients receiving PN. Recommendations for insulin therapy via PN can be found in the hyperglycemia section in chapter 8 ("Complications of Parenteral Nutrition").

Insulin binds (adsorbs) to the surface of the delivery container and the administration set. Binding is particularly problematic with polyvinyl chloride containers. The extent of binding to a particular container is also influenced by the PN formulation within the container. The effect of the PN formulation on the extent of insulin binding to the container surface is as follows (from greatest binding to least)[17]: 0.9% sodium chloride > dextrose > amino acids > albumin. Therefore, the same dose of insulin will have a different amount of activity depending on the vehicle in which it is administered. The higher the concentration of insulin, the lower the extent of adsorption, because the container has a limited number of binding sites.

Iron dextran. Although not recommended by the manufacturer, iron dextran has been administered in PN formulations. Results of studies evaluating iron dextran stability and compatibility in PN solutions have been inconsistent.[18-20] The inconsistency may relate to the use of maintenance compared with replacement iron doses via PN.[17] Most clinicians agree that iron dextran supplementation via 3-in-1 formulations is not recommended because of the risk of altering the stability of the fat emulsion when exposed to the additional cationic properties of iron dextran.[20] If iron dextran is added to the dextrose/amino acid PN formulation, first-dose precautions (monitor vital signs every 15 minutes) should be conducted during the first hour of the PN infusion because of the risk of anaphylaxis.

Heparin. Unfractionated heparin has been added to PN preparations to promote clearance of ILE. It is proposed that heparin can increase serum levels of lipoprotein lipase and lipolytic activity, thereby stabilizing triglyceride levels.[21,22] Heparin should not be added to PN admixtures to reduce risk of central vein thrombosis.[7] Unless unfractionated heparin administration is contraindicated, adding heparin at a dose of 1 unit/mL of neonatal PN solution improves ILE clearance. Unfractionated heparin is not compatible with 3-in-1 formulations.[9]

References

1. Boullata JI, Hudson LM. Drug-nutrient interactions: a broad view with implications for practice. *J Acad Nutr Diet.* 2012;112(4):506–517.

2. Boullata JI. Drug-nutrition interactions and the brain: it's not all in your head. *Curr Nutr Rep.* 2019;8(2):92–98.

3. Mirtallo JM. Drug-nutrient interaction in patients receiving parenteral nutrition. In: Boullata JI, Armenti VT, eds. *Handbook of Drug-Nutrient Interactions.* 2nd ed. New York, NY: Humana Press; 2010:411–424.

4. Chan LN. Drug-nutrient interactions *JPEN J Parenter Enteral Nutr.* 2013;37(4):450–459.

5. Ayers P, Adams S, Boullata J et al; ASPEN. A.S.P.E.N. parenteral nutrition safety consensus recommendations. *JPEN J Parenter Enteral Nutr.* 2014;38(3):296–333.

6. Mirtallo JM, Canada TW, Johnson D, et al; Task Force for the Revision of Safe Practices for Parenteral Nutrition. Safe practices for parenteral nutrition [erratum in JPEN J Parenter Enteral Nutr. 2006;30(2):177]. *JPEN J Parenter Enteral Nutr* 2004;28(6):S39–S70.

7. Boullata JI, Gilbert K, Sacks G, et al; ASPEN. A.S.P.E.N. clinical guidelines: parenteral nutrition ordering, order review, compounding, labeling and dispensing. *JPEN J Parenter Enteral Nutr* 2014;38(3):334–377.

8. Trissel LA, Gilbert DL, Martinez JF, Baker MB, Walter WV, Mirtallo JM. Compatibility of medications with 3-in-1 parenteral nutrition admixtures. *JPEN J Parenter Enteral Nutr.* 1999;23(2):67–74.

9. Trissel LA, Gilbert DL, Martinez JF, Baker MB, Walter WV, Mirtallo JM. Compatibility of parenteral nutrient solutions with selected drugs during simulated Y-site administration. *Am J Health Syst Pharm.* 1997;54(11):1295–1300.

10. Kalikstad B, Skjerdal A, Hansen TW. Compatibility of drug infusions in the NICU. *Arch Dis Child.* 2010;95(9):745–748.

11. Trissel LA. *Handbook on Injectable Drugs.* 16th ed. Bethesda, MD: American Society of Health-System Pharmacists; 2011.

12. Introduction to pharmacokinetics and pharmacodynamics. In: DiPiro JT, Spruill WJ, Wade WE, Blouin RA, Pruemer JM, eds. *Concepts in Clinical Pharmacokinetics.* 5th ed. Bethesda, MD: American Society of Health-System Pharmacists; 2010:1–18.

13. Howard L, Chu R, Feman S, Mintz H, Ovesen L, Wolf B. Vitamin A deficiency from long-term parenteral nutrition. *Ann Intern Med.* 1980;93(4):576–577.

14. Singh BN. Effects of food on clinical pharmacokinetics. *Clin Pharmacokinet.* 1999;37(3):213–255.

15. Williams L, Davis JA, Lowenthal DT. The influence of food on the absorption and metabolism of drugs. *Med Clin North Am.* 1993;77(4):815–829.

16. Gupta DV. Stability of vitamins in total parenteral nutrient solutions. *Am J Hosp Pharm.* 1986;43(9):2132, 2138, 2143.

17. Seres DS. Insulin adsorption to parenteral infusion systems: case report and review of the literature. *Nutr Clin Pract.* 1990;5(3):111–117.

18. Tu Y, Knox NL, Biringer JM, Eichman ML, Schweinsberg PD, Howard JR. Compatibility of iron dextran with total nutrient admixtures. *Am J Hosp Pharm.* 1992;49(9):2233–2235.

19. Vaughn LM, Small C, Plunkett V. Incompatibility of iron dextran and a total nutrient admixture. *Am J Hosp Pharm.* 1990;47(8):1745–1746.

20. Kumpf VJ. Parenteral iron supplementation. *Nutr Clin Pract.* 1996;11(4):139–146.

21. Zaidan H, Dhanireddy R, Hamosh M, Pramanik AK, Chowdhry P, Hamosh P. The effect of continuous heparin administration on Intralipid clearing in very low birth weight infants. *J Pediatr.* 1982;101(4):599–602.

22. Spear ML, Stahl GE, Hamosh M, et al. Effect of heparin dose and infusion rate on lipid clearance and bilirubin binding in premature infants receiving intravenous fat emulsions. *J Pediatr.* 1988;112:94–98.

Home Parenteral Nutrition Support

Introduction

Home nutrition support allows patients with acute and chronic diseases to be managed successfully outside the hospital for the correction of nutrition disorders. The discharge of the first patient receiving home parenteral nutrition (HPN) in 1968 established the advent of "high-tech" home infusion therapy.

In the United States, it has historically been very difficult to ascertain an accurate prevalence of HPN patients. In a recent study, data from 2013 extrapolated that 25,011 US inhabitants received HPN[1] and in summary theorized that HPN utilization has declined since 1992. Most likely, both of these estimates are underestimated because the majority of HPN in the United States has been collectively provided by many smaller, regional, or hospital-owned infusion providers with a wide variety of payers and reimbursement/billing methodologies that are difficult to account for. (Only 3 national infusion providers along with Medicare billing codes were used in the 2013 estimate; in 2019, there were at least 600 infusion pharmacies providing HPN services per the National Home Infusion Association.[2]) The parenteral nutrition (PN) market has been projected to grow at a rate of 5.8% year by year from 2019 to 2026, so one could infer that HPN will continue to increase year by year because of cancer rates, malnutrition, and premature births in the United States.[3]

Advantages and Benefits of HPN Support

The advantages of HPN relate to survival, economic, and quality-of-life (QOL) outcomes.[4-6] Home care services are cost-effective in comparison with typical per day charges in a hospital or skilled nursing facility.[3,7] Technological advances for home care now allow patients to avoid prolonged hospital stays or repeated hospitalizations for nutrition therapies. Home infusion enables patients and their family members to take an active role in their nutrition support therapy.

Patient Selection and Indications for HNS

Standards of practice from the American Society for Parenteral and Enteral Nutrition (ASPEN) specify that home nutrition support (HNS) should be used for patients who cannot meet their nutrient requirements orally and who are able to receive therapy safely outside of an acute care facility.[8] Prior to the initiation of home nutrition support, the primary disease state and clinical condition of the patient should be stabilized. Clinical indications for HPN encompass many more disease states and situations than those specified as reimbursement-eligible under the Centers for Medicare and Medicaid Services (CMS) policy. By contrast, medical necessity for PN is the most common general criterion required for nongovernmental payers. Indications for HPN include intestinal failure or dysfunction, short bowel syndrome, malabsorptive disorders, acute or chronic bowel obstruction, Crohn's disease, radiation enteritis, intestinal and pancreatic fistula, intestinal ischemia, pancreatitis, and severe, life-threatening malnutrition.[9] *International Classification of Diseases, Tenth Revision (ICD-10)* codes for common diagnoses related to HPN are listed in Table 11-1.

Clinicians should evaluate the risks and benefits of home nutrition support on an individual basis, along with relevant cultural and religious values and patient/family preferences.[10] In some situations, the burden of HPN management may outweigh the benefits. Similarly, the benefits and burdens associated with the use of artificial nutrition and hydration in the patient with terminal illness with end-stage disease should be carefully evaluated.[10,11] HPN is rarely covered by insurance if patients are on hospice, and usually a private hospice agency is involved. (Medicare does not cover HPN if the patient has transitioned to hospice.) In these situations, it is important to consider that loss of the desire to eat and drink is a natural part of the dying process.[12]

Table 11-1. *ICD-10* Codes for Common Diagnoses Related to HPN

Code	Anatomic Conditions
D00.1	Carcinoma in situ of esophagus
D0.10	Carcinoma in situ of other and unspecified digestive organs (includes colon, other parts of the intestine)
K22.2	Esophageal stricture or stenosis
J86.0	Tracheo-esophageal fistula
K31.5	Duodenal obstruction
K31.6	Gastrojejunocolic fistula
K63.20	Intestinal fistula
	Motility Disorders
K31.84	Gastroparesis
K31.89	Other functional disorder of the intestine
K56.6	Other and unspecified intestinal obstruction
K91.1	Postgastrectomy dumping syndrome
021.0–021.1	Hyperemesis gravidarum
R13.10	Dysphagia
	Intestinal Disease and Malabsorptive Disorders
C25.0	Malignant neoplasm of the pancreas
E84.9	Cystic fibrosis
K50.0	Regional enteritis
K55.0	Acute vascular insufficiency of intestine (ischemia)
K56.6	Unspecified intestinal obstruction
K91.1	Postvagotomy syndrome
K63.9	Intestinal disorder (unspecified)
K85.0	Acute pancreatitis
K86.1	Chronic pancreatitis
K91.2	Short bowel syndrome
K90.3	Pancreatic steatorrhea
K90.89	Malabsorption: other specified intestinal
K90.9	Intestinal malabsorption, unspecified
K52.9	Other and unspecified noninfective gastroenteritis and colitis

Table 11-1 continued on next page

Code	Anatomic Conditions
	Nutrition Disorders
E44.1	Malnutrition of mild degree
E44.0	Malnutrition of moderate degree
E46	Unspecified protein calorie malnutrition
E43	Unspecified severe protein calorie malnutrition
E78.-	Disorders of lipoprotein metabolism and other lipidemias
E84.30	Magnesium disorder
E83.51	Hypocalcemia
E86.9	Volume depletion
E87.0	Other disorders of fluid, electrolyte, and acid-base balance
E66.-	Overweight and obesity
D50.8	Iron deficiency anemia (dietary)
D64.9	Anemia: unspecified
R63.4	Abnormal weight loss

HPN, home parenteral nutrition; *ICD-10, International Classification of Diseases, Tenth Revision.* World Health Organization. (2004). ICD-10: international statistical classification of diseases and related health problems : tenth revision, 2nd ed. World Health Organization. https://apps.who.int/iris/handle/10665/42980

Discharge Planning

Patients receiving HPN support are usually discharged from an acute care or rehabilitation care facility; however, a considerable subset of patients may be stable enough to initiate PN in the home with the support of an experienced HPN team.[13] Figure 11-1 provides a checklist to facilitate the transition to home care.[14] In addition to nutrition needs, other factors that should be assessed as part of the discharge planning process include financial and insurance considerations, central venous access and availability of nursing support, home safety, physical and psychological needs assessment, as well as patient/caregiver willingness to learn and self-administer HPN.

Figure 11-1. HPN Discharge Checklist

- ○ Documentation of valid indication for HPN
- ○ Documentation of expected length of therapy
- ○ Confirmation of appropriate central venous access
- ○ Confirmation of reimbursement
- ○ Establishment of home infusion pharmacy
- ○ Establishment of home health agency
- ○ Completion of psychosocial assessment
- ○ Completion of patient education (including HPN instructions, CVL care, self-monitoring)
- ○ Evaluation of home environment
- ○ Dissemination of pertinent home health contact information
- ○ Verification that home infusion pharmacy and home health agency have received orders
- ○ Documentation of follow-up appointment(s)

CVL, central venous line; HPN, home parenteral nutrition.

Reimbursement Eligibility Criteria

Investigation into the patient's individual insurance coverage is second only to the decision that nutrition support is needed after hospital discharge. Understanding the reimbursement process includes knowledge of coverage restrictions or limitations for services, equipment, and supplies under individual policies. In situations of limited, pending, or no insurance coverage, discharge may be delayed until sufficient home health and infusion benefits are available.

Insurance coverage for HPN varies by type of program as well as individual plans. Government programs (ie, Medicare and Medicaid) have very strict coverage criteria and require specific diagnoses, detailed medical history, objective studies, laboratory values, and other clinical data to determine eligibility. Coverage policies and reimbursement for HPN vary with private payers and managed care organizations and frequently require preauthorization or precertification. Many require that the therapy be "medically necessary" and the "sole source of nutrition." Some insurance policies establish their own criteria for HPN, whereas others follow the policy set forth by CMS.[15] Regardless of the type of insurance, it is also important to determine whether the patient has home health nursing, infusion, or durable medical equipment benefits of sufficient scope for therapies that may be needed indefinitely. Plans vary greatly if additional home nursing visits are needed; if non–nutrition-related needs such as wound care, tracheostomy or ostomy care are indicated; or if disease/ medication management services are required. All of this could be a potential financial burden for patients and families if insurance coverage is lacking.

HPN is covered under the Prosthetic Device benefit of Medicare Part B and is intended for a "beneficiary with permanent, severe pathology of the alimentary tract which does not allow absorption of sufficient nutrients to maintain weight and strength commensurate with the beneficiary's general condition."[15,16]

Prosthetic device benefits require a permanent dysfunction of a body part or organ, which means short-term nutrition support would not be covered. Under CMS, HPN is the "provision of sufficient nutrients to maintain weight and strength commensurate with the patient's overall health status," and the condition must have a "permanent impairment of long and indefinite duration" of ≥3 months.[15] Some Medicare Part D plans (which are intended as oral prescription drug plans) may pay a small percentage of the cost of an individual nutrient or drug within a PN prescription, such as an amino acid or an electrolyte; however, Part D does not pay for the equipment, supplies, or professional services associated with the provision of PN or any other infusion therapy.[15]

Table 11-2 lists the requirements for eligibility and documentation required for PN coverage PN under Medicare.[15-17] Because of the requirement for permanent dysfunction of the alimentary tract under Medicare, conditions such as swallowing disorders, psychological disorders (eg, depression), anorexia (eg, secondary to cancer), dyspnea of severe pulmonary or cardiac disease, medication side effects, or renal failure are not covered.[15,16] The PN prescription must also meet specified calorie, protein, and fat guidelines. These guidelines may be in excess of actual needs for some patients, which would require the physician to provide additional documentation as to why the nutrients are out of the designated range.[16] Infusion pumps and supplies are covered for patients who meet PN eligibility criteria. Medicare Part A covers nursing care for HPN if the patient is homebound and the agency is a Medicare-certified home health agency. This restriction on homebound status is slated to be changed in the near future.

Table 11-2. CMS/Medicare Policy for HPN Coverage

Category	Coverage Requirements
General	• Condition will require PN for >3 mo • Condition is severe enough that patient cannot maintain weight and strength on oral intake or a combination of oral nutrition and EN • Diagnosis (*ICD-10* code) pertinent to need for PN (see Table 11-1) • Weight and weight history • Serum albumin within 1 wk of HPN • Specific disease criteria and supporting documentation
Massive small bowel resection within 3 mo, leaving 5 feet (≈1.5 m) or less of small bowel beyond the ligament of Treitz	• Operative report with evidence of ≤5 feet (≈1.5 m) of small bowel • Radiographic reports
Short bowel syndrome with net GI fluid and electrolyte malabsorption on an oral diet of 2.5–3 L/d, enteral losses >50% of the oral/enteral intake, and urine output of <1 L/d	• Operative report indicating extent of resection • Radiographic reports • Motility studies • Intake and output records demonstrating net fluid loss • Signs of dehydration and electrolyte imbalance • Results of 72-h fecal fat test • List of medications used to control diarrhea • Documentation of nutrient modification and/or failed tube trial
Severe exacerbation of regional enteritis requiring bowel rest for ≥3 mo	• Operative report • Pathology report • Radiographic reports • Indication for bowel rest
Pancreatitis with or without pseudocyst requiring bowel rest for >3 mo	• Operative report • Radiographic report • Indication for bowel rest
Enterocutaneous fistula requiring bowel rest for >3 mo during which feeding distal to the fistula is not possible	• Operative report • Radiographic report • Motility studies • Contraindication to EN • Evidence of inability to place tube distal to fistula
Complete mechanical small bowel obstruction for which surgery is not an option	• Operative report that confirms obstruction • Radiographic report that confirms obstruction • Evidence of inability to place tube distal to obstruction
Severe fat malabsorption and malnutrition in which fecal fat is >50% of oral/enteral intake on a diet of ≥50 g/d as measured by a 72-h fecal fat test	• Fecal fat test results • Operative report • Radiographic report • Pharmacologic approaches tried • Evidence of EN failure • Nutrition assessment with evidence of malnutrition defined as >10% weight loss in ≤3 mo and serum albumin level of ≤3.4 g/dL

Table 11-2 continued on next page

Category	Coverage Requirements
Severe motility disorder that is unresponsive to prokinetic medication	• Radiographic report • Motility studies • Medications used to attempt to improve motility • Result of tube trial or contraindication to tube feeding • Nutrition assessment with evidence of malnutrition defined as >10% weight loss in ≤3 mo and serum albumin level of ≤3.4 g/dL

Malnutrition NOS	• Weight loss >10% in ≤3 mo and serum albumin level of <3.4 g/dL
	• One of the following:
	  ◦ Moderate fat malabsorption documented by 72-h fecal fat ≥25% of oral/enteral on ≥50 g fat/d
	  ◦ Malabsorption confirmed by objective test other than 72-h fecal fat (eg, D-xylose test, Sudan stain of stool, etc)
	  ◦ Gastroparesis confirmed with studies or failure of material to reach jejunum in 3–6 h or manometric motility studies unresponsive to prokinetic medication
	  ◦ Small bowel resection leaving >5 feet of small bowel beyond ligament of Treitz
	  ◦ Small bowel syndrome not as severe in previous small bowel category
	  ◦ Mild to moderate exacerbation of enteritis or enterocutaneous fistula
	  ◦ Partial mechanical small bowel obstruction for which surgery is not an option

CMS, Centers for Medicare and Medicaid Services; EN, enteral nutrition; GI, gastrointestinal; HPN, home parenteral nutrition; *ICD-10, International Classification of Diseases, Tenth Revision*; NOS, not otherwise specified; PN, parenteral nutrition.

Safety Evaluation

The Joint Commission Home Care Accreditation Program has included some National Patient Safety Goals for the home patient. Although they are not specific for HPN, they are related and include the following: improving accuracy of patient identification, improving the safety of using medications, reducing the risk of healthcare-associated infections, and reducing the risk of patient harm resulting from falls.[18] Once it is determined that the criteria for medical necessity and benefit coverage are met, the next step is to evaluate the safety of the home environment and the capability for learning to use necessary equipment.[19] The following questions should be explored to determine the safety of the home environment[8]:

1. Is the neighborhood accessible to the home healthcare provider for delivery and professional visits?

2. Is the environment clean with reliable utilities (sanitary water, electricity, refrigeration, storage space, electrical outlets, telephone)? Note: Special provisions should be made if electricity or phone are not culturally accepted.

3. Can the patient move safely around the house and to the bathroom (stairs, carpeting)?

4. Is the patient/caregiver willing and able to learn the home infusion procedures and operation of the equipment?

5. Is the caregiver willing and able to provide additional needed assistance for care within the home?

6. Is the patient/caregiver able to learn to recognize problems and contact help from the home healthcare provider or emergency services?

7. Is laboratory monitoring available as frequently as needed to prevent fluid and electrolyte complications?

Needs Assessment

Assessment for home care suitability includes evaluation of the skilled nursing needs, performance of activities of daily living, medication management, wound and skin care, and the patient's ability to recognize when to seek medical attention. When beginning HPN, the patient and caregiver additionally should be assessed for their ability to learn how to reliably monitor weight, hydration status, oral intake, ostomy output, and blood glucose levels if indicated; to recognize early signs and symptoms of infection; and to manage the PN access device and site.

Patients and caregivers should be prepared for the necessary time commitment for administration of PN. Although this will become easier with repetition, the responsibility may initially be overwhelming. Reassurance and patience on the part of the home healthcare professionals can inspire confidence. Although leaving an institutional environment usually indicates health improvement, this new responsibility may add to the stress of illness. Continuity of care and trusting supportive home care clinicians can assist with handling feelings of stress associated with HPN and related conditions, such as high-output stomas associated with short bowel syndrome.

HPN requires the use of complex technical equipment. When possible, demonstration of the equipment prior to discharge will provide both an opportunity for teaching and insight into the patient and caregiver's ability to learn. If mastering the use of equipment and learning procedures is not possible in the acute care or rehabilitation setting, extra teaching time should be allotted for the initial home visits. Various teaching methods should be utilized with patients. Ensuring willingness and ability to safely manage equipment and procedures can prevent complications and hospital readmission.[20] Initial and additional ongoing education related to central line care and independent management of the nutrition support results in increased patient satisfaction and compliance.[21]

Social changes due to loss of job or family role, disconnection from friends, and limitation in physical stamina all may contribute to stress after hospital discharge. Cultural and religious beliefs can also influence health-related practices and should be considered in the overall patient assessment. The patient's perception of health and illness will affect behaviors, tolerance of discomfort, knowledge of options, and expectations of change and outcome. Ensuring appropriate follow-up in the form of appointments and telephone numbers of providers may be beneficial. Providing information regarding available local or national organizations for peer support and education has been shown to improve outcomes associated with home nutrition support.[21]

Selection of Home Care and Infusion Provider Services

A variety of organizations may participate in the delivery and management of HPN services, including durable medical equipment companies, home infusion providers, and nursing care agencies. Home care providers specializing in nutrition support are available to assist with the transition from the hospital to the home. These agencies may provide all home care services needed or coordinate with other organizations for home nursing visits, medical equipment, PN/infusion pharmacy needs, and supplies. A predischarge teaching visit familiarizes the patient with what he or she is expected to learn and provides the home care clinician a chance to assess the patient's or caregiver's receptiveness and ability to manage at home. Because HPN is often administered as an overnight or cycled infusion, the home care providers need to be readily available by telephone 24 h/d, 7 d/wk and have capability for nursing support whenever needed.

Role of Nutrition Support Clinicians

Continuity of care and communication within and among all organizations participating in the care of the patient receiving HPN should be frequent, structured, in-depth, and ongoing.[8] The home care provider should coordinate needs for PN with other professional services providing wound care, ostomy care, respiratory care, physical therapy, or home health aide services.

Frequently, the hospital-based nutrition support team or home infusion provider takes responsibility for the safe delivery, administration, and ongoing monitoring of the HPN. These activities should be coordinated with the patient's primary care physician (if he or she is not the prescribing physician) and all other medical specialists involved. It is not uncommon for a patient who is receiving HPN to receive regular follow-up care from a gastroenterologist, oncologist, or surgeon. A psychologist or psychiatrist may also be involved for treatment of anxiety or depression. Regular communication with the primary care physician is essential for new or ongoing cardiac, respiratory, renal, or neurological concerns. Collaboration by all specialists including the home nutrition support provider can be achieved through active communication and documentation.

The ASPEN home care standards recommend interdisciplinary collaboration by the referring physician, nutrition support practitioners, and home care provider.[8] Ideally, a physician with expertise in HPN should be available for the management of the patient's nutrition care plan, interpretation of diagnostic testing, and evaluation of changes in medical condition. The roles, responsibilities, and required competencies of the home care pharmacist, nurse, and dietitian are detailed in the ASPEN discipline-specific standards of professional practice, and these may overlap depending on the availability of each professional in the home care setting.[22-25]

The home care pharmacist has an essential role in evaluating the nutrition therapy prescription, compounding of PN formulations, evaluating drug-nutrient interactions, dispensing medical supplies and equipment, and monitoring laboratory results in conjunction with the home nutrition support dietitian if one is available. Assuring that the HPN dispensed is consistent with the acute care PN discharge prescription is essential when the patient is transitioning between institutions.[26] A study in a pediatric cohort identified discrepancies between acute care–prescribed PN and delivered/administered HPN as a topic of concern.[27] Changes to the inpatient PN order are often needed for the home setting to accommodate the initiation of cycling or changing from a 2-in-1 admixture with lipids piggybacked in the hospital, to a 3-in-1 or total nutrient admixture for home. If appropriate, this makes the process easier and more convenient for the patient and caregiver. This requires communication and clarification of orders between the home care pharmacist and the hospital team. Verification of accuracy is particularly important given that HPN is almost always compounded in a batch supply and not 1 day at a time as it is in the hospital setting, making adherence to national standards for compatibility and stability even more crucial in the home setting.[26]

The home care nurse has an active role in teaching the patient and caregiver, conducting in-home patient physical and psychosocial assessment, performing dressing changes and access site care, collecting blood or other specimens, providing medication instruction and reconciliation, evaluating compliance, and monitoring the response to nutrition support.

The home care dietitian assists in the development of the nutrition care plan; recommends energy, macronutrient, and micronutrient requirements; performs and evaluates the nutrition-focused physical examination; assesses the ongoing adequacy and appropriateness of nutrient delivery and intake; and assists with the transition to tube feeding and/or oral diet. The dietitian may also be involved in evaluating reimbursement eligibility prior to onboarding, assisting with securing clinical documentation required for coverage. A process for timely communication among the physician, nutrition support practitioners, home care provider, patient, caregiver, and any other healthcare professionals is essential.

Nutrition Care Plan

Short- and Long-Term Goals

Short-term goals include basic patient education and the safe provision and administration of HPN ordered. At the onset of care, patients and caregivers should be provided with contact information for all providers; review of administration of PN therapy including setup, flushing, and troubleshooting the pump; and initial teaching on prevention of PN complications. Long-term goals would include the achievement of desired clinical/nutrition outcomes, independence with PN administration, and prevention of rehospitalization and other HPN complications. Independence is achieved through comprehensive patient and family education addressing care of the vascular access device (VAD), troubleshooting high-tech equipment, and emphasis on adherence to medication regimens and restrictions in diet or activity. Optimizing the organization and safety of the home environment should decrease therapy-related anxiety, facilitate learning, and promote independence.

Barriers to achieving short- and long-term nutrition support goals can be overcome with intensive patient and family teaching, ongoing assessment of compliance, and monitoring for early signs and symptoms of problems. Identifying and communicating areas of individual patient risks will assist the members of the healthcare team who are managing the patient to anticipate special needs. Information regarding safety, community resources, and ways to improve the ability to manage within the home environment will promote satisfaction and QOL and reduce complications.

Route and Access for Home Nutrition Support

Decisions about the route and access device for HPN should be made early in the discharge planning process. The access device chosen should be one that the patient/caregiver can safely manage and minimizes risk of complications (see chapter 3 on parenteral access devices). Information on device insertion date, type, tip location, length, patency, and site condition must be made available to the home care provider prior to the start of care.

Long-term PN requires a central venous access device. Central venous catheter (CVC) placement is defined by the final catheter tip location in the superior or inferior vena cava. HPN catheters may be placed into either a large peripheral vein, such as the basilic or cephalic vein, or into the subclavian or internal jugular (IJ) vein. The catheter is then advanced to the distal portion of the superior vena cava or the cavoatrial junction. A peripherally inserted central catheter is readily placed, replaced, or removed and is at low risk for insertion complications. Subclavian or IJ catheters are either tunneled or implanted. Tunneled catheters, known as Hickman, Broviac, or Groshong catheters, enter the vein and are then tunneled subcutaneously to exit lower on the chest wall. The purpose of the tunnel is to decrease the risks of infection and accidental removal. On the basis of ASPEN guidelines, it is recommended that tunneled CVCs be used for patients who require daily, long-term HPN.[28]

An implanted device, or port, is a disk with a self-sealing silicone septum and a rigid titanium or plastic base. It is surgically placed into a subcutaneous pocket and connected to a catheter that is inserted into a vein using a medical wire and advanced into the central venous system. The most common location of an implanted port is on the chest wall, but in some situations, the upper arm may be the site of choice. The port is accessed using a specially designed right-angle tapered noncoring needle with a side opening, known as a Huber needle. Because the entire port is under the skin, minimal nursing care is needed, and unrestricted bathing is permitted after the incision heals, unless the port is accessed with a Huber needle; in that case, weekly Huber needle changes are needed when the port is in use. Tunneled or implanted devices on the chest wall are usually not visible under clothing and allow the full range of arm and hand movement.

External catheters (those not completely under the skin like ports), which include tunneled catheters, require regular, direct nursing care or patient/

caregiver training for proper catheter and site care. Catheter dressings and tubing should be clean and dry at all times. Implanted ports require professional care and training for needle placement, site care, and catheter flushing.

Nutrient Requirements

Nutrient requirements are developed following a nutrition assessment (see chapter 1 on nutrition assessment). Energy requirements are determined by predictive equations or are measured using indirect calorimetry, if available. Nutrient and total fluid requirements should be determined while considering whether PN therapy is providing total or partial nutrition support. Goals of therapy should be determined with the patient and caregiver and should be individualized based on assessment of nutrition status, body composition, and performance status and function, while taking into account any preexisting nutrition deficits. The overall goals of nutrition therapy are to restore macro- and micronutrients, replete and maintain normal serum electrolyte levels, maintain euglycemia, and improve or maintain lean body mass, performance status, and function. In situations in which a patient's body weight is either above or below the preferred value, a maximum or minimum weight goal may be set.

Patients who are either taking nothing by mouth or experiencing abnormal fluid losses will likely need additional fluid or water. For the HPN patient, the PN volume is based on the desired total daily fluid volume, inclusive of fluid losses. A period of evaluation to assess tolerance of PN as well as to achieve fluid and electrolyte stability is invaluable for determining the home nutrition support prescription. Desired tolerance includes achieving normal blood glucose and acceptable urine output. Careful supervision of changes to the formula in the inpatient setting may minimize changes and maximize uncomplicated delivery in the home setting.

Administration Schedule

The patient's and caregiver's preferences should be carefully considered in determining the infusion cycle. PN always requires controlled infusion pump delivery. Although most PN regimens begin as a 24-hour infusion, decreasing the number of hours of infusion allows for freedom to resume normal activities and prevents liver and gallbladder complications in the long term. By increasing the flow rate, the total infusion time is decreased, giving the patient time off the pump. This is referred to as a cyclic infusion or cyclic feeding. Fluid tolerance can be assessed by monitoring urine volume and frequency. The convenience of a shorter infusion cycle is balanced against the higher volume delivered over a shorter period of time. The cycle should include a tapered rate at the end of the infusion to minimize risk of hypoglycemia.[29] Tapering at home typically includes a 1-hour ramp-up at the beginning of the infusion and a 1–2 hour ramp-down at the end of the infusion. Home PN pumps are preprogrammed to take care of calculating the taper so that there are no additional programming steps for the patient or nurse. Careful monitoring of blood glucose may be needed as the infusion rate is increased, which ideally is done in the hospital prior to discharge. The maximum glucose infusion rate for adults is 4–7 mg/kg/min. The generally accepted rate of glucose infusion is 5 mg/kg/min.[30] In pediatrics, the maximum glucose infusion rate may be greater, as in 14 mg/kg/min for infants.[31] To derive grams of dextrose per day, the formula for this calculation is as follows: weight (kilograms) × desired glucose infusion rate × minutes per day / 1000. For example, to infuse a 60-kg female at 5 mg/kg/min for 12 hours, the grams of dextrose per day equals 60 kg × 5 mg × 770 minutes / 1000 = 231 g.

More rapid infusion rates may cause hyperglycemia, particularly for patients with blood glucose issues. If indicated, blood glucose checks should be scheduled within the first 2 hours, 4–6 hours later, and at the end of the cycle. Insulin therapy should be initiated and advanced cautiously, and blood glucose monitoring should be continued until acceptable blood glucose levels are achieved. Regimens for home insulin administration may be set up as either a sliding scale or the addition of regular insulin to the PN solution. Appropriate blood glucose control is a goal to prevent complications from HPN. Patients with diabetes should have basal insulin requirements met by longer-acting insulin outside of the PN, whereas breakthrough elevations in blood glucose are covered with subcutaneous sliding-scale injections. The risk vs benefit of having a patient add regular insulin to the PN bag daily should be evaluated carefully.

Prevention of Complications

Complications related to HPN can be summarized as mechanical, infectious, or metabolic.[5] Mechanical complications include occlusion, leakage, malposition or accidental removal of the access device, or equipment failure or malfunction. Infectious complications relate to the access device, exit site, and surrounding skin. Metabolic complications include blood glucose or fluid and electrolyte abnormalities, gastrointestinal (GI) intolerance, organ system dysfunction, and vitamin, mineral, and trace element deficiencies or toxicities (see chapter 8 on the complications of PN therapy).

In patients receiving HPN, catheter infection is the most common complication of PN therapy and the most common reason for hospital readmission.[32,33]

Definitions of terms should be clear. A central line–associated bloodstream infection (CLABSI) is a serious infection that occurs when germs (usually bacteria or viruses) enter the bloodstream through the central line. A catheter-related bloodstream infection (CRBSI) is a rigorous clinical definition, based on precise laboratory findings that identify the CVC as the source of the bloodstream infection (BSI) and is used to determine diagnosis, treatment, and possibly epidemiology of BSI in patients with a CVC. The term *CRBSI* is not typically used for surveillance purposes, and there are few data available for comparison. Using the CRBSI definition requires more resources than use of the CLABSI definition because hospitals must have the capacity to correctly collect and label blood culture sets drawn from the CVC and peripheral phlebotomy, as well as from the CVC segment/tips. *CLABSI* is a term used only for surveillance purposes to identify BSIs that occur in the population at risk (patients with central lines). Use of this term and the CLABSI definition from the Centers for Disease Control and Prevention's National Healthcare Safety Network may lead to an overestimation of the infection rate compared with the use of the rigorous CRBSI criteria.[33] Signs and symptoms of a CRBSI may include fever, lethargy, chills, rigors, elevated leukocytes, and hyperglycemia. Redness, tenderness, or discharge at the skin site may indicate catheter exit site infection. Immediate evaluation and intervention is necessary for suspected or actual infection.[34] On the basis of ASPEN guidelines, it is suggested that a line with the fewest number of lumens needs to be used to reduce the risk of CLABSIs.[28] Secondary to insufficient evidence, there are no recommendations regarding the ideal type of central venous access device material to reduce CLABSI incidence.[28] If a patient experiences a CRBSI, follow-up monitoring should include a home visit for reassessment of the patient and/or caregiver's compliance with technique and administration procedures. This visit serves as a review of the proper handling of PN access and equipment, as well as an opportunity for reevaluation of the home environment.

Catheter occlusion may occur because of a mechanical obstruction such as a kink in the catheter or from thrombus or precipitation of PN components. Diagnostic studies may be indicated when catheter flushing or aspiration is difficult. Patients requiring long-term HPN and those who have had multiple catheters are at increased risk of catheter-related venous thrombosis, and some patients may require anticoagulation therapy for prevention.[35]

Abnormal liver function is not uncommon in patients requiring long-term HPN.[36] The mechanism for liver dysfunction is not completely understood and is thought to be multifactorial.[5] Potential causes of PN-associated liver dysfunction include overfeeding, excessive intravenous (IV) fat or carbohydrate dosage, lack of enteral stimulation, infection, choline deficiency, and aluminum toxicity.[37] If signs of cholestasis occur, ultrasonography should be performed to rule out extrahepatic causes. The PN formulation should be routinely evaluated to be sure that the patient is not receiving excessive calories or excess fat emulsion for his or her weight.[38] Cycling of the PN infusion, if the patient is receiving continuous therapy, may be beneficial. Every attempt should also be made to encourage oral intake or a transition to enteral nutrition (EN) if possible.

Metabolic bone disease is seen in patients receiving long-term HPN.[39] The cause of osteopenia and osteoporosis is also multifactorial and may include preexisting disease, malabsorption, use of steroids, inactivity, mineral deficiency (calcium, phosphorus, magnesium), or vitamin D deficiency or excess.[40] Annual bone mineral-density testing should be performed.

Micronutrient deficiencies can be less common in patients receiving long-term PN because of the routine addition of multivitamin and trace element additives to the PN admixture. However, as a result of many PN component shortages over the last decade, along with less-than-ideal doses of some nutrients in the multivitamin and trace element combination products, long-term HPN patients do require regular monitoring for micronutrient deficiencies.[37] Further, patients should be monitored for iron deficiency because iron is not routinely added to PN. Monitoring of serum levels of trace elements should be conducted to prevent deficiency and toxicity. Refer to Table 11-3 for suggested laboratory monitoring time frames. Because serum values are not always representative of deficiency and toxicity, patients should also be examined for physical signs.[41]

Table 11-3. Laboratory Monitoring for HPN

Parameter	New Patients Baseline	New Patients Weeks 1–4	Monthly	Long-term Patients Every 3–12 mo[a]
Basic metabolic panel	X	X	X	
Hepatic panel	X	X	X	
Magnesium	X	X	X	
Phosphorus	X	X	X	
CBC with differential	X	X	X	
Trace elements	X			X
Phospholipid fatty acid profile	X			X
Water soluble vitamins B_6, B_{12}, MMA, RBC folate	X[b]			X
Fat soluble vitamins A, 25(OH)D, E	X[b]			X
Iron indices	X[c]			X

25(OH)D, 25-hydroxyvitamin D; CBC, complete blood cell count; HPN, home parenteral nutrition; MMA, methylmalonic acid; RBC, red blood cell.
Source: Adapted with permission from Mueller CM, ed. *The ASPEN Adult Nutrition Support Core Curriculum.* 3rd ed. Silver Spring, MD: ASPEN; 2017.
[a]Repeat blood work as warranted based on previous results, nutrition-focused physical examination findings, and national product shortages. Repeat less frequently if results are normal (eg, 12 months).
[b]Check other micronutrients if deficiencies are suspected based on nutrition-focused physical examination findings.
[c]Only check at baseline in the absence of recent surgery, blood transfusion, or major blood loss.

Prevention of Rehospitalization

Because hospital readmission is discouraging, disruptive, and costly to the patient and healthcare system, the Medicare Hospital Readmissions Reduction Program may prompt hospitals to develop strategies to help decrease readmissions by preventing complications. Although clearly not all complications can be prevented, there are known strategies that minimize risk.[42] Reasons for complications within the first 90 days of HPN include inadequate training, patient and caregiver noncompliance, prescription errors or incorrect dosing of nutrients, healthcare worker error, and equipment malfunction.[43]

Early recognition of the signs and symptoms of complications promotes early treatment intervention. Regular measurement of weight and awareness of output are essential for early detection of dehydration or volume overload. A standardized protocol for diagnosis and management of common complications facilitates obtaining the vital information the home care clinician needs for treatment decisions. One example is the use of protocols to obtain blood cultures and complete blood counts in the event of a fever >38.6°C (101.5°F).

Community resources provide peer support to enhance independence and promote a sense of well-being.[44] Patients who participate in peer support groups report less depression, anxiety, and worry; fewer rehospitalizations; and increased self-care and satisfaction with the care given by their healthcare professionals.[21]

Patient Education

The goal of patient education is to provide needed information to enable patients to be responsible for their own therapy. Patients are sent home with complex therapy regimens requiring skilled procedures such as dressing changes, catheter access, and medication administration. Education is the foundation for success and helps prevent procedure- and therapy-related complications.[45] Empowering patients with verbal and written references to recognize signs and symptoms can enable appropriate action in the event of serious complications such as fever, thirst, or bleeding. When available, involvement of a significant other in education sessions will provide a backup, a second set of hands, and support for administration of nutrition support. All methods of teaching should be considered to provide the patients and caregivers with the power to succeed at home.

Educational Materials

According to the National Assessment of Health Literacy in the United States, at least one-third of Americans have limited reading comprehension.[46] To meet the recommended reading grade level of fifth to sixth grade, all words should be familiar and <3 syllables, and medical and technical terms should be limited or avoided altogether.[47] If complex or medical language is used, this should be explained using familiar words.

Printed patient education material should be selected on the basis of content and complexity. The written style should be simple, casual, and conversational. Additionally, materials should bridge language barriers or be printed in the patient's primary language. Content should be relevant to the specific type of nutrition support as well as to the age and culture of the patient. All information should be accurate and reflect current standards of practice.[48] The most important information should be highlighted or otherwise easy to locate. Key points should be repeated as a means of reinforcement. Terms used should be consistent throughout the document. Although medical equipment may be identified by the manufacturer's names or abbreviations, only one term should be used within an educational guide.

All steps for any skilled procedures should be organized, precise, and easy to read. Active verbs are preferred in directions. Any excess wording should be minimized to present the important points concisely. Steps should be kept simple, and too much information should be avoided. Suggested content for printed education materials includes the following: why the HPN therapy is being recommended, how PN therapy is expected to work in the body, step-by-step directions for skilled procedures, common pitfalls to avoid, signs and symptoms of complications, and telephone numbers of all healthcare providers.

The use of lists and graphic illustrations help clarify written text, emphasize skills presented, and provide cues for future reference. Drawings and photographs illustrate important points of information. All illustrations should focus on patient action and be simple, realistic, and relevant.[49] Use of mnemonics will reinforce learning new concepts.

The new ASPEN PN safety consensus recommendations document has a PN label specifically for HPN patients based on United States Pharmacopeia general chapter <17>, which organizes the prescription label in a patient-centered manner (see Figure 11-2 for this label template).[50]

Learning Assessment

A patient's readiness to learn is affected by physical or emotional conditions. Physical limitations such as pain, fatigue, and immobility will need to be taken into account when scheduling teaching sessions. Emotional anxiety or stress apart from the task of learning the necessary skills for delivery of nutrition support will interfere with learning concentration. A 1-on-1 session conducted in a private and quiet environment may enhance learning readiness. Teaching sessions should be scheduled at the patient's convenience and during a time of day free from other family obligations; however, this may not be possible because visits are usually set up at PN startup and disconnect times to better evaluate the patient and caregiver techniques. Accommodations will need to be made to address physical limitations such impaired dexterity, mobility, vision, or hearing.

After an initial demonstration, the patient or family should be asked to use return demonstration of the required procedure to assess learning. For new learners, this will most likely require repeated demonstration. The goal

Figure 11-2. Standard HPN Label Template: Adult Patient (as an example)

Patient Information

PATIENT NAME   BIRTH DATE/AGE

PATIENT HOME ADDRESS   HEIGHT (CM)   WEIGHT (KG)

VAD/CVC TYPE   LOCATION

Administration date/time/indication

Infuse 1 bag/d for nutrition.

Infuse at _____ mL/h over _____ h   Start at _____ (time)   Stop at _____ (time)

Macronutrients	Amount per day
Amino acids[a]	_____ g
Dextrose	_____ g
ILE[a]	_____ g

Electrolytes	Amount per day
Sodium phosphate	_____ mmol of phosphate (sodium _____ mEq)
Sodium chloride	_____ mEq
Sodium acetate	_____ mEq
Potassium phosphate	_____ mmol of phosphate (potassium _____ mEq)
Potassium chloride	_____ mEq
Potassium acetate	_____ mEq
Magnesium sulfate/chloride	_____ mEq
Calcium gluconate	_____ mEq

Vitamins, trace elements	Amount per day
Multicomponent vitamins[a]	_____ mL

Add prior to administration

Multicomponent trace elements[a]   _____ mL *to be added immediately prior to administration*

Other additives

Insulin _____ *units to be added immediately prior to administration*

Medications _____ *medication-specific units (mcg, mg, g).*
Specify if requires adding immediately prior to administration.

Total Volume: _____ mL, Overfill volume: _____ mL
Do not use after date/time: _____

Prescriber and contact information:

Institution/pharmacy name: _____
Institution/pharmacy address: _____
Pharmacy telephone number:

CVC, central venous catheter; HPN, home parenteral nutrition; ILE, lipid injectable emulsion; VAD, vascular access device. aSpecify product name.
Source: Adapted with permission from Ayers P, Adams S, Boullata J, et al; ASPEN. A.S.P.E.N. parenteral nutrition safety consensus recommendations. *JPEN J Parenter Enteral Nutr.* 2014:38(3):296–333.

Home Parenteral Nutrition Support

CHAPTER 11

is to have the patient become independent with HPN to improve QOL and make living with daily infusions as normal as possible.[51]

Teaching and Evaluation Strategies

High-tech home care equipment both contributes to nutrition support delivery and at the same time imposes significant constraints on patients' lives.[52,53] A patient's perception of how this technology impacts his or her private and social life will influence acceptance.[54] Factors such as motor noise, light, misunderstood digital messages, alarms, and tubing attachment are physical barriers to acceptance. Fear of exposure to illness, anxiety over equipment malfunction, and altered body image interfere with normal family and social activities.[55] Use of appropriate technology and proper education on the use of equipment will increase compliance with and acceptance of home therapy.[56]

The objective of the initial home visit is to teach and reinforce correct technique for HPN infusion. The home care nurse should use this training period to assess knowledge and explain the reasons behind the procedures and techniques. Issues such as storage of supplies, refrigeration of formulas, and disposal of medical waste can be addressed efficiently within the home. Corrections to the patient's technique can be made immediately while observing the patient and caregiver within the home environment. Selection of an appropriate work area with adequate lighting, proper hand hygiene, use of clean or disposable toweling, and restricted pet access are issues that should be addressed. Preparation of PN requires that the patient or caregiver demonstrates competence in the use of needles and syringes. Management of a VAD requires sterile techniques for flushing or dressing change. The goals of this visit and ongoing teaching are for the patient and caregiver to demonstrate a solid understanding of the procedures and techniques and to become proficient in the care of PN equipment, access devices, and the site.

Along with physical assessment, subsequent visit objectives are to promote adherence to the regimen and to support compliance with procedures and handling techniques. Repeated demonstration of processes should be consistent. Follow-up home visits provide reassurance to the patient and caregiver that continued assistance and support are available. Using a printed guide of steps for new procedures adds a readily available reference that will reduce procedure-related anxiety and promote confidence as the patient works toward independence. Every effort should be made to anticipate and respond to the patient's physical and emotional needs through interdisciplinary communication among the prescribing physician, members of the nutrition support team (if applicable), the home infusion provider, and home nursing agencies.

Consistent reassessment at regular intervals can be readily accomplished through telephone contact. Focused questions should target known issues or problems. Special needs can also be addressed on an individual and ongoing basis to eliminate barriers to achieving the goals of therapy. Developing a relationship with the patient and family will initially reduce therapy-related anxiety and result in increased satisfaction and enhanced compliance with nutrition support–related procedures. Strategies for relationship building include the following: consistently reinforcing goals, making regular and frequent contact, providing encouragement, demonstrating respect for others and their concerns, expressing understanding of circumstances, anticipating needs, dealing with limitations, and ensuring services are available for all needs.

Clinical Monitoring in the Home

Home care visits are used to obtain the patient's vital signs, record weight, assess hydration status, note any pertinent physical examination findings, observe and assess the VAD site, review medication use, and, if applicable, evaluate readiness to transition to oral nutrition.

Easily obtained, objective physical assessments are blood pressure, pulse, temperature, and weight. Keeping a record of these in the home facilitates communication among various home care providers. Additionally, this record can be brought to office visits or referenced during telephone calls to the primary care provider. Dehydration can be recognized by blood pressure and pulse changes, especially when measured with the patient in both lying and standing positions (orthostatic vital sign measurement). Elevations of temperature and pulse may be early signs of infection. Rapid weight loss or gain reflects a change in fluid status and should be assessed in the context of other symptoms of fluid retention (edema, shortness of breath) or dehydration (low urine output, dry mouth). Recording of output (ostomy, emesis, urine, and stool) can be difficult in the home and should be limited to special situations requiring evaluation of volume or significant electrolyte imbalance or as a means to prevent rehospitalization. Patients/caregivers should be educated about reporting significant changes in the character or volume of output.

Observation of the VAD site should be done at each home visit. Early signs and symptoms of infectious problems may be recognized by visual inspection of the insertion site, dressing, and surrounding skin for inflammation. Signs of mechanical malfunction of the device include leaking, difficulty flushing, or frequent pump alarm. Pain or swelling may indicate vascular access catheter damage and subcutaneous infiltration.

Adequacy and tolerance of therapy is assessed through functional status, physical examination, and laboratory values. Functional status is how well a patient performs the activities of daily living. These include ambulation, bathing, dressing, and meal preparation. The level of independence with household chores, hobbies, and recreational activities are other performance indicators. Physical examination will reveal changes in weight, anthropometrics, or signs of nutrient deficiencies.

All laboratory results should be documented at baseline on discharge or at the beginning of home nutrition support and then regularly throughout the course of therapy. Suggested collection of laboratory parameters includes blood glucose, blood urea nitrogen and creatinine, and electrolytes, including magnesium and phosphorus on a weekly basis for 4 weeks or until stable. Additionally, a complete blood count, serum proteins, liver function, triglycerides, vitamins, minerals, and trace elements should be monitored. Table 10-3 lists laboratory parameters and frequency of assessment for PN.[9] Laboratory tests ordered may vary depending on shortages of PN additives or other medications prescribed for the patient; for example, if a blood thinner is ordered, the patient may require a regular prothrombin time and international normalized ratio. Ongoing quarterly follow-up should include all parameters mentioned, unless a change in clinical condition occurs that necessitates more frequent monitoring on an individual, which is determined on a case-by-case basis.[9] To facilitate processing and correct billing, it is helpful to inform the laboratory of the diagnosis, clinical condition, or *ICD-10* codes that correlate with the requested diagnostic test (see Table 10-1).

Emergency Planning

It is important that emergency planning information be provided to HPN patients, such as in the event of a hurricane, fire, or earthquake. It is suggested that HPN patients have 3–4 days of HPN plus essential supplies (syringes, flushes, tubing, etc) at home. If indicated, it is also suggested that HPN patients have 3–4 days of IV fluids available if they require supplemental fluids. Standardized, commercially available bags of PN products may be a viable option because they do not require refrigeration and have a longer shelf life (up to 2 years if the bag is unactivated) compared with compounded PN. Other items of importance include, but are not limited to, an emergency/disaster plan, a copy of pertinent health information, bottled water for hand washing, hand sanitizer, battery-operated flashlights, extra batteries for the infusion pump, and a list of emergency contacts/local hospitals.[57]

QOL, Outcomes Management, and Resources

Tools to Monitor QOL

QOL is a multidimensional concept that includes evaluation of physical health status, psychological well-being, social and cognitive function, illness, and treatment. Because expectations regarding health and the ability to cope with limitations and disability can greatly affect a person's perception of health and satisfaction with life, people with the same objective health status may have very different QOLs. The World Health Organization defines QOL as "An individual's perception of their position in life in the context of the culture and value system in which they live and in relation to their goals, expectations, standards, and concerns."[21] Good QOL is generally accepted as a "state of complete physical, mental, and social well-being and not merely the absence of disease."[58] QOL may also be defined as the subjective perception of satisfaction or happiness with life in domains of importance to an individual. HPN-dependent adults define QOL as "how much one enjoys life, being happy and satisfied with life, and being able to do what you want to do when you want to do it."[59]

Historically, the most frequently used generic instruments for measuring the QOL of HPN patients were the Short Form 36 Questionnaire, Quality of Life Index, Sickness Impact Profile, and Nottingham Health Profile.[59] Consequently, most published studies use generic measures of health status or disease-specific questionnaires to study the QOL of home EN and PN patients.[60,61] Published research demonstrates poor QOL in patients receiving HPN that is influenced by age, self-esteem, drug and narcotic usage, depression, coping skills, family and peer support systems, financial insecurity, and underlying disease.[60-64] Qualitative reviews of HPN-dependent adults identify disturbed social life, inability to eat normally, diarrhea, ostomy bag rupturing and leaking, pain, polyuria, sleep disruption, and a need for psychosocial support as factors influencing QOL.[59,65-70] Despite technological inconveniences associated with infusion therapy, patients do, however, recognize and report the benefit of being kept alive with HPN.[59,62,70]

Baxter and colleagues[71] designed the first patient-based treatment-specific QOL questionnaire for HPN (HPN-QOL). The instrument includes 8 functional scales (general health, travel, physical function coping, ability to eat and drink, employment, sexual function, and emotional function), 2 HPN items, and 9 symptom scales (body image, weight, immobility, fatigue, sleep pattern, GI symptoms, pain, presence of stoma, and financial issues). The HPN-QOL differentiates between QOL affected by HPN therapy and the underlying illness or disease. Benefits of using a therapy-specific

QOL instrument for individual patient care include providing information for therapy management and identifying problems requiring intervention.[71] Subsequently, a shorter QOL questionnaire has been developed that demonstrates good correlation with the HPN-QOL questionnaire in regard to the patient's social state, mental state, and everyday functioning. There is also good correlation in relation to the patient's general health, level of independence, and experience with handling PN.[72]

Clinicians and patients should discuss QOL at routine intervals, whether a validated instrument is used or not. We know from studies and discussion with individuals requiring long-term HPN that it is important to know that one can live a "normal" life even with HPN dependency.[59,70] Patients have a strong desire for information to help them better understand the prognosis of their condition and the rationale for the therapy.[73-76] Because these individuals face potentially long-term therapies requiring substantial lifestyle adaptations with known risks and complications, a frank and open conversation about goals and expectations is necessary. Open communication between clinician and patient can help identify how a patient defines QOL and what makes QOL poor or good. When introducing these therapies, provide a realistic image of what will occur at home and adequately portray the complexity of the technology.[53] Continue a dialogue with the patient to help them adapt and adequately cope with the lifestyle adjustments associated with HPN.

Patient Support

Many organizations provide important outreach services, free educational materials, and emotional support to patients, families, and caregivers.[53,77] The Oley Foundation (www.Oley.org), established in 1983, is a national nonprofit, educational advocacy, and support organization for consumers of home EN and PN. Networking may occur through regional Oley Ambassadors, who provide information regarding support groups and meetings in their geographic area, or through Oley-sponsored regional and national consumer conferences, which provide inspiration, support, advocacy and education. Educational resources available from the Oley Foundation include video libraries; the bimonthly *Lifeline Letter* newsletter with relevant articles about medical advances and therapies, disease states, and legislative and reimbursement updates, along with shared personal experiences; and the "My HPN" online education modules (Take Charge, Catheter-Associated Infection, Fluid Balance, and Glucose Control). The Oley Foundation website also offers Internet links to other national and international organizations related to nutrition support and homecare: disease- and condition-specific societies and foundations, home care agencies, equipment supply and exchange programs, infection control groups, insurance and disability benefits, discount and free prescription services, government agencies, and parenting and caregiver resources. Table 11-4 lists selected online social media that provide additional opportunities for networking between HPN patients and their families.

Table 11-4. Selected Online Social Media for Networking Among HPN Consumers

Website	Description
http://www.inspire.com/groups/oley-foundation/	The Oley Foundation Support Community connects patients, families, friends and caregivers for support and inspiration.
www.shortbowelfoundation.org	A nationally based foundation providing education, support, and advocacy services to patients, families, and healthcare providers who deal with short bowel syndrome or similar medical conditions.
Living Life on Total Parenteral Nutrition (TPN) – Facebook group	A place for parents of children receiving PN or a place for anyone who lives by receiving PN to share tips and ideas, or to vent if one is struggling with PN-related issues.

HPN, home parenteral nutrition; PN, parenteral nutrition.

Summary

Home care involves more than simply transferring nutrition support from the acute care setting to the home. Home care providers are required to teach therapy-related management skills and provide education to ensure the technology used is safe and effective. Ongoing clinical monitoring is essential to prevent complications and promote successful achievement of nutrition outcomes, as well as patient satisfaction and QOL. Interdisciplinary collaboration among the case manager or discharge planner, prescribing and primary care physician, hospital-based nutrition support team, home infusion provider, and nursing agency, along with the patient and caregiver, is necessary for successful transition from the inpatient setting to the home.

References

1. Mundi M, Pattinson A, McMahon M, Davidson J, Hurt RT. Prevalence of home parenteral and enteral nutrition in the United States. *Nutr Clin Pract*. 2017;32(6):799–805.

2. National Home Infusion Association website. http://nhia.org/provider_search/provider_search.cfm. Accessed December 4, 2019.

3.   Grand View Research. *Parenteral Nutrition Market Size, Share & Trends Analysis Report By Nutrient Type (Carbohydrates, Lipid Emulsion, Single Dose Amino Acid Solution, Trace Elements), By Region, And Segment Forecasts, 2019 – 2026*. San Francisco, CA: Grand View Research; 2019. https://www.grandviewresearch.com/industry-analysis/parenteral-nutrition-market. Accessed December 10, 2019.

4.   Howard L, Ament M, Fleming CR, Shike M, Steiger E. Current use and clinical outcome of home parenteral and enteral nutrition therapies in the United States. *Gastroenterology*. 1995;109(2):355–365.

5.   DiBaise JK, Scolapio JS. Home parenteral and enteral nutrition. *Gastroenterol Clin North Am*. 2007;36(1):123–144.

6.   Howard L. Home parenteral nutrition: survival, cost, and quality of life. *Gastroenterology*. 2006;130(2 suppl 1):S52–S59.

7.   The National Association for Home Care. Basic statistics about home care. https://www.nahc.org/assets/1/7/10HC_Stats.pdf. Updated 2010. Accessed November 10, 2019.

8.   Kovacevich DS, Frederick A, Kelly D, Nishikawa R, Young L; ASPEN Board of Directors and the Standards for Specialized Nutrition Support Task Force. Standards for specialized nutrition support: home care patients. *Nutr Clin Pract*. 2005;20(5):579–590.

9.   Konrad D, Mitchell R, Hendrickson E. Home nutrition support. In: Mueller CM, ed. The *ASPEN Nutrition Support Core Curriculum*. Silver Spring, MD: ASPEN; 2017:767–782.

10. Barrocas A, Geppert C, Durfee SM, et al; ASPEN Ethics Position Paper Task Force; ASPEN Board of Directors; ASPEN. A.S.P.E.N. ethics position paper. *Nutr Clin Pract*. 2010;25(6):672–679.

11. Monturo C. The artificial nutrition debate: still an issue … after all these years. *Nutr Clin Pract*. 2009;24(2):206–213.

12. Palecek EJ, Teno JM, Casarett DJ, Hanson LC, Rhodes RL, Mitchell SL. Comfort feeding only: a proposal to bring clarity to decision-making regarding difficulty with eating for persons with advanced dementia. *J Am Geriatr Soc*. 2010;58(3):580–584.

13. Newton AF, DeLegge MH. Home initiation of parenteral nutrition. *Nutr Clin Pract*. 2007;22:57–65.

14. Kumpf VJ, Tillman EM. Home parenteral nutrition: safe transition from hospital to home. *Nutr Clin Pract*. 2012;27(6):749–757.

15. Allen P. Medicare coverage for home parenteral nutrition – an oxymoron? Part 1. *Practical Gastroenterol*. 2016;158:34–50.

16. Bonnes SL, Salonen BR, Hurt RT et al. Parenteral and enteral nutrition – from hospital to home: will it be covered? *Nutr Clin Pract*. 2017;32(6):730–738.

17. Centers for Medicare and Medicaid Services. Parenteral nutrition therapy appendices draft R1.0d. https://www.cms.gov/Research-Statistics-Data-and-Systems/Computer-Data-and-Systems/Electronic-Clinical-Templates/Downloads/Parenteral-Nutritional-Therapy-Appendices-Draft-20180520-R10d.pdf. Accessed November 11, 2019.

18. The Joint Commission. National patient safety goals effective January 2020. Home Care Accreditation Program. https://www.jointcommission.org/-/media/tjc/documents/standards/national-patient-safety-goals/npsg_chapter_ome_jan2020.pdf. Accessed November 26, 2019.

19. Bonifacio R, Alfonsi L, Santarpia L, et al. Clinical outcome of long-term home parenteral nutrition in non-oncological patients: a report from two specialised centres. *Intern Emerg Med*. 2007;2(3):188–195.

20. Shepperd S, Doll H, Angus RM, et al. Avoiding hospital admission through provision of hospital care at home: a systematic review and meta analysis of individual patient data. *CMAJ*. 2009;180(2):175–182.

21. Smith CE, Curtas S, Werkowitch M, Kleinbeck SV, Howard L. Home parenteral nutrition: does affiliation with national support and educational organization improve patient outcomes? *JPEN J Parenter Enteral Nutr*. 2002;26(3):159–163.

22. Mascarenhas MR, August DA, DeLegge MH, et al; ASPEN Task Force on Standards for Nutrition Support Physicians; ASPEN Board of Directors; ASPEN. Standards of practice for nutrition support physicians. *Nutr Clin Pract*. 2012;27(2):295–299.

23. Rollins C, Durfee SM, Holcombe BJ, Kochevar M, Nyffeler MS, Mirtallo J; ASPEN Task Force for Revision of Nutrition Support Pharmacist Standards. Standards of practice for nutrition support pharmacists. *Nutr Clin Pract*. 2008;23(2):189–194.

24. DiMaria-Ghalili RA, Bankhead R, Fisher AA, Kovacevich D, Resler R, Guenter PA. ASPEN Board of Directors; Nurses Standards Revision Task Force. Standards of practice for nutrition support nurses. *Nutr Clin Pract*. 2007;22(4):458–465.

25. Russell M, Stieber M, Brantley S, et al; ASPEN Joint Standards Task Force; American Dietetic Association Dietitians in Nutrition Support Dietetic Practice Group; ASPEN; American Dietetic Association. Standards of practice and standards of professional performance for registered dietitians (generalist, specialty, and advanced) in nutrition support. *Nutr Clin Pract*. 2007;22(5):558–586.

26. Kumpf V. Challenges and obstacles of long-term home parenteral nutrition. *Nutr Clin Pract*. 2019;34(2):196–203.

27. Raphael BP, Murphy M, Gura KM, et al. Discrepancies between prescribed and actual pediatric home parenteral nutrition solutions. *Nutr Clin Pract*. 2016;31(5):654–658.

28. Kovacevich DS, Corrigan M, Ross VM, et al. American Society for Parenteral and Enteral Nutrition guidelines for the selection and care of central venous access devices for adult home parenteral nutrition administration. *JPEN J Parenter Enteral Nutr*. 2019;43(1):15–31.

29. Metheny NM. Parenteral nutrition. In: Metheny NM, ed. *Fluid & Electrolyte Balance: Nursing Considerations*. Sudbury, MA: Jones & Bartlett Learning; 2012:169–178.

30. ASPEN Board of Directors and the Clinical Guidelines Task Force. Guidelines for the use of parenteral and enteral nutrition in adult and pediatric patients [erratum in *JPEN J Parenter Enteral Nutr*. 2002;26(2):144]. *JPEN J Parenter Enteral Nutr*. 2002;26(1 suppl):1SA–138SA.

31. Crill CM, Gura KM. Parenteral nutrition support. In: Corkins MR, ed. *The A.S.P.E.N. Pediatric Nutrition Support Core Curriculum*. 2nd ed. Silver Spring, MD: ASPEN; 2015:593–614.

32. Bozzetti F, Mariani L, Bertinet DB, et al. Central venous catheter complications in 447 patients on home parenteral nutrition: an analysis of over 100,000 catheter days. *Clin Nutr*. 2002;21(6):475–485.

33. Association for Professionals in Infection Control and Epidemiology. *Guide to the Elimination of Catheter-Related Bloodstream Infections*. Washington, DC: Association for Professionals in Infection Control and Epidemiology; 2009. http://www.apic.org/Resource_/EliminationGuideForm/259c0594-17b0-459d-b395-fb143321414a/File/APIC-CRBSI-Elimination-Guide.pdf. Accessed December 10, 2019.

34. Mermel LA, Farr BM, Sherertz RJ, et al; Infectious Diseases Society of America; American College of Critical Care Medicine; Society for Healthcare Epidemiology of America. Guidelines for the management of intravascular catheter-related infections. *Clin Infect Dis*. 2011;32(9):1249–1272.

35. Steiger E. Dysfunction and thrombotic complications of vascular access devices. *JPEN J Parenter Enteral Nutr*. 2006;30(1 suppl):S70–S72.

36. Dray X, Joly F, Reijasse D, et al. Incidence, risk factors, and complications of cholelithiasis in patients with home parenteral nutrition. *J Am Coll Surg*. 2007;204(1):13–21.

37. Cavicchi M, Beau P, Crenn P, Degott C, Messing B. Prevalence of liver disease and contributing factors in patients receiving home parenteral nutrition for permanent intestinal failure. *Ann Intern Med*. 2000;132(7):525–532.

38. Fulford A, Scolapio JS, Aranda-Michel J. Parenteral nutrition-associated hepatotoxicity. *Nutr Clin Pract*. 2004;19(3):274–283.

39. Seidner DL. Parenteral nutrition-associated metabolic bone disease. *JPEN J Parenter Enteral Nutr*. 2002;26(5 suppl):S37–S42.

40. Pironi L, Tjellesen L, De Francesco A, et al; ESPEN-Home Artificial Nutrition Working Group. Bone mineral density in patients on home parenteral nutrition: a follow-up study. *Clin Nutr*. 2004;23(6):1288–1302.

41. Howard L, Ashley C, Lyon D, Shenkin A. Autopsy tissue trace elements in 8 long-term parenteral nutrition patients who received the current U.S. Food and Drug Administration formulation. *JPEN J Parenter Enteral Nutr*. 2007;31(5):388–396.

CHAPTER 11

42. Smith CE, Curtas S, Kleinbeck SV, et al. Clinical trial of interactive and videotaped educational interventions reduce infection, reactive depression, and rehospitalizations for sepsis in patients on home parenteral nutrition. *JPEN J Parenter Enteral Nutr.* 2003;27(2):137–145.

43. de Burgoa LJ, Seidner D, Hamilton C, Stafford J, Steiger E. Examination of factors that lead to complications for new home parenteral nutrition patients. *J Infusion Nurs.* 2006;29(2):74–80.

44. Dakof GA, Taylor SE. Victims' perceptions of social support: what is helpful from whom? *J Pers Soc Psychol.* 1990;58(1):80–89.

45. Cox JA, Westbrook LJ. Home infusion therapy. Essential characteristics of a successful education process—a grounded theory study. *J Infusion Nurs.* 2005;28(2):99–107.

46. National Center for Education Statistics. *National Assessment of Adult Literacy of America's Adults in the 21st Century.* NCES Pub. NO. 2006470. Washington, DC: National Center for Education Statistics; 2003. http://nces.ed.gov/naal/pdf/2006470.pdf. Accessed November 26, 2019.

47. Sand-Jecklin K. The impact of medical terminology on readability of patient education materials. *J Community Health Nurs.* 2007;24(2):119–129.

48. Clayton LH. Strategies for selecting effective patient nutrition education materials. *Nutr Clin Pract.* 2010;25(5):436–442.

49. Doak LG, Doak CC, Meade CD. Strategies to improve cancer education materials. *Oncol Nurs Forum.* 1996;23(8):1305–1312.

50. Ayers P, Adams, Boullata J, et al; ASPEN. A.S.P.E.N. parenteral nutrition safety consensus recommendations. *JPEN J Parenter Enteral Nutr.* 2014;38(3): 296–333.

51. Gifford H, Delegge M, Epperson LA. Education methods and techniques for training home parenteral nutrition patients. *Nutr Clin Pract.* 2010;25(5):443–450.

52. Marden SF. Technology dependence and health-related quality of life: a model. *J Adv Nurs.* 2005;50(2):187–195.

53. Winkler MF, Ross VM, Piamjariyakul U, Gajewski B, Smith CE. Technology dependence in home care: impact on patients and their family caregivers. *Nutr Clin Pract.* 2006;21(6):544–556.

54. Lehoux P. Patients' perspectives on high-tech home care: a qualitative inquiry into the use-friendliness of four technologies. *BMC Health Serv Res.* 2004;4(1):28. doi:10.1186/1472-6963-4-28

55. Lehoux P, Saint-Arnaud J, Richard L. The use of technology at home: what patient manuals say and sell vs. what patients face and fear. *Sociol Health Illn.* 2004;26(5);617–644.

56. Huisman-de Waal G, van Achterberg T, Jansen J, Wanten G, Schoonhoven L. 'High-tech' home care: overview of professional care in patients on home parenteral nutrition and implications for nursing care. *J Clin Nurs.* 2011;20(15–16):2125–2134.

57. Ireton-Jones C, Nishikawa K, Nishikawa R. Home parenteral and enteral nutrition during natural disasters: a guide for clinicians and consumers. *Nutr Clin Pract.* 2019;34(2):216–219.

58. Orley J. The World Health Organization (WHO) quality of life project. In: Trimble MR, Dodson WE, eds. *Epilepsy and Quality of Life.* New York, NY: Raven; 1994:99–133.

59. Winkler MF, Hagan E, Wetle T, Smith C, Maillet JO, Touger-Decker R. An exploration of quality of life and the experience of living with home parenteral nutrition. *JPEN J Parenter Enteral Nutr.* 2010;34(4):395–407.

60. Baxter JP, Fayers PM, McKinlay AW. A review of the instruments used to assess the quality of life of adult patients with chronic intestinal failure receiving parenteral nutrition at home. *Br J Nutr.* 2005;94(5):633–638.

61. Winkler MF. Quality of life in adult home parenteral nutrition patients. *JPEN J Parenter Enteral Nutr.* 2005;29(3):162–170.

62. Baxter JP, Fayers PM, McKinlay AW. A review of the quality of life of adult patients treated with long-term parenteral nutrition. *Clin Nutr.* 2006;25(4):543–553.

63. Fortune DG, Varden J, Parker S, Harper L, Richards HL, Shaffer JL. Illness beliefs of patients on home parenteral nutrition (HPN) and their relation to emotional distress. *Clin Nutr.* 2005;24(6):896–903.

64. Persoon A, Huisman-de Waal G, Naber TA, et al. Impact of long-term HPN on daily life in adults. *Clin Nutr.* 2005;24(2):304–313.

65. Silver HJ. The lived experience of home total parenteral nutrition: an online qualitative inquiry with adults, children, and mothers. *Nutr Clin Pract.* 2004;19(3):297–304.

66. Brotherton AM, Judd PA. Quality of life in adult enteral tube feeding patients. *J Hum Nutr Diet.* 2007;20(6):513–522; quiz 523–525.

67. Brotherton A, Abbott J. Clinical decision making and the provision of information in PEG feeding: an exploration of patients and their cares' perceptions. *J Hum Nutr Diet.* 2009;22(4):302–309.

68. Walker A. In the absence of food: a case of rhythmic loss and spoiled identity for patients with percutaneous endoscopic gastrostomy feeding tubes. *Food Cult Soc.* 2005;8(2):161–180.

69. Huisman-de Waal G, Naber T, Schoonhoven L, Persoon A, Sauerwein H, van Achterberg T. Problems experienced by patients receiving parenteral nutrition at home: results of an open interview study. *JPEN J Parenter Enteral Nutr.* 2006;30(3):215–221.

70. Thompson CW, Durrant L, Barusch A, Olson L. Fostering coping skills and resilience in home enteral nutrition (HEN) consumers. *Nutr Clin Pract.* 2006;21(6):557–565.

71. Baxter JP, Fayers PM, McKinlay AW. The clinical and psychometric validation of a questionnaire to assess the quality of life of adult patients treated with long-term parenteral nutrition. *JPEN J Parenter Enteral Nutr.* 2010;34(2):131–142.

72. Theilla M, Kagan I, Chernov K, Cohen J, Kagan I, Singer P. Self-evaluation of quality of life among patients receiving home parenteral nutrition: a validation study. *JPEN J Parenter Enteral Nutr.* 2018;42(3):516–521.

73. Mansilla ME. Benefits from artificial nutritional support: a testimonial. *Nutrition.* 2003;19(1):78–80.

74. Kindle R. Life with Fred: 12 years of home parenteral nutrition. *Nutr Clin Pract.* 2003;18(3):235–237.

75. Ireton-Jones C, Lang RK, Gravenstein ME, Schimel S. Home nutrition support from the patient's perspective: the real reality story! *Nutr Clin Pract.* 2006;21(6):542–543.

76. Fairman J, Compher C, Morris J, Mullen JL. Living long with short bowel syndrome: a historical case of twenty-nine years of living with home parenteral nutrition. *JPEN J Parenter Enteral Nutr.* 2007;31(2):127–134.

77. Kovacevich DS. Parenteral and enteral nutrition support groups. *Nutr Clin Pract.* 2003;18(3):238–239.

Multichamber-Bag Parenteral Nutrition Products

Introduction

Standardized, commercially available parenteral nutrition (PN) products, more commonly referred to by clinicians as multichamber-bag PN (MCB-PN) products, can provide an alternative to traditional compounded PN admixtures. MCB-PN products are available as 2-chamber bag systems that provide dextrose and amino acids with or without electrolytes and as 3-chamber bag systems containing electrolytes, dextrose, amino acids, and lipid injectable emulsion (ILE).[1] These products are often referred to as *premixed* in older literature. The term *premixed* should be abandoned because these products require activation and the addition of other nutrients to deliver an appropriate PN regimen.

MCB-PN products have an additive port that allows for the addition of multivitamins, multi-trace elements, and other additives needed in PN. MCB-PN products are commercially produced under current United States Pharmacopeia (USP) and US Food and Drug Administration regulations.

Advantages

MCB-PN products can provide health systems with a PN option that can be safer and have less strain on financial and employee resources.[1-6] MCB-PN products allow for minimal transcription errors and may decrease errors associated with admixture preparation. A systematic review of the literature noted emerging evidence suggesting that MCB-PN products may be associated with a lower risk of infectious complications. It was noted that data are limited in quality and quantity.[2,7] A 3-chamber MCB-PN product may provide additional benefit compared with a 2-chamber MCB-PN by reducing the risk of infection due to additional manipulation.[8] MCB-PN products also may help health system and home infusion pharmacies avoid issues with shortages of PN components used in compounding PN admixtures.[3] Unactivated MCB-PN products have a long shelf life, and they can be used for home PN patients when they are traveling or during emergencies.[1]

Disadvantages

MCB-PN products may be easier to use, but individuals prescribing and preparing MCB-PN products must be adequately trained. The labeling of MCB-PN products does not align with the current ASPEN PN Safety Consensus Recommendations.[9] Pharmacists involved with the preparation of MCB-PN products should be trained on proper activation and additive techniques. These pharmacists should also be knowledgeable about how additives can effect stability and sterility.[9] MCB-PN products may be an option for facilities with a small number of PN patients (<15 bags per day), but facilities with large PN volumes and patients with significant electrolyte or macronutrient needs may not be able to meet patients' needs with MCB-PN products.[6] These products may not be appropriate for patients with decreased electrolyte clearance (eg, renal insufficiency).[1]

Safety and Errors

Two safety advantages for MCB-PN products over compounded PN admixtures have been proposed[3]:

1. Reduction in potential errors related to simplified prescribing and compounding and

2. Potential for reduction in PN-related blood stream infections.

Using MCB-PN product does come with opportunities for error. The internal membrane seals must be broken prior to administration. Policies and procedures must be developed to ensure that pharmacy staff activate these products and that any additives are admixed in accordance with USP general chapter <797> standards.[3]

Results of recent studies seem to indicate MCB-PN products may reduce the rates of bloodstream infections. However, the reduction may be seen only in those patients for whom MCB-PN products were administered intact or minimally altered. A study by Turpin et al[10] showed an increased infection rate when compounded PN admixtures were manipulated on the patient care area.

Current Formulations

There are 2 formulations for MCB-PN. Two-chamber MCB-PN products (Table 12-1, Figure 12-1) provide dextrose and amino acid solutions with or without electrolytes. Two-chamber MCB-PN products are available in 1-L and 2-L bags with a variety of dextrose and amino acid combinations. The maximum amount of protein is 100 g in a 2-L bag. ILEs can be added directly to the bag, or they can be piggybacked in a 2-in-1 fashion. This MCB-PN system can be used in pediatric and adult patients.[10]

Three-chamber MCB-PN products provide dextrose, amino acids, and ILEs in one bag (Figure 12-2). This formulation is available in 4 presentations that can be administered via a central vein (Table 12-2) and 3 presentations that can be administered via a central or peripheral vein (Table 12-3). The maximum amount of protein is 85 g in a 2566-mL bag. Three-chamber MCB-PN products are not recommended for use in patients <2 years of age because of the inability to meet nutrition requirements in this patient population.[11]

Table 12-1. Two-Chamber MCB-PN Products Available in 1–2 L[a]

Product (Amino Acid %/ Dextrose %)	Available With Electrolytes	Protein (g/L)	Kcal/L	Osmolarity (mOsm/L), Including Electrolytes[b]
2.75/5	Yes	27.5	280	665
4.25/5	Yes	42.5	340	815
4.25/10	Yes	42.5	510	1070
5/15	Yes	50	710	1395
5/20	Yes	50	880	1650

[a]Values are from Clinimix and Clinimix E.[12]
[b]Values are from Clinimix E

Table 12-2. Three-Chamber MCB-PN Products Available (Central Vein Administration)[a]

	1026	1540	2053	2566
Amino acids (g)	34	51	68	85
Dextrose (g)	100	150	200	250
Fats (g)	40	60	80	100
Total energy (kcal)	870	1310	1745	2180

[a]Values are from Kabiven, Fresenius Kabi.[13]

Table 12-3. Three-Chamber MCB-PN Products (Peripheral or Central Vein Administration)[a]

Volume (mL)	1440	1920	2400
Amino acid (g)	34	45	57
Dextrose (g)	97	130	162
Fats (g)	51	68	85
Total energy (kcal)	970	1300	1620

[a]Values are from Perikabiven, Fresenius Kabi.[13]

Figure 12-1. Example of 2-chamber Bag

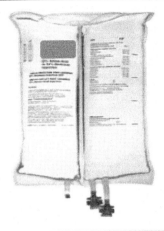

Source: Reprinted with permission from Curtis C, Nystrom E. PN shortages and use of multi-chamber bag PN products. Webinar presented for: ASPEN; December 11, 2018; Silver Spring, MD.

Figure 12-2. Example of 3-chamber Bag

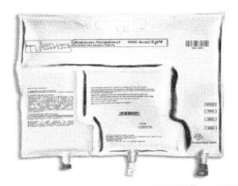

Source: Reprinted with permission from Curtis C, Nystrom E. PN shortages and use of multi-chamber bag PN products. Webinar presented for: ASPEN; December 11, 2018; Silver Spring, MD.

Determining Appropriateness

There are numerous factors to consider before determining if MCB-PN is appropriate. A recent publication[3] included a decision chart to help guide selection of PN products (Figure 12-3). Applying a method similar to that used in this tool may prove to be a useful for facilities using MCB-PN products and compounded PN admixtures.

Figure 12-3. MCB-PN Decision Chart[3]

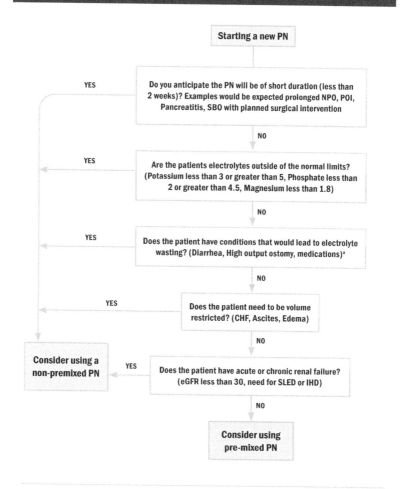

CHF, congestive heart failure; eGFR, estimated glomerular filtration rate; IHD, ischemic heart disease; NPO, nothing by mouth; PN, parenteral nutrition; POI, postoperative ileus; SBO, small bowel obstruction; SLED, sustained low-efficiency dialysis.

POI = Post-op Ileus

SBO = Small Bowel Obstruction

[a]Examples include: Foscarnet, Amphotericin B, Cisplatin, Ifosphamide

Summary

MCB-PN products provide an alternative to traditional compounded PN admixtures. The appropriate role of MCB-PN products in the nutrition support clinician's therapy should be based on patient-specific and institutional requirements. The advantages and disadvantages must be weighed to determine whether MCB-PN products will meet the needs of an institution's patient population. When MCB-PN is used in an appropriate patient population, it provides a safe and effective alternative to compounded PN admixtures. However, nutrition support clinicians must use recommendations from ASPEN, the Institute for Safe Medication Practices, and other national organizations to ensure patient safety.

References

3. Patel R. Parenteral nutrition formulations. In: Mueller CM, ed. *The ASPEN Adult Nutrition Support Core Curriculum.* 3rd ed. Silver Spring, MD: ASPEN; 2017: 297–320.

4. Alfonso JE, Berlana D, Ukleja A, Boullata J. Clinical, ergonomic and economic outcomes with multichamber bags compared with (hospital) pharmacy compounded bags and multibottle systems: a systematic literature review. *JPEN J Parenter Enteral Nutr.* 2017;41(7):1162–1177.

5. Hall JW. Safety, cost and clinical considerations for the use of premixed parenteral nutrition. *Nutr Clin Pract.* 2015;30(3):325–330.

6. Miller SJ. Commercial premixed parenteral nutrition: is it right for your institution? Nutr Clin Pract. 2009;24(4):459–469.

7. Beattie C, Allard J, Raman M. Comparison between premixed and compounded parenteral nutrition solutions in hospitalized patients requiring parenteral nutrition. *Nutr Clin Pract.* 2016;31(2):229–234.

8. Blanchette LM, Huiras P, Papadopoulos S. Standardized versus custom parenteral nutrition: impact on clinical and cost-related outcomes. *Am J Health Syst Pharm.* 2014;71(2):114–121.

9. Bozat E, Korubuk G, Onar P, Abbasoglu O. Cost analysis of premixed multichamber bags versus compounded parenteral nutrition: breakeven point. *Hosp Pharm.* 2014;49(2):170–176.

10. Pontes-Arruda A, Dos Santos MC, Martins LF, et al; EPICOS Study Group. Influence of parenteral nutrition delivery system on the development of bloodstream infections in critically ill patients: an international, multicenter, prospective, open-label, controlled study-EPICOS Study. *JPEN J Parenter Enteral Nutr.* 2012;36(5):574–586.

11. Gervasio J. Compounding vs standardized commercial parenteral nutrition product: pros and cons. *JPEN J Parenter Enteral Nutr.* 2012;36(2 suppl):40S–413.

12. Ayers P, Adams S, Boullata J, et al. A.S.P.E.N. parenteral nutrition safety recommendations. *JPEN J Parent Enteral Nutr.* 2014;38(3):296–333.

13. Turpin RS, Solem C, Pontes-Arruda A, et al. The impact of parenteral nutrition preparation on bloodstream infection risk and cost. *Eur J Clin Nutr.* 2014;68(8):953–958.

14. CLINIMIX (Amino Acid in Dextrose) injections and CLINIMIX E (amino acid with electrolytes in dextrose with calcium) injections. Baxter website. http://www.baxtermedicationdeliveryproducts.com/nutrition/clinimix.html. Accessed December 3, 2019.

15. KABIVEN, PERIKABIVEN. Fresenius Kabi website. https://kabivenusa.com/. Accessed December 3, 2019.

CHAPTER 12

Optimizing Electronic Health Records for Nutrition Care[i]

Introduction

Electronic health records (EHRs) offer access to patient information locally, regionally, and nationally and facilitate coordination of care across healthcare settings. Healthcare clinicians who frequently provide direct patient care that influences nutrition care — nurses; pharmacists; medical providers, including physicians and advanced practice providers; and dietitians — will be referred to here as nutrition clinicians. Nutrition care of the patient in the inpatient, ambulatory, or long-term healthcare setting commences with screening and assessment. Known or suspected nutrition deficiencies or problems are addressed with information from nutrition screening and assessment.

The first Nutrition Care Process flowchart was published in 1994 to propose nutrition care indicators to The Joint Commission on Accreditation of Healthcare Organizations (now referred to as The Joint Commission) for patient care with paper-based workflows.[1] More recently, the Academy of Nutrition and Dietetics (the Academy) published the Nutrition Care

i **Source:** Adapted with permission from Kight CE, Bouche JM, Curry A, et al; Academy of Nutrition and Dietetics, ASPEN; Association of Clinical Documentation Improvement Specialists. Consensus recommendations for optimizing electronic health records for nutrition care. Nutr Clin Pract. 35(1):12-23. Note that minor edits have been made to the original article to conform with ASPEN style.

Process, which is a systematic framework and language to guide nutrition and dietetics practitioners in documenting delivery of nutrition care.[2,3] The American Society for Parenteral and Enteral Nutrition (ASPEN) developed Nutrition Care Pathways to provide the interprofessional nutrition clinician a framework to guide nutrition care for pediatric (Figure 13-1) and adult patients (Figure 13-2).[4]

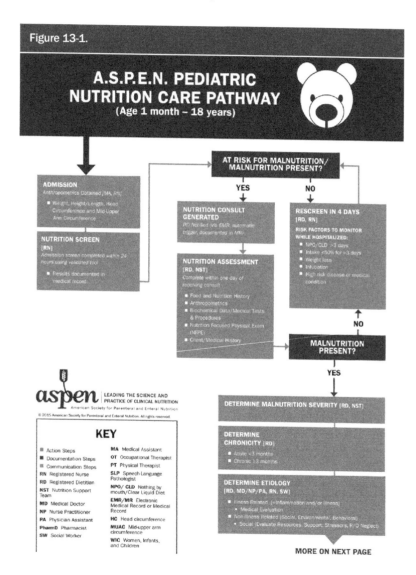

Figure 13-1.

A.S.P.E.N. PEDIATRIC NUTRITION CARE PATHWAY
(Age 1 month – 18 years)

MORE ON NEXT PAGE

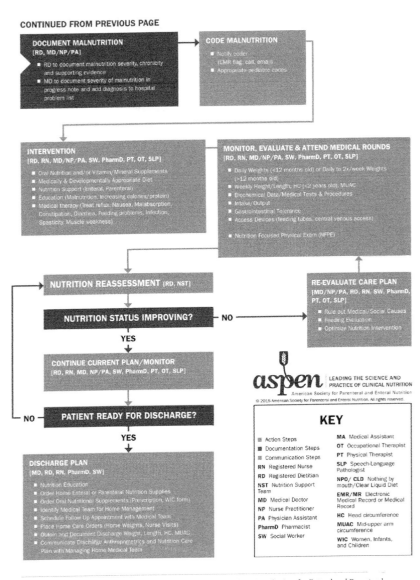

EMR/MR as used in this figure is equivalent to EHR. A.S.P.E.N., American Society for Enteral and Parenteral Nutrition; EHR, electronic health record; EMR, electronic medical record; MR, medical record.
Source: Reprinted with permission from the American Society for Enteral and Parenteral Nutrition, Copyright 2015.

The pathways illustrate recommended steps from screening through discharge from a healthcare setting with a focus on malnutrition. However, the provision of nutrition care for any nutrition condition in any healthcare setting follows the pathway steps: identification, assessment, intervention, monitoring, and discharge planning.

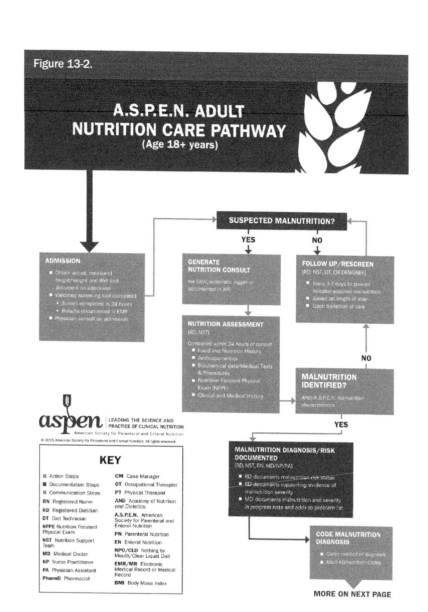

Figure 13-2.

A.S.P.E.N. ADULT NUTRITION CARE PATHWAY
(Age 18+ years)

SUSPECTED MALNUTRITION?

YES | NO

ADMISSION
- Obtain actual, measured height/weight and BMI and document on admission
- Validated screening tool completed
  - Screen completed in 24 hours
  - Results documented in EMR
- Physician consult on admission

GENERATE NUTRITION CONSULT
The EMR automatic trigger or documented in MR

FOLLOW UP/RESCREEN
[RD, NST, DT, OR DESIGNEE]
- Every 3-7 days to prevent hospital acquired malnutrition
- Based on length of stay
- Upon transition of care

NUTRITION ASSESSMENT
[RD, NST]
Completed within 24 hours of consult
- Food and Nutrition History
- Anthropometrics
- Biochemical data/Medical Tests & Procedures
- Nutrition Focused Physical Exam (NFPE)
- Clinical and Medical History

MALNUTRITION IDENTIFIED?
AND/A.S.P.E.N. malnutrition characteristics

NO

YES

MALNUTRITION DIAGNOSIS/RISK DOCUMENTED
[RD, NST, RN, MD/NP/PA]
- RD documents malnutrition risk status
- RD documents supporting evidence of malnutrition severity
- MD documents malnutrition and severity in progress note and adds to problem list

CODE MALNUTRITION DIAGNOSIS
- Coder notified of diagnosis
- Adult Malnutrition Codes

MORE ON NEXT PAGE

aspen | LEADING THE SCIENCE AND PRACTICE OF CLINICAL NUTRITION
American Society for Parenteral and Enteral Nutrition
© 2015 American Society for Parenteral and Enteral Nutrition. All rights reserved.

KEY

- Action Steps
- Documentation Steps
- Communication Steps

RN Registered Nurse
RD Registered Dietitian
DT Diet Technician
NFPE Nutrition Focused Physical Exam
NST Nutrition Support Team
MD Medical Doctor
NP Nurse Practitioner
PA Physician Assistant
PharmD Pharmacist

CM Case Manager
OT Occupational Therapist
PT Physical Therapist
AND Academy of Nutrition and Dietetics
A.S.P.E.N. American Society for Parenteral and Enteral Nutrition
PN Parenteral Nutrition
EN Enteral Nutrition
NPO/CLD Nothing by Mouth/Clear Liquid Diet
EMR/MR Electronic Medical Record or Medical Record
BMI Body Mass Index

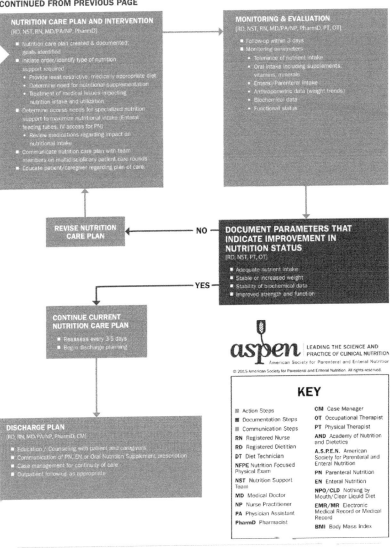

NUTRITION CARE PLAN AND INTERVENTION
[RD, NST, RN, MD/PA/NP, PharmD]

- Nutrition care plan created & documented; goals identified
- Initiate order/identify type of nutrition support required
  - Provide least restrictive, medically appropriate diet
  - Determine need for nutritional supplementation
  - Treatment of medical issues impacting nutrition intake and utilization
- Determine access needs for specialized nutrition support to maximize nutritional intake (Enteral feeding tubes, IV access for PN)
  - Review medications regarding impact on nutritional intake
- Communicate nutrition care plan with team members on multidisciplinary patient care rounds
- Educate patient/caregiver regarding plan of care.

MONITORING & EVALUATION
[RD, NST, RN, MD/PA/NP, PharmD, PT, OT]

- Follow-up within 3 days
- Monitoring parameters
  - Tolerance of nutrient intake
  - Oral intake including supplements, vitamins, minerals
  - Enteral/Parenteral intake
  - Anthropometric data (weight trends)
  - Biochemical data
  - Functional status

REVISE NUTRITION CARE PLAN

← NO —

DOCUMENT PARAMETERS THAT INDICATE IMPROVEMENT IN NUTRITION STATUS
[RD, NST, PT, OT]

- Adequate nutrient intake
- Stable or increased weight
- Stability of biochemical data
- Improved strength and function

— YES →

CONTINUE CURRENT NUTRITION CARE PLAN

- Reassess every 3-5 days
- Begin discharge planning

DISCHARGE PLAN
[RD, RN, MD/PA/NP, PharmD, CM]

- Education / Counseling with patient and caregivers
- Communication of PN, EN or Oral Nutrition Supplement prescription
- Case management for continuity of care
- Outpatient follow-up as appropriate

aspen LEADING THE SCIENCE AND PRACTICE OF CLINICAL NUTRITION
American Society for Parenteral and Enteral Nutrition

© 2015 American Society for Parenteral and Enteral Nutrition. All rights reserved.

KEY

- Action Steps
- Documentation Steps
- Communication Steps

RN Registered Nurse
RD Registered Dietitian
DT Diet Technician
NFPE Nutrition Focused Physical Exam
NST Nutrition Support Team
MD Medical Doctor
NP Nurse Practitioner
PA Physician Assistant
PharmD Pharmacist

CM Case Manager
OT Occupational Therapist
PT Physical Therapist
AND Academy of Nutrition and Dietetics
A.S.P.E.N. American Society for Parenteral and Enteral Nutrition
PN Parenteral Nutrition
EN Enteral Nutrition
NPO/CLD Nothing by Mouth/Clear Liquid Diet
EMR/MR Electronic Medical Record or Medical Record
BMI Body Mass Index

EMR/MR as used in this figure is equivalent to EHR. A.S.P.E.N., American Society for Enteral and Parenteral Nutrition; EHR, electronic health record; EMR, electronic medical record; MR, medical record.
Source: Reprinted with permission from ASPEN, Copyright 2015.

Optimizing Electronic Health Records for Nutrition Care

Nutrition clinicians address inadequate or excessive food intake; nutrient deficiencies or nutrient excesses related to fluid, vitamins, and/or minerals; alterations in gastrointestinal function from the mouth to the colon, malnutrition, and food insecurity; and education and counseling for nutrition and health issues. Healthcare costs in the United States in 2017 were $3.5 trillion.[5] Diagnoses with nutrition therapy as an important component include obesity, with healthcare costs of $147 billion to $210 billion per year[6]; diabetes, with annual costs of $327 billion[7]; and gastrointestinal, liver, and pancreatic diseases, with an estimated annual cost of $135.9 billion.[8] The direct medical costs for disease-associated malnutrition based on the National Health and Nutrition Examination Survey, excluding institutionalized participants, were estimated to be $15.5 billion annually.[9] The estimated costs of inpatient stays related to malnutrition accounted for nearly $49 billion, or 12.6% of aggregate hospital costs, compared with $389.1 billion for all nonmaternal and nonneonatal inpatient stays.[10] It is imperative that nutrition clinicians document the identification of nutrition conditions with associated interventions to allow communication of the treatment plan to all clinicians in any healthcare setting. Nutrition diagnoses left unrecognized by lack of identification or treatment and follow-up care contribute to the high costs of medical care.

The following consensus recommendations from a work group of ASPEN, the Academy, and the Association of Clinical Documentation Improvement Specialists outline opportunities for EHR optimization for various interprofessional activities presented within the framework of the ASPEN Nutrition Care Pathways. Although the steps are identical for both pediatric and adult patients, the separate pathways vary in timeline and tools for each population during hospitalization. Therefore, the consensus recommendations apply to both pediatrics and adults, but differences between the patient populations will be identified, where appropriate. The consensus recommendations are appropriate for the patient at any entry point into the healthcare system. The task force, using this pathway, has provided recommendations for (1) nutrition screening and assessment; (2) nutrition diagnosis; (3) nutrition care plan and interventions; (4) monitoring, reassessment, and nutrition goals; and (5) discharge plan.

Each healthcare discipline documents information in the EHR in both structured and unstructured data formats. Structured data are data that reside in a fixed field, are stored in a database, and can be easily retrieved for reports, flowsheets, or graphs. Structured data are unambiguous, specific, and defined, usually within allowed parameters ranging from anthropometric data to specific parenteral nutrition (PN) components. The nutrition clinician enters structured data directly into the EHR with information such as vital signs, nutrition assessment findings, orders, medications, procedures, and diagnoses and views structured data in many forms, such as the above, and problem lists, allergies, and laboratory findings. Structured data options for entering information in the EHR can include checkboxes, drop-down lists, and radio buttons. The advantage to the end user of having structured data for nutrition care is to visually depict a patient's nutrition history within 1 view, such as a flowsheet report or graph. Structured data also enable increased semantic interoperability between EHR systems.[11] Unstructured data include text in clinical notes or comment boxes or scanned documents. Both data forms reflect the patient's nutrition history for communication to other providers and to the patient. There are small variations in the structured vs unstructured forms contained within different EHR platforms; however, this permits the end user to integrate both types of data into 1 report while developing the patient care plan.

The vendor and institution EHR implementation analysts are familiar with typical provider and care team workflows and understand the documentation requirements for providing patient care and appropriate billing. Build, implementation, and optimization of an EHR system should be a clinical project and not just an Information Systems project. Nutrition clinicians are the experts for content and workflows and should be part of the EHR implementation and ongoing maintenance teams. ASPEN, the Academy, and the Association of Clinical Documentation Improvement Specialists have developed these consensus recommendations to guide EHR and related developers and implementation teams on the optimal build for documentation and treatment interventions involved in patient nutrition care to maximize the quality of patient care and healthcare team effectiveness and efficiency.

ASPEN Consensus Recommendations for EHR optimization

The recommendations found in this chapter do not constitute medical or other professional advice and should not be taken as such. To the extent that the information published herein may be used to assist in the care of patients, this is the result of the sole professional judgment of the attending healthcare professional whose judgment is the primary component of quality medical care. The information presented here is not a substitute for the exercise of such judgment by the healthcare professional. Circumstances in clinical settings and patient indications may require actions different from those recommended in this document, and, in those cases, the judgment of the treating professional should prevail.

Nutrition Screening

Nutrition screening is the first step in the ASPEN Nutrition Care Pathways to identify individuals at risk for malnutrition.[4] The Joint Commission promotes the use of standards of care for hospitals to provide safe and high-quality patient care. Its standards pertaining to nutrition screening and assessment are located in the section "Provision of Care, Treatment, and Services (PC.01.02.01)"[12]:

> The goal of assessment is to determine the care, treatment, and services that will meet the patient's initial and continuing needs. Patient needs must be reassessed throughout the course of care, treatment, and services. Identifying and delivering the right care, treatment, and services depends on the following three processes:
>
> 1. Collecting information about the patient's health history as well as physical, functional, and psychosocial status.
>
> 2. Analyzing the information in order to understand the patient's needs for care, treatment, and services.
>
> 3. Making care, treatment, and services decisions based on the analysis of information collected.

The depth and frequency of assessment depends on a number of factors, including the patient's needs, program goals, and the care, treatment, and services provided. Assessment activities may vary between settings, as defined by the hospital's leaders. Information gathered at the patient's first contact might indicate the need for more data or a more intensive assessment. At a minimum, the need for further assessment is determined by the care, treatment, and services sought; the patient's presenting condition(s); and whether the patient agrees to the recommended care, treatment, and services.

The Elements of Performance state:

> The hospital defines, in writing, the scope and content of screening, assessment, and reassessment. Patient information is collected according to these requirements.
>
> In defining the scope and content of the information it collects, the organization may want to consider information that it can obtain, with the patient's consent, from the patient's family and the patient's other care providers, as well as information conveyed on any medical jewelry.
>
> Assessment and reassessment information includes the patient's perception of the effectiveness of, and any side effects related to, his or her medication(s).

The hospital defines, in writing, criteria that identify when additional, specialized, or more in-depth assessments are performed. Note: Examples of criteria could include those that identify when a nutritional, functional, or pain assessment should be performed for patients who are at risk.

The hospital has defined criteria that identify when nutritional plans are developed.[12]

The nutrition screening tool in all healthcare settings should be easy and quick to score, as well as standardized and validated. There are several standardized and validated nutrition screening tools available for adults,[13-16] but the availability of these tools is more limited for pediatric patients.[17,18] The nutrition screen is typically performed by a nurse or dietitian and is incorporated into the required office visit or hospital admission documentation for the patients who require nutrition screening.

The generation of scores from screening tools in the EHR enables triggering of further workflow steps in the pathway through reports and alerts. Clinical Decision Support is a process that provides guidance to clinicians during patient care with configuration by the Information Systems staff of alerts to release at appropriate times in the workflow to improve efficiency and outcomes and avoid errors.[19] Clinical Decision Support interventions associated with nutrition screening include creation of a nutrition consult order when the screen value indicates risk or display of screen scores on the dietitian's daily patient unit reports.

A structured data element for nutrition screening allows an organization to report their screening compliance during The Joint Commission's regularly scheduled audits and advises clinical nutrition managers and clinic managers whether there is adequate staffing to provide nutrition services. The Joint Commission has no requirements regarding a time frame for rescreening hospitalized patients for nutrition risk if the initial screen was normal. However, ASPEN recommends a repeat nutrition screen every 3-7 days for adults and every 4 days for pediatric patients if the hospital admission nutrition screen determines the patient is not at risk for malnutrition.[14,20] A longer period before rescreening may be appropriate for patients in other care settings.

Nutrition Assessment

The next step in the Nutrition Care Pathway is nutrition assessment.[4] A positive nutrition screen result should trigger an automatic notification to the dietitian for a nutrition assessment to be completed within the time frame specified at each institution, as described here. Nutrition assessment data include food- or nutrition-related history, biochemical data, medical tests, procedures, anthropometric measurements, client history, and nutrition-focused physical examination findings.

Nutrition Care Pathway steps should be incorporated into the EHR build and workflow following the guidelines set forth by Health Level 7 (HL7) and the newly revised standards of the Electronic Nutrition Care Process Record System guidelines. HL7 International has undertaken a project in conjunction with the Academy to create an Electronic Nutrition Care Process Record System.[21] The goal is to develop a standard list of functions and criteria for integration of the Academy's Nutrition Care Process to align with the HL7 International EHR System Functional Model that provides a standard description and common understanding of functions for healthcare settings. The Academy has also developed the Consolidated Clinical Document Architecture *R2.1 Nutrition Transitions of Care Implementation Guide*, an HL7 standard that identifies what nutrition data should be included in an EHR in any transitions-of-care setting.[22] Transitions-of-care settings include home health agencies, inpatient rehabilitation facilities, long-term acute care hospitals, skilled nursing facilities, and community-based clinics or nonprofits, such as those for diabetes prevention and treatment.

Nutrition Diagnosis

The nutrition screening and assessment steps of the Nutrition Care Pathway result in identification of nutrition problems that require treatment by nutrition clinicians. The Academy's Nutrition Care Process utilizes nutrition diagnosis to standardize nutrition diagnostic terminology.[2] A nutrition diagnosis as defined by the Academy describes a specific nutrition problem that can be improved or resolved through nutrition interventions. The domains of nutrition diagnosis include *intake*, which is defined as too much or too little of a food or nutrient compared with actual or estimated needs; clinical, which is defined as nutrition problems that relate to medical or physical conditions; and *behavioral-environmental*, which is defined as knowledge, attitude, beliefs, physical environment, access to food, or food safety.[23] A medical diagnosis, on the other hand, is used by healthcare providers and coders as described in the *International Statistical Classification of Diseases and Related Health Problems*, 10th Revision (*ICD-10*)[24] codes. Documentation of the nutrition diagnosis used by dietitians and *ICD-10* codes used by providers both describe problems that require nutrition intervention and treatment to resolve to improve patient health and well-being.

Malnutrition is 1 nutrition (clinical domain) and medical diagnosis (*ICD-10 code*) that affects patient care as well as appropriate coding, billing, and reimbursement.[25] Patients can be diagnosed with malnutrition in any healthcare setting. Organizations should adopt explicit malnutrition criteria that all healthcare professionals can apply consistently. Developing malnutrition criteria that include representatives from nutrition and medicine with clinical documentation integrity and coding departments improves malnutrition documentation required for billing. The Academy and ASPEN published recommended criteria for the identification of adult[26] and pediatric[27] malnutrition. The malnutrition diagnoses have been mapped to *ICD-10* codes: mild protein-calorie malnutrition is E44.1, moderate protein-calorie malnutrition is E44.0, and (unspecified) severe protein-calorie malnutrition is E43. Many hospitals have adopted the Academy and ASPEN consensus criteria for malnutrition as written, or developed their own clinical indicators by addition or removal of criteria.

Comprehensive documentation by the nutrition care clinician and the medical providers to support compliant coding and capture of the nutrition diagnosis includes (1) the diagnosis and its severity (eg, severe protein-calorie malnutrition) documented by a provider (physician, advanced practitioner provider); (2) the clinical indicators to support the diagnosis (eg, weight loss of 10% in a 3-month time frame); (3) development of a treatment plan to address the diagnosis of malnutrition (eg, initiation of enteral nutrition [EN]); and (4) progress and/or changes in a patient's status in reassessment notes (eg, patient tolerating goal EN and weight loss stopped). Malnutrition is a secondary diagnosis that can affect the Medicare-Severity Diagnosis-Related Group Complications or Comorbidities and Major Complications or Comorbidities.[28]

Although nutrition clinicians usually diagnose malnutrition, it is imperative that this diagnosis is documented in structured data format for automatic inclusion in the attending physician/team documentation templates to document how the diagnosis impacted treatment, nursing care, and length of stay.[29] Addition of the malnutrition diagnosis to the problem list by the physician, or nutrition clinician if allowed by organizational policies, facilitates transfer of the diagnosis across and between healthcare systems.

The nutrition diagnosis section of the EHR incorporates information from nutrition screening and assessment to generate the plan of care to treat nutrition problems that will be described in the nutrition interventions. Documenting a nutrition diagnosis has the potential to direct nutrition interventions and the resources required to care for the patient. Accurate documentation by physicians and advanced practice providers must be present to support coding, reimbursement, benchmarking, and high-quality patient care.[29]

Nutrition Care Plan and Intervention

A nutrition care plan based on data gathered in the nutrition assessment will address identified nutrition diagnoses. The care plan defines specific nutrition interventions to alter or eliminate the etiologies of nutrition problems. It also includes goals to describe the anticipated response to these interventions. Interventions are a planned set of specific behaviors or actions performed, which are delegated, coordinated, or recommended by a nutrition clinician who facilitates achievement of the desired goals, such as improved intake with nutrition support, weight stabilization, or improved wound healing.

Nutrition care plans are documented by all nutrition clinicians, although they are typically discipline-specific and not integrated. Appropriate documentation and ordering in the EHR will help improve the likelihood that patients receive the indicated nutrition intervention and treatment. Documentation of the treatment care plan helps ensure that all members of the healthcare team know the interventions needed to address a patient's nutrition diagnoses.

Nutrition interventions include oral diets, oral nutrition supplements (ONS), EN, and PN. Nutrition interventions also include nutrition-related medications or supplements, such as vitamin or mineral preparations, as well as assessing for and making changes in nutrition therapies to prevent or treat drug-nutrient interactions. Nutrition education and nutrition counseling for the patient and family, as well as coordination of nutrition care, are other types of nutrition interventions that can be vital to improving or maintaining nutrition status.[23] The EHR system should accommodate and be configured within an organization to allow the appropriate ordering and documentation of these interventions.

Diet orders can be simple or complex, with multiple modifications. The order functionality in the EHR should promote easy and clear application of necessary diet restrictions, including dysphagia modifications and assistance with feeding or environmental alterations. The Academy's Nutrition Care Manuals include appropriate diets for many nutrition care settings.[30,31] The diet orders in the Nutrition Care Manuals provide guidance for the naming convention and types of diets to configure in the diet order module. Some diet orders require a single selection, whereas others require multiple select options.

The healthcare organization determines standard definitions for nutrient levels, such as potassium, protein, and fiber, which should be clear to the clinicians ordering and implementing these orders. When the diet order changes because of short-term nothing-by-mouth status or addition of a new modification, the EHR should carry the parameters over from the previous diet to the new diet order with the ability of the clinician to modify these parameters as needed. For example, if a patient is on a consistent carbohydrate diet and the cardiology consultant subsequently changes the diet to a heart-healthy one, the consistent carbohydrate restriction should remain by default. ONS orders should be configured to allow flexibility on the type of supplement and timing of administration of the supplement to meet the patient's needs. HL7 diet order standards are available to assist in the build and implementation of electronic transmission of nutrition orders.[32] Food service computer systems are often integrated with the EHR and employ electronic transmission of nutrition orders using HL7 standards.

The use of standardized electronic EN orders improves patient safety by reducing the opportunities for incomplete, ambiguous, or incorrect EN orders.[33] Critical components of the EN order include the EN formula name, the delivery site (ie, route), the administration method (eg, continuous, cyclic, or bolus), the rate of infusion with goal rate or volume, and water flush instructions. The use of required fields within the EN order for these critical components will prevent order submission until the order is complete. A free text comment box in the EN order allows for entry of order instructions to clarify administration instructions. An EN order set that includes these details for the diet order and orders for laboratory monitoring, assessment of tolerance, and consults could be developed by organizations.[33] Implementation of scanning software with the EHR would increase the accuracy of delivering the right product to the right patient at the right time, as has been demonstrated in neonatal intensive care units[34] and children's hospitals.[35]

PN is a high-alert medication that is best ordered using a computerized provider order entry system.[36] The PN order components should be available in the computerized provider order entry system with all PN ingredients listed by their full generic names with specific ordering amounts per day for adult patients and per kilogram per day for neonatal and pediatric patients. Clinical Decision Support can alert those prescribing PN when order components exceed recommended or safe clinical limits or exceed limits of compatibility. Other important order requirements of the computerized provider order entry include patient dosing weight, indications for PN, route of administration (central vein or peripheral vein), method of administration (continuous vs cyclic), PN administration date and time, and PN instructions for total volume and infusion rate. The EHR should be able to transmit these orders via direct interface to an automated compounding device to avoid manual transcription of the electronic PN orders into the automated compounding device, which increases the chances of a transcription error. ASPEN, the Academy, and the American Society of Health-System Pharmacists have published joint consensus recommendations that address, in more detail, the PN functionality needed in an EHR.[37]

Historically, providers (ie, practitioners with independent prescriptive authority), including physicians, advanced practice nurses, and physician assistants, ordered the nutrition therapies for hospitalized patients, including oral diets, ONS, EN, and/or PN, per Centers for Medicare and Medicaid Services regulations. However, in 2014, the Centers for Medicare and Medicaid Services Conditions of Participation were revised to allow dietitians and other qualified nutrition clinicians to independently order therapeutic diets, ONS, EN, PN, and nutrition-related laboratory and imaging tests, if within the clinician's scope of practice per the state laws and regulations and within the hospital's medical staff rules, regulations, and bylaws.[38] In 2016, these conditions were extended to long-term care settings.[39]

These privileges may require a nutrition clinician consult from the provider requesting that they order these therapies. If the nutrition clinician is unable to place the nutrition support order per their healthcare privileges, options include pending or holding the order for prescribing providers to review and sign. Other considerations would be to implement electronic notifications to review, advance, or change an order based on laboratory values, intake and output, medications, and physical assessment findings. Electronic order sets may enhance the order process, as well as providing consistent treatment plans among providers and organizations.[33,36]

Nutrition Monitoring and Evaluation

The monitoring and evaluation (reassessment) step of the Nutrition Care Pathway is vital to resolution of the nutrition diagnoses. It is the step in which a nutrition clinician determines whether the Nutrition Care Plan is helping to resolve nutrition problems or if it needs revision. ASPEN recommends follow-up within 3 days for hospitalized patients with a diagnosis of malnutrition.[40] During initial hospital assessment, the nutrition clinician should designate a time for reassessment(s) in accordance with hospital policies. If the patient is seen in an ambulatory setting, follow-up appointments are typically scheduled when the initial reason for visit cannot be resolved in 1 visit. Data in the nutrition reassessment include information that has accrued since the initial assessment, including oral diet, ONS, EN, PN, and other nutrient intake; new or changed biochemical results; medical tests and procedures; serial anthropometric measurements; and nutrition-focused physical findings. When the nutrition clinician documents the reassessment findings, the previously established nutrition diagnoses and goals should autopopulate, ensuring consistency in care. Language to describe the status of the nutrition goals may include *resolved, unresolved, improvement shown, or no longer appropriate.*

The use of structured data to capture nutrition reassessment parameters improves efficiency of the clinician's daily tasks with integration of intake data with anthropometrics and biochemical data to revise nutrition orders, such as for EN or PN. Structured data at the facility level are key to data-driven quality improvement initiatives to meet organizational missions, goals, and strategic plans. Consistency among healthcare facilities is key to conducting large-scale nutrition outcomes research, such as the Malnutrition Quality Improvement Initiative, which includes recommendations for electronic clinical quality measures for all steps of the Nutrition Care Pathway.[41] The clinical quality measures developed include those for nutrition screening, assessment, diagnosis, and interventions.

In monitoring nutrition and evaluation, the use of a template format, such as the Consolidated Clinical Document Architecture, will not only create a standardized approach to nutrition documentation but will also promote nutrition interoperability across the care spectrum.[22] The template will improve transition of nutrition care on discharge from the hospital to the next care setting.

Discharge Plan

Discharge planning is an interdisciplinary approach to provide continuity of care. It is a process that begins at admission when the provider determines anticipated posthospital services and planning that includes the patient and family,[42] development of a structured discharge plan tailored to meet the individual's needs,[43] and discharge coordination rounds with interdisciplinary participants to ensure completion of discharge teaching.[44,45]

Inclusion of resolved and unresolved nutrition diagnoses, especially malnutrition, in the hospital discharge summary provides valuable information to the primary care, referring, or next-setting physician for ongoing treatment. Electronic discharge orders and instructions should include ongoing nutrition support as appropriate, frequency of follow-up evaluation by the healthcare team for laboratory studies, nutrition reassessment, and physical examination.

Patients should receive after-hospital or clinic visit summaries, which are generated from structured data and embedded clinical documentation, such as care instructions. Components of the nutrition plan include the interventions recommended by the nutrition clinician, along with recommendations for follow-up care. If nutrition education was an intervention to address a nutrition diagnosis, the EHR should provide a link to the educational material for future reference.

When patients need EN or PN, the EHR should generate a form with the patient's prescription or order for the home infusion company or durable medical equipment agency. The home nutrition support company will need the same information discussed here under nutrition interventions for EN and PN, such as product, formulation, rate and time of administration, and the name of the physician who will provide postdischarge care. Vitamins and minerals and other medications appropriate to the Nutrition Care Plan prescribed through the medication administration module will be transmitted electronically to the patient's pharmacy or next facility.

The Joint Commission has standards that address transitions of care and has an initiative underway to offer various interventions and resources to improve these transitions of care. The Joint Commission requires that the active issues, diagnoses, medications, required services, warning signs of worsening conditions, and whom to contact 24 h/d, 7 d/wk in case of an emergency be provided to the patient and/or caregivers in an alternate care setting on hospital discharge.[46] When a patient is being discharged to an alternative care setting, many hospitals send a Continuity of Care form along with the patient that documents these items and other pertinent information. The Continuity of Care form should be integrated into the EHR, such that it is easy to find and review. Paper Continuity of Care forms may get lost or delayed in getting scanned into the EHR and, once scanned, may be difficult to find for review.

Summary

An EHR presents patient data in digital format to be used for the provision of medical care, shared across healthcare settings within and between organizations, for the patient's personal health record, and for population health studies. The technology of EHRs is ever-changing, so that now clinicians can take patient photographs and store to their medical record to document muscle and fat depletion or vitamin and mineral deficiencies using their personal telephone, for example. EHRs offer the nutrition clinician the ability to track important steps in the provision of nutrition care that follow the ASPEN Nutrition Care Pathways—nutrition screening and assessment, documentation of the nutrition diagnosis, the nutrition care plan and associated interventions, reassessment of data to determine whether nutrition goals are improving the nutrition diagnosis, and the nutrition discharge plan for ongoing treatment of unresolved nutrition problems. The EHR can provide tools for the nutrition clinician to document nutrition data in structured and unstructured forms that communicate the patient's nutrition history from 1 clinician to the next.

The nutrition leaders in an organization should ensure their technologically savvy clinicians advocate for the needs of their colleagues with the Information System teams who are responsible for the build and maintenance of the system for their department. The appointed technologically savvy clinicians should also participate in ongoing improvement and maintenance to meet the ever-changing best practices of nutrition care.

References

1. Kushner RF, Ayello EA, Beyer PL, et al. National Coordinating Committee for Nutrition Standards clinical indicators of nutrition care. *J Am Diet Assoc.* 1994;94(10):1168–1177.

2. Swan WI, Vivanti A, Hakel-Smith NA, et al. Nutrition Care Process and Model Update: toward realizing people-centered care and outcomes management. *J Acad Nutr Diet.* 2017;117(12):2003–2014.

3. Swan WI, Pertel DG, Hotson B, et al. Nutrition Care Process (NCP) Update Part 2: developing and using the NCP terminology to demonstrate efficacy of nutrition care and related outcomes. *J Acad Nutr Diet.* 2019;119(5):840–855.

4. Adult and pediatric nutrition care pathways. ASPEN website. http://www.nutritioncare.org/guidelines_and_clinical_resources/Malnutrition_Solution_Center/. Accessed March 3, 2019.

5. National health expenditure data. Centers for Medicare and Medicaid Services website. https://www.cms.gov/research-statistics-data-and-systems/statistics-trends-and-reports/nationalhealthexpenddata/nationalhealthaccountshistorical.html. Accessed May 3, 2019.

6. The healthcare costs of obesity. The State of Obesity website. https://www.stateofobesity.org/healthcare-costs-obesity/. Accessed May 3, 2019.

7. The cost of diabetes. American Diabetes Association website. http://www.diabetes.org/advocacy/news-events/cost-of-diabetes.html. Accessed May 3, 2019.

8. Peery AF, Crockett SD, Murphy CC, et al. Burden and cost of gastrointestinal, liver, and pancreatic diseases in the United States: update 2018. *Gastroenterology.* 2019;156(1):254–272.e211.

9. Goates S, Du K, Braunschweig CA, Arensberg MB. Economic burden of disease-associated malnutrition at the state level. *PLoS One.* 2016; 11(9):e0161833. doi:10.1371/journal.pone.0161833

10. Barrett ML, Bailey MK, Owens PL. *Non-Maternal and non-Neonatal Inpatient Stays in the United States Involving Malnutrition, 2016.* US Agency for Healthcare Research and Quality website. https://www.hcup-us.ahrq.gov/reports/HCUPMalnutritionHospReport_083018.pdf. Published August 30, 2018. Accessed March 7, 2019.

11. Interoperability and health information exchange. HIMSS website. https://www.himss.org/library/interoperability-health-information-exchange. Accessed May 3, 2019.

12. The Joint Commission E-dition. https://e-dition.jcrinc.com. Accessed January 7, 2019.

13. Anthony PS. Nutrition screening tools for hospitalized patients. *Nutr Clin Pract.* 2008;23(4):373–382.

14. Mueller C, Compher C, Ellen DM; ASPEN Board of Directors. A.S.P.E.N. clinical guidelines: nutrition screening, assessment, and intervention in adults. *JPEN J Parenter Enteral Nutr.* 2011;35(1):16–24.

15. Correia MITD. Nutrition screening vs nutrition assessment: what's the difference? *Nutr Clin Pract* 2018;33(1):62–72.

16. Academy of Nutrition and Dietetics, Evidence Analysis Library. Nutrition screening in adults, 2016-2018. https://www.andeal.org/topic.cfm?menu=5382. Accessed March 5, 2019.

17. White M, Lawson K, Ramsey R, et al. Simple nutrition screening tool for pediatric inpatients. *JPEN J Parenter Enteral Nutr.* 2016;40(3):392–398.

18. Academy of Nutrition and Dietetics, Evidence Analysis Library. Nutrition screening pediatrics. https://www.andeal.org/topic.cfm?menu=5767. Accessed March 5, 2019.

19. What is clinical decision support (CDS)? HealthIT.gov website. https://www.healthit.gov/topic/safety/clinical-decision-support. Accessed June 4, 2019.

20. Ukleja A, Gilbert K, Mogensen KM, et al. Standards for nutrition support: adult hospitalized patients. *Nutr Clin Pract.* 2018;33(6):906–920.

21. Project Summary for Electronic Nutrition Care Process Record System (ENCPRS) Functional Profile. HL7 International website. http://www.hl7.org/special/committees/projman/searchableprojectindex.cfm?action=edit&ProjectNumber=706. Accessed March 5, 2019.

22. Project Summary for HL7 CDA R2 Implementation Guide: C-CDA R2.1 Supplemental Templates for Nutrition, Release 1 (US Realm). HL7 International website. http://www.hl7.org/special/Committees/projman/searchableProjectIndex.cfm?action=edit&ProjectNumber=1371. Accessed March 5, 2019.

23. *Electronic Nutrition Care Process Terminology (eNCPT) Reference Manual: Dietetics Language for Nutrition Care.* Academy of Nutrition and Dietetics website. www.ncpro.org. Accessed June 7, 2019.

24. World Health Organization. *International Statistical Classification of Diseases and Related Health Problems, 10th Revision.* Geneva, Switzerland: World Health Organization; 2012.

25. Giannopoulos GA, Merriman LR, Rumsey A, Zwiebel DS. Malnutrition coding 101: financial impact and more. *Nutr Clin Pract.* 2013;28(6):698–709.

26. White JV, Guenter P, Jensen G, et al. Consensus statement: Academy of Nutrition and Dietetics and American Society for Parenteral and Enteral Nutrition: characteristics recommended for the identification and documentation of adult malnutrition (undernutrition). *JPEN J Parenter Enteral Nutr.* 2012;36(3):275–283.

27. Becker P, Carney LN, Corkins MR, et al; Academy of Nutrition and Dietetics; ASPEN. Consensus statement of the Academy of Nutrition and Dietetics/American Society for Parenteral and Enteral Nutrition: indicators recommended for the identification and documentation of pediatric malnutrition (undernutrition). *Nutr Clin Pract.* 2015;30(1):147–161.

28. Phillips W. Accurate documentation of malnutrition diagnosis reflects increased healthcare resource utilization. *Nutr Clin Pract.* 2015;30(5):604–608.

29. Phillips W, Browning M. A clinician's guide to defining, identifying and documenting malnutrition in hospitalized patients. *Pract Gastroenterol.* 2017;41(11):19–33.

30. Academy of Nutrition and Dietetics. *Nutrition Care Manual.* https://www.nutritioncaremanual.org/. Accessed January 7, 2019.

31. Academy of Nutrition and Dietetics. *Pediatric Nutrition Care Manual.* https://www.nutritioncaremanual.org/. Accessed January 7, 2019.

32. HL7 version 3 domain analysis model: diet and nutrition orders, release 2. HL7 International website. http://www.hl7.org/implement/standards/product_brief.cfm?product_id=289. Accessed June 5, 2019.

33. Boullata JI, Carrera AL, Harvey L, et al; ASPEN Safe Practices for Enteral Nutrition Therapy Task Force, ASPEN. ASPEN safe practices for enteral nutrition therapy. *JPEN J Parenter Enteral Nutr.* 2017;41(1):15–103.

34. Oza-Frank R, Kachoria R, Dail J, Green J, Walls K, McClead RE Jr. A quality improvement project to decrease human milk errors in the NICU. *Pediatrics* 2017;139(2):e20154451. doi:10.1542/peds.2015-4451

35. Steele C, Bixby C. Centralized breastmilk handling and bar code scanning improve safety and reduce breastmilk administration errors. *Breastfeed Med.* 2014;9(9):426–429.

36. Ayers P, Adams S, Boullata J, et al; ASPEN. A.S.P.E.N. parenteral nutrition safety consensus recommendations. *JPEN J Parenter Enteral Nutr.* 2014;38(3):296–333.

37. Vanek VW, Ayers P, Kraft M, et al; ASPEN; Academy of Nutrition and Dietetics; American Society of Health-System Pharmacists. A call to action for optimizing the electronic health record in the parenteral nutrition workflow: executive summary. *Nutr Clin Pract.* 2018;33(5):594–596.

38. Centers for Medicare and Medicaid Services. Medicare and Medicaid programs; regulatory provisions to promote program efficiency, transparency, and burden reduction; part II. Federal Register website. https://www.federalregister.gov/documents/2014/05/12/2014-10687/medicare-and-medicaid-programs-regulatory-provisions-to-promote-program-efficiency-transparency-and. Accessed March 5, 2019.

39. Centers for Medicare and Medicaid Services. Medicare and Medicaid programs; reform of requirements for long-term care facilities. Federal Register website. https://www.federalregister.gov/documents/2016/10/04/2016-23503/medicare-and-medicaid-programs-reform-of-requirements-for-long-term-care-facilities. Accessed March 5, 2019.

40. ASPEN. *Improve Patient Outcomes: A.S.P.E.N.'s Step-by-Step Guide to Addressing Malnutrition.* Silver Spring, MD: ASPEN; 2015.

41. McCauley SM. Malnutrition care: preparing for the next level of quality. *J Acad Nutr Diet.* 2016;116(5):852–855.

42. Mennuni M, Gulizia MM, Alunni G, et al. ANMCO position paper: hospital discharge planning: recommendations and standards. *Eur Heart J Suppl.* 2017;19(suppl D):D244–D255.

43. Shepperd S, McClaran J, Phillips CO, et al. Discharge planning from hospital to home. *Cochrane Database Syst Rev.* 2010;(1):CD000313. doi:10.1002/14651858.CD000313.pub3

44. Bobay K, Bahr SJ, Weiss ME, Hughes R, Costa L. Models of discharge care in Magnet® hospitals. *J Nurs Adm.* 2015;45(10):485–491.

45. Weiss ME, Bobay KL, Bahr SJ, Costa L, Hughes RG, Holland DE. A model for hospital discharge preparation: from case management to care transition. *J Nurs Adm.* 2015;45(12):606–614.

46. The Joint Commission. Transitions of care: the need for a more effective approach to continuing patient care. https://www.jointcommission.org/assets/1/18/Hot_Topics_Transitions_of_Care.pdf. Accessed March 7, 2019.

CHAPTER 13

Contributors to Previous Editions

Stephen Adams, MS, RPh, BCNSP
Geisinger Medical Center
Danville, PA

Jorge Albina, MD
Rhode Island Hospital
Providence, Rhode Island

Debra A. Andris, ANP, MSN
Medical College of Wisconsin
Milwaukee, WI

Joseph Boullata, PharmD, RPh, BCNSP, FASPEN
University of Pennsylvania
Philadelphia, PA

Charlene Compher, PhD, RD, LDN, CNSC, FADA, FASPEN
University of Pennsylvania
Philadelphia, PA

Sharon Durfee, RPh, BCNSP
Poudre Infusion Therapy-Columbine Health
Fort Collins, CO

Charles E. Edmiston, PhD
Medical College of Wisconsin
Milwaukee, WI

Jane Gervasio, PharmD, BCNSP, FCCP
Butler University College of Pharmacy and Health Science
Indianapolis, IN

Elizabeth Hagan RN, CNSC
Rhode Island Hospital
Providence, Rhode Island

Gordon L. Jensen, MD, PhD, FASPEN
Pennsylvania State University
University Park, PA

Michael D. Kraft, PharmD, BCNSP
University of Michigan
Ann Arbor, MI

Elizabeth A. Krzywda, ANP, MSN
Medical College of Wisconsin
Milwaukee, WI

Vanessa Kumpf, PharmD, BCNSP
Vanderbilt University Center for Human Nutrition
Nashville, TN

Ainsley M. Malone, MS, RD, LD, CNSD
Mt. Carmel West Hospital
Columbus, OH

Neil Marshall, RN, BSN, CRNI, CNSC
Walgreens Infusion Services,
Sun Valley, CA

Nilesh Mehta, MD
Boston Children's Hospital
Boston, MA

Jay M. Mirtallo, MS, RPh, BCNSP, FASHP
The Ohio State University Medical Center
Columbus, OH

Charles Mueller, PhD, RD, CNSC
Weill/Cornell Medical College
New York, NY

Antoinette Neal, RN, CRNI, CNSC, VA-BC
Infusion Pharmacy, Cleveland Clinic at Home
Independence, Ohio

Gordon S. Sacks, PharmD, BCNSP, FCCP
Auburn University
Auburn, AL

David S. Seres, MD, ScM, PNS
New York Presbyterian Hospital–Columbia University Medical Center
New York, NY

Marion Winkler PhD, RD, CNSC, FASPEN
Rhode Island Hospital
Providence, Rhode Island

Patricia Worthington, RN, MSN, CNSC
Thomas Jefferson University Hospital
Philadelphia, PA

Index

Competency validation, 64,
149–150, 227
Complete blood count (CBC), 265,
270
Compounded sterile product
(CSP), 120–121, 121*t*
Computerized prescriber order
entry (CPOE) system, 97, 102,
103*f*, 149–150
Congestive heart failure (CHF),
12, 284*f*
Consolidated Clinical Document
Architecture, 296, 301
Continuity of Care, 255–256,
301–302
Copper, 81, 81*t*, 179, 192*t*
deficiency, 191
C-reactive protein, 8, 8*t*, 17*t*
Creatinine, 161*t*, 270
Cremophor, 242
Crohn's disease, 34, 188*t*, 248
Cyclic feeding, 260
Cyclic infusion, 157–158, 186, 189,
260
Cyclosporine A, 242
Cysteine, 76, 85, 98*t*, 99*f*, 100*f*, 135
Cystic fibrosis, 249*t*
Cytokine, 7, 17*t*, 181

D

Dacron cuff, 50
Deep vein thrombosis (DVT), 42*t*,
49, 53*t*, 58
Deficiencies
choline, 263
chromium, 174
copper, 191
essential fatty acid deficiency
(EFAD), 109, 175, 182
iron, 132, 250*t*, 263
magnesium, 190
of minerals, 263
nutrient, 142*t*, 292
selenium, 179
thiamin, 146
zinc, 179
Degludec, 244
Dehydration, 176, 264, 269
Denosumab, 191

Dermatitis, 175
Desorption, 242
Detemir, 244
Dextrose, 25, 73, 83, 111*f*, 119, 128.
See also Total nutrient admixture
(TNA)
acid-base balance and, 82
amino acids and, 61, 74, 236,
239*t*, 240*t*, 244–245, 279, 281
hypertonic, 149
infusions, 108
medication compatibility with,
239*t*, 240*t*, 243
in multichamber-bag parenteral
nutrition (MCB-PN), 279
Di-2-ethylhexyl phthalate (DEHP),
157, 242
Diabetes, 261, 292
mellitus, 104
prevention and treatment of, 296
Dialysis catheters, 46
Diazepam, 236
Diet orders, 298
Diethylhexyl phthalate (DEHP),
157, 242
Dieticians, 205–206, 258
Digoxin, 236
Drug and nutrition interactions
(DNIs), 233, 235*t*, 241
Dry weight, 104
Durable medical equipment
companies, 256
Dyspnea, 252
Dysrhythmias, 145

E

Edema, 158, 243, 269
Education, patient, 265–266, 267*f*,
268–269
Egg
allergy, 176
phospholipid emulsifier, 127, 176
Electrocardiogram, 153
Electrolytes, 25, 82, 101, 112*f*, 270
clearance, 280
daily adult guidelines, 105*t*
disturbances, 146
fluids and, 177
intake of, 104